Traditional Foods Are Your Best Medicine

Let your food be your medicine, and your medicine be your food.

HIPPOCRATES,
FATHER OF MEDICINE

TRADITIONAL FOODS
ARE YOUR
BEST MEDICINE

**Health and Longevity
With the Animal
Sea and Vegetable
Foods of Our Ancestors**

by Ronald F. Schmid, N.D.

With a Foreword by Michael B. Schachter, M.D.

Ballantine Books • New York

A unique and visionary individual set out over fifty years ago on the first of his several journeys to the far corners of the earth. He believed physical and moral problems developing in America were not a part of the natural order of life, and he sought to determine the underlying causes.

His thesis: fundamental changes in nutrition and ways of living were the reason many modern people had lost their resistance to disease, their ability to reproduce normal children, and their traditional moral values.

He found and studied cultures where people still lived according to the wisdom of their ancestors. He discovered the nature of the nutrition and ways of living that for thousands of years had prevented our modern problems in traditional societies.

Dr. Weston Price's classic book *Nutrition and Physical Degeneration* was first published in 1939. Elegant proof of his basic premises, it remains a blueprint for recovery from the diseases plaguing modern cultures. Dr. Price's work has influenced thousands of men and women involved in efforts to provide better health care through natural means. This book is dedicated to his memory, and to their future.

Photographs by Weston Price, courtesy of the Price-Pottenger Nutrition Foundation.

Library of Congress Catalog Card Number: 88-91985

ISBN: 0-345-35737-X

This edition published by arrangement with Ocean View Publications.

Cover design by Andrew Newman

Manufactured in the United States of America

First Ballantine Books Edition: January 1989
10 9 8 7 6 5 4 3 2 1

Contents

Foreword   *xiii*

Preface   *xv*

Introduction   *xvii*

I

TRADITIONAL FOODS

History
Anthropology
Research
Clinical Experience

1. *Traditional Diets and Natural Health Care*   3
2. *Dr. Weston Price and Traditional Societies*   6
3. *Benefits of Raw Foods*   34
4. *Evolution, Food, and Health: From Ancient Ancestors to Contemporary Hunter-Gatherers*   45
5. *Long-Lived People of Vilcabamba, Hunza, and Georgian Russia*   52
6. *Protective Characteristics of Traditional Diets*   66
7. *Fish, Fat-Soluble Nutrients, and Health*   75
8. *A Review of Several Well-Known Diets*   87
9. *Creating a Traditional Diet for Health and Longevity*   99
10. *Recovery Through Nutrition: Dietary Considerations for Specific Conditions*   106
11. *Relationships: Individuals, Physicians, and Health Goals*   132

II

TRADITIONAL VERSUS MODERN FOODS

A Guide to Natural Eating

12.	Fish and Shellfish	139
13.	The Production of Modern Meat, Fowl, and Eggs	144
14.	Naturally Raised Meat, Fowl, and Eggs	156
15.	Conventional Milk and Milk Products	163
16.	Certified Raw Milk, Butter, and Raw Milk Cheeses	167
17.	Chemical Versus Organic Farming	172
18.	Vegetables	175
19.	Whole Grain Foods	180
20.	Fruits, Nuts, and Seeds	183
21.	Other Foods, Seasonings, and Beverages	186
22.	Vitamins, Minerals, and Food Supplements	197

Epilogue   Toward a Philosophy of Natural Living   204

Appendix 1   Seafood: Characteristics and Habitat of Popular Fish and Shellfish   207

Appendix 2   Understanding Laboratory Tests   234

Appendix 3   Food Irradiation: The Latest Threat to Our Foods   241

Appendix 4   An Explanation of California's Organic Food Act of 1982   244

Appendix 5   Exercise and Sports   246

Bibliography   251

Index   261

Acknowledgments   270

Expanded Contents

Foreward by *Michael B. Schachter, M.D.*   *xiii*

Preface   *xv*

Introduction   *xvii*

I

TRADITIONAL FOODS

History
Anthropology
Research
Clinical Experience

1 Traditional Diets and Natural Health Care   3
    How Nature Cures   *3*
    Getting Well Naturally   *4*

2 Dr. Weston Price and Traditional Societies   6
    EUROPE (1931)   *8*
        Swiss of the Loetschental Valley   *8*
        Gaelics on the Islands of the Outer Hebrides   *9*
    NORTH AMERICA (1933)   *11*
        Eskimos of Alaska and Northern Canada   *11*
        Indians of North America   *13*
    MELANESIA, POLYNESIA, AND HAWAII (1934)   *16*
    AFRICA (1935)   *18*
    AUSTRALIA, THE TORRES STRAIT ISLANDS, AND NEW ZEALAND (1936)   *22*
        Aborigines of Australia   *22*
        Torres Strait Islanders   *23*
        New Zealand Maori   *24*
    ANCIENT AND PRESENT-DAY PERU (1937)   *25*
        Ancient Civilizations   *25*
        Andes Mountain and Amazon Jungle Indians   *27*
    PHOTOGRAPHS FROM *NUTRITION AND PHYSICAL DEGENERATION*   *29*

3 Benefits of Raw Foods   34
    Dr. Francis M. Pottenger   *34*

Pottenger's Cats and Raw Foods: The Ten-Year Study   35
Parallels Between Pottenger's and Price's Work   39
Raw Foods and Calcium Metabolism   40
Raw Foods and Chronic Diseases   41
Raw Foods and the Digestive System   41
Safety, Convention, and Tastes   42

4 *Evolution, Food, and Health: From Ancient Ancestors to
Contemporary Hunter-Gatherers*   **45**
Evolution and Diet   45
Contemporary Hunter-Gatherers   48
Implications For Post-Agricultural Revolution Diets   50

5 *Long-Lived People of Vilcabamba, Hunza, and Georgian Russia*   **52**
Verifying Ages and Health Status   52
Georgian Russia   57
Vilcabamba   57
Hunza   60
Conclusions About Long-Lived People   63
The Traditional American Diet   64

6 *Protective Characteristics of Traditional Diets*   **66**
Fat-Soluble Nutrients in Foods of Animal Origin   67
Fiber   69
Minerals   70
Raw Food Proteins and Enzymes   71
Using Protective Nutrients   73

7 *Fish, Fat-Soluble Nutrients, and Health*   **75**
Essential Fatty Acids and EPA   75
The More Fish, The Less Heart Disease: A Twenty-Year Study   78
Fish Oils Dramatically Lower High Blood Fats   79
Fishermen and Farmers in Japan: A Comparison   80
The Effects of a Mackerel Diet on Blood Platelets   81
Fish Oils in Vision and Intellectual Function   82
Fatty Acids and Linseed Oil   83
Fat-Soluble Nutrients in Dairy Products   83
Fresh Greens in the Diet   84
Cod Liver Oil   85

8 *A Review of Several Well-Known Diets*   **87**
The Pritikin Diet   87
High-Protein Weight Loss Diets   89
The Gerson Diet   90
Raw Foods Diets and Fasting   93
The Macrobiotic Diet   94

9 *Creating a Traditional Diet For Health and Longevity*   **99**
The Dynamic State of an Optimal Diet   99
Proportions and Balance   101
Nutrition in Pregnancy   104

10 Recovery Through Nutrition: Dietary Considerations For Specific Conditions   **106**
    Colds, Flus, Mononucleosis: When and How to Fast   *106*
    Allergies   *108*
    Chronic Fatigue and Thyroid Problems   *110*
    Arthritis and Back Problems   *112*
    Heart and Circulatory Disorders   *114*
    Malignancies   *117*
    Rheumatoid Arthritis   *122*
    Herpes   *123*
    Skin Problems   *124*
    Gastrointestinal Diseases   *125*
    Hypoglycemia, Diabetes, and Weight Problems   *126*
    Headaches   *127*
    Anxiety, Emotional Disturbances, and Mental Illness   *128*
    Candidiasis   *129*
    Other Conditions   *130*

11 Relationships: Individuals, Physicians, and Health Goals   **132**
    Working With a Physician   *133*
    The Significance of the Medical History and the Physical Exam   *134*
    Health Goals   *135*

II

TRADITIONAL VERSUS MODERN FOODS

A Guide to Natural Eating

12 Fish and Shellfish   **139**
    Water Pollution   *139*
    Quality and Flavor   *142*

13 The Production of Modern Meat, Fowl, and Eggs   **144**
    The Production of Meat   *145*
    Antibiotics   *146*
    Hormones   *147*
    The Feeding of Modern Animals   *150*
    Veal Calves   *151*
    Pig Factories   *152*
    The Egg Industry   *152*
    Inspection   *152*

14 Naturally Raised Meat, Fowl, and Eggs   **156**
        Defining Organic   *156*
        Natural Diet For Animals   *157*
        Fowl and Eggs   *157*
        Beef   *158*
        Organ Meats   *158*
        Lamb   *159*
        Vilhjalmur Stefansson's 1928 Experiment   *160*

15 Conventional Milk and Milk Products   **163**
        Pasteurization   *163*
        Toxic Residues and Fat Composition   *164*
        Homogenization   *164*
        Synthetic Vitamin D   *165*

16 Certified Raw Milk, Butter, and Raw Milk Cheeses   **167**
        Milk in History and Evolution   *167*
        Utilizing Raw Dairy Foods   *168*
        Availability, Certification, and Safety   *170*
        The Superiority of Raw Milk   *170*

17 Chemical Versus Organic Farming   **172**
        Chemical Agriculture   *172*
        Organic Farming and Living Soil   *173*

18 Vegetables   **175**
        Green Vegetables   *175*
        Using Indigenous Foods   *176*
        Sprouts   *176*
        Sea Vegetables   *177*
        Other Vegetables   *178*
        The Nightshades   *178*
        Raw Vegetable Juices   *179*

19 Whole Grain Foods   **180**
        Whole Grains   *180*
        Foods Made From Whole Grains   *181*

20 Fruits, Nuts, and Seeds   **183**
        Fruits   *183*
        Nuts and Seeds   *185*

21 Other Foods, Seasonings, and Beverages   **186**
        Vegetable Oils   *186*
        Vinegar and Lemon Juice   *187*
        Honey and Other Sweeteners   *188*
        Herbs and Seasonings   *189*
        Alcoholic Beverages   *191*
        Caffeine-Containing Drinks   *193*
        Refined Flour and Sugar   *195*

22 *Vitamins, Minerals, and Food Supplements* 197
    Vitamins in Foods Versus Laboratory Vitamins—How Natural Are
      "Natural" Vitamins? *197*
    Antioxidants—Vitamin E, Vitamin C, and Selenium *198*
    Food Supplements *200*
    Megavitamin Supplements Versus Traditional Foods *201*

Epilogue   *Toward a Philosophy of Natural Living* 204

Appendix 1   *Seafood: Characteristics and Habitat of Popular Fish and Shellfish* 207
    SALTWATER FISH *207*
      Anchovies, Bluefish, Butterfish, The Cod Family, Dolphin (Mahi-
      mahi), Halibut, Herring, Mackerel, Pompano, Salmon, Sardines,
      Sea Trout, Shad, Shark, Smelt, Snapper, Sole and Flounder,
      Steelhead, Striped Bass, Swordfish, Tilefish, Tuna, and Whitebait
    SHELLFISH *221*
      Abalone, Clams, Crab, Lobster, Mussels, Octopus, Oysters, Scallops,
      Shrimp, and Squid
    FRESHWATER FISH *228*
      Bass, Trout, and Whitefish
    SOME GENERAL CONSIDERATIONS *230*
      Sushi and Sashimi, Smoked and Salted Fish, Roe, Stocks, and Preser-
      vatives Sometimes Used on Fresh Fish and Shellfish

Appendix 2   *Understanding Laboratory Tests* 234
    Complete Blood Count (CBC) *234*
    Urinalysis *235*
    Erythrocyte Sedimentation Rate (ESR) *236*
    Blood Chemistry: Cholesterol, Triglycerides, Fasting Glucose, Glyco-
      hemoglobin, Glucose Tolerance Test, and Thyroid Hormones *236*

Appendix 3   *Food Irradiation: The Latest Threat to Our Foods* 241

Appendix 4   *An Explanation of California's Organic Food Act of 1982* 244

Appendix 5   *Exercise and Sports* 246
    Walking and Running *246*
    How Sports Can Help You *248*

Bibliography 251

Index 261

Acknowledgments 270

IMPORTANT NOTICE

A serious study of nutrition and health care explains what is reasonable and what is not, what is safe for one to do on one's own, and when one should see a competent physician. This book is written in such a manner, but to protect fully the interests of each reader as well as those of the author and the publisher, a clear statement of what this book is, and what it is not, must be made.

The book is sold with the understanding that the author and the publisher are not rendering medical, health care, or other professional service. If one has any indication that health care or other expert assistance is required, a competent professional should be sought. This important advice is repeated in several pertinent places.

All of the available information about the subjects covered is not contained herein; rather, this book complements, amplifies, and supplements other published information. For more information, see the many references in the bibliography.

The intent is to educate and entertain. Every effort was made to be accurate and complete. However, there may be errors. This book should be used only as a general guide and not as an ultimate source of information.

Many references to raw foods are made. The reader should recognize that although the author presents evidence that raw foods of the highest quality are beneficial to health, the use of tainted raw foods may result in serious illness, including hepatitis, parasitic diseases, tuberculosis, and brucellosis. It is the responsibility of the consumer to assure himself that all foods eaten are of a quality that will not cause disease. The author and Ocean View Publications shall have neither liability nor responsibility to any person or entity with respect to any loss or damage caused, or alleged to be caused, directly or indirectly, by the information contained in this book.

Foreword

Dr. Ron Schmid taught me a great deal about recovery from chronic diseases and the attainment of superior health through nutrition, and I believe he can do the same for you. From 1981 to 1983, he worked as a nutritional consultant at Mountainview Medical Associates in Nyack, New York. Under my direction, he saw and consulted with hundreds of our patients. I was frequently amazed by the rapid and lasting improvement many of these chronically ill people experienced when following the traditional diets Dr. Schmid individually worked out with each. This book contains the principles underlying his success with patients.

In skillfully analyzing the work of Drs. Weston Price and Francis Pottenger—the two nutritional giants of the first half of the twentieth century—Dr. Schmid shows clearly how changing agricultural practices and the trend toward ever more refined and fractionated foods have contributed to the emergence of degenerative diseases—heart disease, cancer, arthritis, diabetes, gastrointestinal disease, and others—as major health problems in western civilization. In a scholarly, yet easy to understand manner, he guides us to an understanding of the relationship between what we eat, the development of chronic diseases, and how we feel.

Insights gained from an understanding of the work of Price and Pottenger are used in an exciting review of the long-lived people of Vilcabamba, Hunza, and Georgian Russia. Recent medical research about the effects of nutrients in fish and naturally raised meats on human health, and about the health and nutrition of our ancient ancestors and of contemporary hunter-gatherers, is presented in several fascinating chapters.

From this wealth of information come the elements needed to forge a lifestyle that can lead to health and longevity. Practical, succinct chapters on the details of what to look for in choosing foods take us from theory to practical application; we emerge with both understanding *and* a useful everyday guide to healthy eating.

We do not live in a vacuum; individual health in many ways depends on government policy and economics. Dr. Schmid contrasts the methods modern agriculture uses to raise animals and plants with the more natural methods of traditional cultures, demonstrating how the differences may drastically affect our health. An appendix carefully documents the dangers of a new threat—the insufficiently tested plan to irradiate foods with nuclear waste products. Few stones are left unturned; another appendix details the life habits of fish and shellfish, enabling one to choose wisely from this important but sometimes tainted source of important nutrients.

This is a fascinating, practical, and inspiring book that clearly demonstrates the vital importance of our traditional foods not only for the individual but for the future of our culture. A glance at the bibliography indicates the quality of the evidence Dr. Schmid has compiled. A thorough reading and the implementation of the principles presented will set one well along toward that most elusive of goals—optimal health.

Mountainview Medical Associates   MICHAEL B. SCHACHTER, M.D.
Nyack, New York

Confusion reigns when the subject turns to nutrition. Every popular diet book presents a different expert's opinion on food. What should we eat and how much? What are the effects of meat, cholesterol, fruit, animal fats, vegetables, vegetable oils, fish, eggs, milk, cheese, grains, raw foods? How much damage does sugar do? Refined flour?

Which experts are right—those who say cholesterol is killing us, or those who tell us it is not the real culprit in heart disease?

Do food additives and pollutants cause cancer? Sweets and fats? Or might modern foods lack nutrients protective against cancer?

What foods help prevent chronic disease?

What foods will enable us to enjoy the robust good health we sense has been partly lost to modern living and modern foods?

These questions have no simple answers.

In seeking answers, several other questions might first be asked:

What was the health of people in traditional and primitive cultures existing into the early twentieth century, people eating only their traditional foods? What about isolated traditional cultures still surviving, and the three hundred thousand remaining hunter-gatherers still living and eating primitively?

If the health of such people is superior to ours, could this be directly related to their foods? If so, what foods did and do such people eat? What differences exist between their foods and modern foods? How do their meats, fish, milk products, fruits, vegetables, and grains differ from the foods we use? Do the differences help explain our modern problems?

What is the effect of traditional kinds of foods on people with chronic diseases? What evidence has been published in the medical literature?

Facts from historical records and recent medical research provide answers to these questions. With the understanding the answers provide, confusion about nutrition can be clarified. Answers to many seemingly unanswerable questions become clear.

This book demonstrates that the healthiest, strongest, and most disease resistant cultures ever known lived on natural foods—fish, meat, fowl, vegetables, fruits, and sometimes grains and unprocessed dairy products. How and why modern foods differ, the effects of the difference, and steps that may be taken to build health with superior foods will be explained.

Vegetables, and in some cases grains and fruits, were important foods for most of these cultures, and for many provided more calories than animal source foods. Invariably, however, the latter were considered of prime importance and great efforts were made to secure them. You'll discover why.

This book shows how a common sense approach to diet enables one to use traditional foods to prevent and often reverse disease.

* * *

Our genes and the structure of our enzymes have been passed down through thousands of generations. The building-block molecules of genes are identical in all living things. Biological laws unite all life forms.

Laws of physics govern the movement of planets, the changing of seasons, the coming and going of tides; biological laws govern the ways the human body reacts to different foods. People once argued the earth was flat, that blood did not circulate in the human body...some now argue that our ills are not intimately connected with food.

Illness weighs heavily, but those willing to give nature's methods an honest try can be helped to help themselves. To be frank at the outset: traveling a path to good health requires disciplined eating. The body requires natural foods in order to function well. Most are readily available. Some shopping in special places may be needed—seafood markets, natural foods stores, places with high quality fresh vegetables, and if possible, stores with naturally raised beef and fowl. Refined foods must be largely avoided.

By making an effort and accepting elements of a natural diet and lifestyle, one may rebuild one's birthright—good health. Notice the words "elements of;" this is not an all or nothing proposition. A willingness to work on change will yield results. Understand the principles, and apply what is reasonable now. The foundation is commitment and disciplined application; benefits follow proportionately.

If intuitively you have turned to nutrition as a means to better health, if you want to understand how and why foods affect us and the place of food in the human story...then this book may become very important to you.

* * *

Without the love and support through the years of my mother, grandmother, and stepfather, good health would have been impossible for me to achieve. My friends and my patients have taught me, and encouraged my efforts. Mike Schachter provided guidance in my development as a physician and in writing this book. Most of all, Ellen Schmid gave me the reason, inspiration, and time to conceive and complete the book, which simply would not have happened without her love.

Introduction

Preventing and Reversing Disease With Natural Foods

A Path to Health. An understanding of food can lead to increased health and happiness, two conditions that are not the same but may be thought of concurrently.

Though people often appear jovial despite poor health, this is often a mask used in attempting to hide underlying unhappiness. Others who are very ill truly do adapt, and lead emotionally fulfilling lives in the face of great pain and suffering. Perhaps they think one must accept one's lot in life, that they have no alternative. But this sadly relegates to fate a small part of the world one may control—one's own body.

A good friend taught me the saying, "God grant me the serenity to accept the things I cannot change, the courage to change the things I can, and the wisdom to know the difference." Such serenity and wisdom may bring a measure of happiness. But without the courage to change the things one can, a greater measure does not come. A path to health involves that greater measure.

Health may be thought of as largely physical, a matter of the body and the brain functioning well. Happiness is more a matter of the human spirit. Many definitions of health refer to finely tuned interrelationships between the physical, the mental, and the spiritual. Perhaps if we define health more simply, we may achieve it more readily.

A healthy body functions easily, as does a healthy mind. Desires for food, sex, exercise, mental challenges, and family life—for a full life— are strong. No signs of distress are present—no colds, aches or pains, undue fatigue, or allergies, much less more serious conditions. There is a feeling of physical strength, endurance, and vigor, and a nonchalant assumption that one's body should function perfectly and effortlessly.

There is much to learn from those who lived before us, especially those who lived simpler and healthier lives. A hint from Havelock Ellis, anthropologist and pioneer sexologist: "People have forgotten what the savage instinctively knows—that a perfect body is the supreme instrument of life."

* * *

Is a long and healthy life possible...free of the degenerative diseases plaguing modern people? Where does one begin?

Taking control is the first step. Eat according to an understanding of what foods and proportions are best for you.

Food involves constant choice. A cheerful attitude, an upright posture, breathing deeply in a tense situation—these too are choices. We often grant control of such things to those around us, coming to believe our lives are not our own, the responsibility not ours. We may think that much of what we accept is of little consequence. Indeed, our culture urges us to accept things that our forefathers would have found abhorrent.

Simple changes like walks regularly taken, whatever the weather, can become a reflex activity one can count on to bring good feelings. Time outdoors is missing from too many lives.

Dietary changes are best achieved gradually, as an understanding of food and of one's own needs deepens. Trying to change too much abruptly may create physical and psychological difficulties. Yet without discipline and commitment, no progress is made. A reasonable middle course allows the flexibility to make a diet work. Dietary changes are best based on understanding and gradually changing tastes; the reasons for eating certain foods provide the basis for resolutions.

Natural foods become more comfortable as one grows accustomed to them; eventually, one may lose all desire for refined foods which once were irresistible. Changes in habits lead to changes in tastes and inclinations.

For people seeking to correct troubling conditions, the foundation of success is a commitment to change. This commitment and a thorough understanding of our traditional foods may enable one to reach the simple but elusive goal of radiant and lasting health.

I

TRADITIONAL FOODS

History
Anthropology
Research
Clinical Experience

1

Traditional Diets and Natural Health Care

How Nature Cures

*T*he human body has an inherent ability to heal. Think of a cut, or a broken bone. Given time, the cut heals, the bone mends. What accomplishes these small miracles?

Nature. Nature cures. This is the basis of lasting healing and lasting health.

The same intrinsic force mending a broken bone can heal arthritis; in both cases, the body can react to disturbances in its natural balance in a way that restores the natural balance. The bone is more easily repaired, for trauma created the problem suddenly, and no deep-seated underlying problem must be corrected for healing to occur. Arthritis is not so simple.

Arthritis develops primarily because of years of faulty dietary habits. The broken bone heals even with somewhat faulty nutrition, but to heal arthritis, conditions causing it must be changed.

For nature to cure, one must understand what nature is—what is natural—and live by it. Even when this is accepted, a problem remains: few modern people understand what constitutes natural diet.

This is no surprise. A systematic investigation of the issue takes years of study; research in a broad range of related fields is necessary. Relentless and constant experimentation with one's own diet is required. Clinical work adds experience. Other methods besides diet may be tried in attempts to build health and alleviate disease, but one learns that no other approach holds the power and potential for healing of food. Then one must learn which foods and in what proportions.

In biology, one classic stands out—Charles Darwin's *On the Origin of Species*, his treatise on the evolution of life on earth. Darwin demonstrated that in nature there are no accidents; for every effect there is a cause. Could human evolution have been shaped by food such that each of us

3

is most suited for a certain kind of diet? This is a reasonable possibility; for each person there would be differences, of course, depending on the geographical origins of his forefathers and the foods shaping them.

Perhaps through study, observation, and trial and error, one may discover one's own best diet. But the questions are endless, the dilemma seemingly unsolvable. Without the guide of traditional wisdom—the accumulated knowledge about foods passed on for thousands of generations—crucial elements needed for a deep understanding of human health and disease are missing.

In his classic book *Nutrition and Physical Degeneration*, first published in 1939 and based on years of studying the nutrition and health of primitive traditional cultures throughout the world, Weston Price provides knowledge necessary to achieve this understanding. His studies taught him the natural laws governing human nutrition and health. Research and clinical experience since have confirmed and enlarged Dr. Price's work.

Getting Well Naturally

Since the author has worked both together with medical doctors as a staff nutritional consultant and independently as a naturopathic physician, a few words are in order about the interwoven history of natural health care in America and naturopathic medicine.

Naturopathic physicians (pronounced nature-oh-pathic) are currently licensed as health care practitioners in the states of Connecticut, Washington, Oregon, Arizona, Alaska, and Hawaii, and in most of the Canadian provinces. In several other states formerly licensing the profession, individuals who were granted licenses in the past still practice. To become licensed, one must graduate from a naturopathic medical school recognized by states granting licenses and pass the state licensing examination.

Naturopathic medicine is a separate and distinct branch of the healing arts. From nineteenth century European roots, the movement grew and became popular in America in the earlier part of this century. One of the founding principles is found in the writings of Hippocrates: "Let your food be your medicine, and your medicine be your food." Given proper conditions, the human body contains the power to heal itself; food is the most basic of those conditions.

Many other states once licensed naturopathic physicians. Under the influence of the American Medical Association, state legislatures began in the 1930's repealing the licensing laws, limiting the practice to those already holding licenses. The influence of the medical monopoly since established has made illegal in most states the diagnosis and treatment of health problems unless one is a medical doctor.

The influence of pharmaceutical companies on medical school curricula has meanwhile made it difficult for medical students to learn the underlying causes of disease and the fundamental steps leading to health; the vast majority of medical schools do not require courses in nutrition.

Students learn to use drugs to alleviate symptoms, and surgery to remove diseased parts, rather than learning to use an understanding of health as the basis for guiding people to natural recovery.

Many people who choose surgery or drugs over the lifestyle changes required in natural therapy or who suffer from certain acute conditions are best served by surgical or pharmaceutical treatment. Naturopathic physicians work cooperatively with other physicians or make an appropriate referral when an individual needs such treatment or requires specialized diagnostic procedures.

In states where the practice of naturopathic medicine is not licensed, any individual may call himself an N.D. (naturopathic doctor), though he holds no license in any state. Both the public and the medical profession often confuse these people, who usually have a mail-order or correspondence degree of some sort, with licensed naturopathic physicians, whose legitimate title is N.D. The confusion of terms is unfortunate, for fifty years ago, thousands of competent and well trained individuals were licensed N.D.'s. As did some conventionally trained physicians who believed in natural methods of health care, they provided an alternative for people preferring such treatment.

The burden of achieving competence as a physician rests with the individual. Practicing medicine is an art; teachers only point the way. Ultimately the artist-physician must develop and fine-tune his skills—as a diagnostician, as a scientist and investigator, and as a communicating and caring human being—and apply them on his canvas, his patient. Many conventional physicians provide this kind of care. A natural health care alternative should incorporate these qualities with an understanding of natural healing. Such an alternative gives interested people real choices about treatment.

This book provides ways of participating in one's own care through nutrition. This is no substitute for a physician's care if needed. Many physicians are sympathetic to the idea that nature cures; hopefully such a doctor may be found by anyone wishing to heal himself through careful diet.

The greatest experts in health have often not been physicians, but rather people possessed of a certain wisdom about the human body, a wisdom understood, lived, and taught to the next generation. Some of this book is about such wisdom.

This traditional wisdom can be researched, written down, and studied; yet it is beyond the words in any book. References in this book provide evidence, but something outside the proven must play a role. Knowledge and understanding of health as part of the human condition may be grounded in observations, published information, and years of personal and clinical experience. Yet conclusions of lasting value must, when practiced, feel intuitively right; the body's response is the final arbiter. One does what works. The subject of the next chapter concerns what has worked in traditional societies for countless generations.

2

Dr. Weston Price
and
Traditional Societies

*T*he name Weston Price is not familiar, ironic in a world in need of the wisdom and knowledge the man uncovered before his death in 1948. *Nutrition and Physical Degeneration*, the text of his life's work, is not found in all libraries. Available only from the Price-Pottenger Nutrition Foundation, it is seldom found in bookstores and the Foundation does not distribute it through the usual channels.

Controversy surrounded the book when it was first published in 1939. Dr. Price was a dentist, and many in his profession found his work profound and significant. So too did many anthropologists; for years, the book was required reading for anthropology classes at Harvard. But the majority of professionals ignored it, and some attacked it. Among the public, there was some enthusiastic acceptance, but the book is long and somewhat tedious. Not written with an eye to the public, it never became widely read.

Dr. Price was born in Ontario in 1870 and raised on a farm. After receiving his dental degree in 1893, he began practicing and doing research. His many published articles brought him recognition, and his textbooks became standards in dentistry.

During his years in practice, he noticed problems in the children of his patients the parents had not experienced. Besides having more decay, in many children the teeth did not fit properly into the dental arch and were, as a result, crowded and crooked. Various explanations seemed inadequate; Price began suspecting changes in nutrition were responsible.

He noticed the condition of the teeth reflected overall health. Considering possible reasons, a revolutionary idea occurred to him: perhaps some deficiency in modern diets caused the problems. Anthropologists had long observed and written of the excellent teeth found in primitive cultures. While others in his profession continued looking for causative factors in dental decay, Dr. Price decided to search among primitive people for a factor protecting them.

His discoveries may genuinely surprise you. He found entire cultures with neither tooth decay nor children with misshapen dental arches and crowded teeth. He interviewed an American medical doctor living among Eskimos and northern Indians who reported that in thirty-five years of observation, he had never seen a case of cancer among the primitives existing on their native foods. When natives eating the white man's foods developed tuberculosis, this doctor eventually took to sending them back to their native villages and native foods; they then usually recovered. In every culture where the people were immune to dental and degenerative disease, biochemical analysis showed the diet to be rich in nutrients poorly supplied in modern diets.

Dr. Price visited and studied cultures where people following tradi-tional ways and diets lived near kinsmen who were eating the foods of modern civilization. Throughout the world in the 1930's, groups in the early stages of modernization were using foods imported from western countries—sugar, white flour, canned foods, and vegetable oils. These people often lived close to fellow villagers and people of the same ances-try living in nearby villages who still ate entirely according to traditional ways.

Price's time in history was unique. The cultures he observed were still truly indigenous, with groups of people living entirely on the local foods. Photographic emulsion was commonly available for the first time; he could easily record his observations. World travel too was readily avail-able for the first time for anyone able to afford it. This combination of old and new enabled his vision to see and record a picture of a world never to be seen again.

His travels took him to the corners of the earth. He and his wife lived with and studied Swiss in high Alpine valleys; Gaelics on islands of the Outer Hebrides; Eskimos in Alaska; Indians in the far northern, western, and central parts of Canada, and in the western United States and Florida; Melanesians and Polynesians in the southern Pacific; Africans in eastern and central Africa; Aborigines in Australia; Malay tribes on islands north of Australia; Maori in New Zealand; and descendants of ancient civili-zations in Peru. Skeletal remains of ancient people were studied wher-ever available.

Price studied dental health, keeping detailed records, including thou-sands of photographs. He analyzed native and modern foods for content of calories, minerals, and vitamins, and made extensive studies of effects of different foods on the chemistry of the saliva and its relation to dental decay. Scores of his articles were published, including a series in *The Journal of the American Dental Association*. He noted the general health of his subjects, and when possible interviewed medical personnel caring for the people.

His observations were not limited to health and diet, for he sought to understand the nature and character of these thousands of people. He came to know many well, and his insights reveal the strength of character of certain individuals, a trait he found typical in traditional cultures. This chapter chronologically tours Dr. Price's search for health.

EUROPE (1931)

Swiss of the Loetschental Valley

The Loetschental Valley, nearly a mile above sea level in an isolated part of the Swiss Alps, had been for over a dozen centuries the home of some two thousand people when Dr. and Mrs. Price first visited in 1931. The people lived in a series of small villages along a river that wound its way along the valley floor. The completion of an eleven-mile tunnel shortly before made the valley easily accessible for the first time.

The people lived as their forefathers had. Wooden buildings, some centuries old, dotted the landscape, with mottoes expressive of spiritual values artistically carved in the timbers. Snow-capped mountains nearly enclosed the valley, making it relatively easy to defend. Though many attempts had been made, the people had never been conquered.

They had no physician, dentist, policeman, or jail. Sheep provided wool for homespun clothes, and the valley produced nearly everything needed for food.

The land, much of it on steep hillsides rising from the river, produced hay for the cattle in winter, and rye for the people. Most households kept goats and cows; the animals grazed in summer on glacial slopes. Cheese and butter were made from fresh summer milk for use all year, and garden greens were grown in summer. Whole rye bread, made in large, stone, community bake-ovens, was a staple all year, as was milk. Most families ate meat once a week, usually on Sunday, when an animal was slaughtered. Bones and scraps were used to make soups during the week.

Dr. Price examined the teeth of all children in the valley between the ages of seven and sixteen. Those still eating the primitive diet were nearly free of cavities—on the average, one tooth showing evidence of ever having had decay was found for every three children examined.

Many young people examined had experienced a period of rampant tooth decay which suddenly ceased, often having first lost teeth. All had left the valley prior to this period and spent a year or two in some city. Most had never had a decayed tooth before or since.

Tuberculosis at this time took more lives in Switzerland than any other disease. Swiss government officials reported a recent inspection of the valley had not revealed a single case. No deaths had occurred from tuberculosis in the history of the valley.

Upon returning to America, Dr. Price had samples of the dairy products sent to him twice a month throughout the year. A pioneer in developing methods for measuring fat-soluble vitamins in foods in the early 1920's, he had written extensively on the subject and was a recognized authority. His analyses found the samples higher in minerals and vitamins than samples of commercial dairy products from the rest of Europe and America, particularly the fat-soluble D-complex vitamins.

The vitamin D-complex helps regulate utilization of calcium and other minerals. Price believed the D-complex and another unidentified nutrient he called "activator X" played crucial roles in the excellent general health, immunity to dental disease, and splendid physical development of the people of the Loetschental Valley. The quality of the foods was apparently responsible for the presence of rich amounts of these nutrients.

The people recognized the importance of foods. The clergyman told of how they thanked God for the life-giving qualities of butter and cheese made in June when the cows ate grass near the snow line; their worship included lighting a wick in a bowl of the first butter made after the cows reached this summer pasturage. Price's analyses showed butter made then was highest in fat-soluble vitamins and minerals.

Spiritual values dominated life. Part of the national holiday celebration each August was a song expressing the feeling of "one for all and all for one." Dr. Price wrote: "One wonders if there is not something in the life-giving vitamins and minerals of the food that builds not only great physical structures within which their souls reside, but builds minds and hearts capable of a higher type of manhood in which the material values of life are made secondary to individual character." He found intangible evidence of this throughout the world.

Conditions in the valley were in stark contrast with those in the lower valleys and plains country in Switzerland—modernized areas where rampant dental decay, misshapen dental arches with crowding of the teeth, and high incidence of tuberculosis and other chronic health problems were the norm. The people of the valley were protected by the quality of their traditional foods.

Few other traditional groups Price studied used milk, cheese, or butter (the others were certain African tribes, including the Masai). Raw, whole milk (both fresh and cultured), cheese, and butter were used in quantity. The milk, from healthy, well-exercised animals, was unpasteurized and unhomogenized. Such foods apparently may play a major role in a health-building diet for people genetically able to utilize them well. For the people of the Loetschental, the milk products provided fat-soluble nutrients and minerals essential in maintaining health.

Gaelics on the Islands of the Outer Hebrides

The Isle of Lewis and the Isle of Harris, visited by Price after leaving Switzerland, are the chief of these islands off the northwest coast of Scotland. The islands were isolated, inaccessible much of the year because of constant rough seas. Most people lived traditionally, working at fishing, sheep-raising, and farming.

Fish was abundant; many men went to sea daily in fishing vessels. Cod, lobsters, crabs, oysters, and clams were readily available. Oat grain was the only cereal that grew well and was a staple. The islands were covered with peat, providing poor farmland and pasturage; there were few cattle. Sheep were raised more for wool than food.

Oat porridge and oat cakes were eaten at most meals, with fish or often lobster. Vegetables were grown in the summer. Baked cod's head stuffed with chopped cod's liver and oatmeal was considered an important part of the diet, especially for children. Other fish organs and fish eggs were regularly used. Because of the isolation, poor pasturage, and lack of dairy animals, milk was practically unknown. So too were fruits.

Modern foods were available in shipping ports—white breads, jams, marmalades, canned vegetables, vegetable oils, sugar, syrup, chocolate, and coffee. Together with some fish, these foods formed the diet of many in these towns. Their health was in stark contrast with that of the rest of the population.

Children living on seafoods, oats, and vegetables in primitive areas showed less than one tooth out of one hundred with any decay. Tuberculosis, cancer, arthritis, and other degenerative diseases were unknown.

Children eating modern foods in the several shipping ports showed an average incidence of 16.3 to over fifty decayed teeth per one hundred examined; even three-year olds had decay. Tuberculosis was a great problem—some populations had been decimated. Wherever Price investigated, afflicted individuals had been eating modern foods. The authorities blamed fireplace smoke in the thatched-roof houses that for centuries had been the peoples' homes. Yet, former generations had been free of tuberculosis.

* * *

Whole grains—rye in the Loetschental, oats in the Outer Hebrides—formed major parts of these European traditional diets. Grains were important too for a few African tribes Price studied. Everywhere else, fish, animals, and vegetables formed the bulk of traditional diets, and grains played little or no role.

Seafood was the other staple in the Outer Hebrides. Fish organs (especially the liver), fish eggs, the head, and the bones were all used. Since there were no dairy foods, bones were important for calcium and other minerals.

Fish, especially the liver, is a rich source of the vitamin D-complex and other fat-soluble nutrients, supplied in the Loetschental Valley mostly by butter, cheese, and milk. In every culture that Price found free of dental and degenerative disease, a rich source of fat-soluble nutrients formed a substantial part of the diet.

NORTH AMERICA (1933)

Eskimos of Alaska and Northern Canada

A story of primitive Eskimos tells of a time when food ran short during the long winter night north of the Arctic Circle, when for months there is no daylight. An Eskimo man takes to stormy seas in a kayak to hunt seal with a harpoon. In darkness, bitter cold, high winds, and rough seas, he searches the dark waters for food. A wave crashing over a kayak can snap even a strong man's back; as breakers approach, the kayaker rolls the vessel, submerging himself. The tight fit of seal skins between the upper edge of the kayak and his waist keeps water from entering. When the white water passes, he flips upright and continues the hunt, finally killing a seal and returning home with food for his family.

As impressive as Weston Price found the physical strength of primitive Eskimos when visiting Alaska and northern Canada, even more impressive was their character—their courage, honesty and openness, dedication to family and community, and ability to survive and thrive in a harsh northern environment. In village after village, he found among Eskimos living entirely on the native diet virtually no decayed teeth and no evidence of chronic disease. Among those partially subsisting on refined foods, decay and disease increased in direct proportion to the amount eaten.

The plight of the primitives' modernized brethren was bleak. With no medical help to alleviate their suffering in the years immediately following the introduction of refined foods, many had been driven by the pain and misery of progressive tooth decay to take their own lives.

The contrast was stark. In many small native settlements where the white man's food was available, some refused it, subsisting entirely on the primitive diet. No evidence of decay or signs of chronic disease were found in them. Their fellow villagers, living the same life except for eating refined foods, had extensive decay, and some had tuberculosis. Among those eating modern foods for several years, some had arthritis.

In children born of parents eating refined foods, the majority had crowding and malocclusion of teeth because the dental arches were too narrow to accommodate the teeth properly. Several of Dr. Price's photographs at the end of this chapter (Figures 4 and 5) illustrate such changes. In contrast is the breadth of the dental arches and the perfect fit of the teeth shown in Figures 1 through 3; these Eskimos and other primitives show nature's normal form for humans, found wherever people subsisted entirely on native traditional foods.

This hereditary pattern, normally passed on from generation to generation in accordance with nature's laws, was disrupted by refined foods. Problems seen in children of Price's patients were for the first time appearing in primitive cultures. Narrowing of the dental arch and subsequent crowding and displacement of teeth is typical. Because so many people show these characteristics today, we may not readily recognize them as abnormal. But such changes, even when minor, are not part of nature's hereditary pattern.

"Intercepted heredity" was the term Price used: the hereditary pattern of perfect dental form, seen clearly in thousands of his photographs, had been intercepted by poor nutrition. The resultant abnormalities are now taken for granted.

Observation reveals most modern people have crowded teeth, though a small minority have the broad dental arches and perfectly fitting teeth normal in primitive cultures. And while most have the four wisdom teeth (the third molars) removed because of crowding, traditional people nearly always had all thirty-two teeth.

Traditional wisdom enabled successive generations to reproduce nature's pattern. This wisdom in every culture prescribed specific kinds and quantities of foods known to insure fertility, the birth of healthy, perfectly formed babies, and optimal development of growing children.

Salmon was an important food for primitive Eskimos, who almost always had homes near deep water. Much was dried and then smoked a few hours for winter use. When eaten, the fish was dipped in seal oil, shown by analysis rich in vitamin A and used also to preserve sorrel grass and flower blossoms.

Salmon eggs were dried raw and used in quantity, a major part of the nutrition for small children after weaning. Rich in iodine, they were used by women of childbearing age to insure fertility. The milt of male salmon were eaten by men for the same purpose; this too was eaten raw. Other foods included caribou, especially the organs; kelp, gathered in season and stored for winter; the organs of large sea mammals; and certain layers of the skin of one whale species (analysis showed this very high in vitamin C). Wild plants and berries were in the summer gathered and stored.

Dietary Fats.   The medical profession is involved in growing controversy about the role of diet in degenerative diseases. A consensus has emerged that animal fats and foods rich in cholesterol are harmful.

There is a small truth in this assertion, but it has been used to reach faulty conclusions. Excessive amounts of fat in America's meat and dairy animals do contribute to the development of disease. But confusion has resulted from a failure to recognize that the inferior quality of modern animals and their fats is the real problem.

The primitive Eskimo diet, mostly fish and wild animals, was rich in animal fats. But these fats were very different from the fats in meat, chicken, and dairy products from today's domestic animals (the reason for this will be explained in later chapters). The traditional people Price investigated all ate diets rich in animal source foods and animal fats. The quality of these foods and fats was largely responsible for their superior physical development and resistance to disease.

Analysis of the deterioration of the modern diet is complex. Beyond the decline in quality, traditional wisdom about the use of different organs and tissues of animals has been forgotten or ignored. Because the liver filters the blood and commercial animals contain man-made poisons, it is often avoided. But in all traditional cultures, liver is among the most important foods.

The displacement of traditional foods by refined foods is the heart of the problem. Attempts to cite the single issue of animal fats and cholesterol as the chief problem and solution are misdirected and sidestep issues central to a reasonable approach to health and disease.

Close examination of traditional cultures and recent research makes clear the causes of modern problems. While Price was a pioneer, other scientists have studied traditional cultures and concluded food is almost certainly responsible for the nearly complete protection hunter-fisher-gatherers enjoy from dental and chronic disease. Recent publication of this work and research comparing oils and fats in fish and wild game with those in domestic animals will be reviewed shortly, after completing our travels with Dr. Price.

Indians of North America

Great unexplored areas of northern British Columbia and the Yukon Territory were still inhabited by Indians in the 1930's when Price visited. He went also to reservations in Canada where Indians lived under more modernized conditions with modern foods, and to Florida to study present-day Seminoles and remains of pre-Columbian Indians.

Regions inside the Rocky Mountain range in the far north of Canada held groups of Indians unable to obtain any sea animal life, not even migrating salmon. Winter temperatures of seventy degrees below zero precluded the possibility of growing cereal grains or fruits, or of keeping dairy animals. The diet of these Indians was thus almost entirely limited to wild animals, making them of special interest.

One old Indian was asked through an interpreter why Indians did not get scurvy. He replied that scurvy was a white man's disease; while it was a possibility for Indians, they knew how to prevent it and white men did not. When asked why he did not tell white men how, he replied white men knew too much to ask Indians anything. Asked how, he went to his chief for permission to tell. Upon returning he explained that when an Indian kills a moose, he opens it up and finds the small ball in the fat above each kidney. He cuts these balls—the adrenal glands—into pieces that are immediately eaten, one by each Indian in the family.

The adrenal glands are among the richest sources of vitamin C in all animal or plant tissues. Cooking destroys vitamin C. The Indians' empirical knowledge and use of different organs and tissues of animals has certainly been verified by modern methods of analysis. Their wisdom preceded the discovery of vitamin C by thousands of years.

Such wisdom is again demonstrated in a story of a white man running out of supplies while crossing a high plateau in the far north country just before the fall freeze-up. A doctor of engineering and science, he was forced to march out of the wilderness when his prospecting plans went awry. While crossing the plateau, he went almost blind with a violent pain in his eyes which persisted for days. He nearly ran into a grizzly one day, and an old Indian tracking the bear recognized the white man's plight.

The Indian led him to a nearby stream, and with a trap of stones caught some trout. Throwing the fish on the bank, he told the prospector to eat the flesh of the head and the tissues behind the eyes. In a few hours the man's pain was largely gone, in a day his sight was returning, and in two, it was close to normal. He had been suffering from xeropthalmia, due to vitamin A deficiency. The fatty tissue around the eyes is one of the richest sources of vitamin A in any animal's body.

For nine months of the year, the nutrition of these northern Indians was mostly wild game, chiefly moose and caribou. Emphasis was placed on eating organs, including the wall of parts of the digestive tract. Some meat and organs were eaten raw; much muscle meat was fed to dogs. Bone marrow was used, especially in feeding children. Plants were used in summer, and some bark and buds of trees in winter.

The thyroid glands of the male moose, greatly enlarged during mating season (fall), were eaten liberally then by men and women in moose country near the Arctic Circle. The Indians said this caused a large percentage of children to be born in June, the best time to bring infants into the harsh northern environment. A known direct relationship exists between thyroid gland activity and fertility.

No teeth with evidence of decay were found in several primitive groups Price examined. In these and other groups, a total of eighty-seven Indians living on the native diet were examined; only four teeth ever affected by decay were found. There were almost no irregular teeth and no impacted third molars.

Inquiries were made about tuberculosis and arthritis; not a single case was seen or heard of among isolated groups. But many crippling cases of rheumatoid arthritis were seen at the point of contact with refined foods, and tuberculosis was taking a severe toll. Tooth decay was rampant, and crooked teeth with deformed dental arches were typical.

Dr. Josef Romig, a surgeon known then as the most beloved man in Alaska, was interviewed by Price at the government hospital in 1933. He had served primitive and modernized Eskimos and Indians for thirty-six years. Cancer was unknown among truly primitive natives, he stated; he had never seen a case, though when they began eating refined foods, it frequently occurred. Other acute surgical problems common among modernized Eskimos and Indians were similarly rare among primitives.

Such experience led Romig to begin sending modernized natives afflicted with tuberculosis back, when possible, to primitive conditions and a primitive diet. Though the disease was generally progressive and eventually fatal when patients remained on refined foods, he found a great majority recovered when returned to traditional foods.

During those years, a physician in Los Angeles with a keen interest in nutrition was using a strikingly similar diet in treating patients with tuberculosis and other chronic diseases. This physician, Francis M. Pottenger, would soon conduct and publish studies validating the use of a diet rich in high-quality animal source foods, especially raw and lightly cooked organs. Pottenger's investigations into the effects of cooking upon foods and his discoveries about the role of animal source foods in healing chronic diseases will be presented in the next chapter.

Price also interviewed the physician directing the hospital at Canada's largest Indian reservation in Brantford, Ontario. The doctor explained that during his twenty-eight years there, the services required had changed completely. He had had contact with three generations of Indian mothers. The grandmothers of the current generation gave birth without difficulty in wilderness homes. But current mothers often were in labor for days and surgical interference was frequently necessary. The main function of the hospital related to problems of maternity. All reservation Indians used refined foods.

Seminole Indians in Florida were studied and comparisons were made with skeletal material from pre-Columbian Indians in museums. Some Seminoles still lived in relative isolation in the Everglades and Cypress swamps; others lived in contact with modern foods along the Tamiami Trail and near Miami.

Several hundred pre-Columbian skulls from burial mounds of southern Florida were examined; not one decayed tooth nor a single dental arch deformity causing crowded or crooked teeth was found. A comparison of the thickness with that of recent skulls showed the older skulls were much thicker, providing further evidence of superior physical development in the primitive culture. Pre-Columbian skeletons showed no evidence of arthritic joint involvement; many Indians eating modern foods had bony deformities from rheumatoid arthritis, as well as tooth decay.

Primitive Wisdom.   The original inhabitants of this land had great wisdom about its utilization. Several Indian cultures ate quantities of superior quality animals and seafoods to maintain resistance to disease, great physical strength, and perfect, normal reproduction. As with the Eskimos, this was accomplished often on diets of mostly fish and wild animals, supplemented by plant foods.

Primitives had detailed information about using specific parts of animals and the unique importance of each part. Many sources indicate a vast knowledge also of medicinal uses of herbs. The development of these cultures was not simply a matter of people randomly eating what was available. Rather, throughout the world, cultures passed on the accumulated wisdom of the group to the next generation. This wisdom was concerned with laws of nature that when ignored lead to sickness, death, and the degeneration of succeeding generations.

We know not from where this wisdom came. We know only of its loss from the consciousness of the vast majority of people today.

Our culture has mobilized the intelligence and resources to send men to the moon, make color televisions, and plumb the atom's depths. Yet in failing to recognize that the Indians we supplanted knew more than we about maintaining the biological integrity of the human species, we have lost much of our health and strength.

MELANESIA, POLYNESIA, AND HAWAII (1934)

The tropics were of interest to Price because he sought universal factors affecting people everywhere, regardless of climate, race, or environment. Melanesians (on New Caledonia and the Fiji Islands) and Polynesians (on the Hawaiian, Cook, Tongan, and Marquesas Islands, and the Tuamotu group including Tahiti) were visited. Arrangements had been made through government officials, everywhere leading to a cordial reception.

Detailed records were kept for each individual on physical development, the condition of every tooth, the shape of the dental arches and face, and kinds of foods eaten. Special or unusual physical characteristics were photographed. More isolated members of each tribe were compared with those living in the vicinity of the port or landing place of the island.

Government reports revealed exactly what was imported. Nearly always, 90 percent of the total value of imported goods consisted of white flour and sugar.

The magnificence of South Sea Islanders found by early explorers is legend—a strong, beautiful, and kindly people. The islands had been densely populated. But by the time Price arrived, populations had been decimated—mostly by tuberculosis, but also by smallpox and measles.

He paints a distressing picture of the majority of those remaining. Most used little of the seafood staples of ancestral diets and together with some vegetables and fruits ate foods made with white flour and sugar. Decay was found in over one-third of teeth examined. Many individuals suffered from tuberculosis, and dental arch deformities were common in young people.

Relatively isolated groups were found, though on many islands there were few such groups. The native diet was mostly shellfish and fish, eaten together with land plants, fruits, and sea vegetables, all selected according to a definite program. Much shellfish was eaten, often raw, as were many small fish. Underground ovens of hot stones were used for cooking. Taro root was dried and powdered, then mixed with water and fermented. The incidence of decay was about one tooth in every two hundred examined, and dental arches were uniformly broad, with no crowding of teeth.

Viti Levu, one of the Fiji Islands, is one of the larger islands in the Pacific. Price hoped to find natives in the interior living far enough from the sea to be dependent entirely on land foods. He could not. Everywhere in the interior, piles of sea shells were found.

Food from the sea had always been considered essential, his guide told him. Even when at war with coastal tribes, arrangements existed whereby interior tribes sent special plant foods by courier to coastal tribes in exchange for seafoods. The couriers were never harmed. Land animals and freshwater fish supplemented what seafoods inland tribes could get. No places were found where seafoods were not eaten.

The same physical changes seen in natives eating modern foods in Switzerland, the Outer Hebrides, Alaska, northern Canada, and Florida were seen in South Seas Islanders who had abandoned traditional diets. Similarly, tuberculosis and arthritis had become prevalent.

The isolated groups immune to these problems were eating diets rich in animal source foods, providing large supplies of fat-soluble vitamins and other nutrients. The source in the South Seas was seafoods.

Groups maintaining immunity to dental and chronic disease on diets consisting entirely of vegetable matter had been especially sought; none were found. As Price's studies progressed, it emerged ever more clearly that healthy, free-ranging animal life of the land and sea everywhere provided humans with essential nutrients apparently unobtainable in adequate quantities from plants.

* * *

Many individuals have recovered from diseases on vegetarian diets. Most have included dairy foods and at least occasional fish or poultry in their regimes. When well balanced, such natural-foods diets are far superior to the diets rich in commercial meat, white flour, and sugar eaten by most people. Even strictly vegetarian diets which exclude all animal foods (known as vegan diets) often initially result in an improvement in health.

But the success of vegan diets is self-limiting. By avoiding all animal foods and animal fats, nutrients essential for development of optimal strength, resistance to disease, and reproductive capacity are lacking.

The author recalls his first philosophy teacher in naturopathic medical school. Crusty and old-fashioned, the doctor had practiced for many years. Surveying thirty-six rather thin and largely vegetarian students on the first day of classes, he cryptically offered, "Most of you people look like you could use a good steak."

Deciphering reality through the smokescreen of preconceptions is never easy. The idea that all natural foods build good health is a common preconception, but behind it lies reality: even when one eats mostly natural foods, precisely which foods are emphasized may determine the course of health.

AFRICA (1935)

The magnificence of Africa has been partially captured in several films; vast rolling plains, primordial sunsets, thundering herds of wild animals, lilting, billowy clouds of long-necked snow-white birds, lions ripping and tearing at flesh before charging the camera. The Africa Price visited was very beautiful, but like the cultures he studied, the beauty too had begun to vanish. But the land proved more permanent and less quickly damaged than the inhabitants, and even today much of the beauty remains.

Last to receive the benefits of modern civilization, the African continent in 1935 had scores of tribes living according to traditional ways. Many lived in the interior, with no access to seafoods, providing an opportunity for a comparison of the health of inland tribal people with that of modernized people living in the interior of other continents.

Price's travels in Africa covered over six thousand miles. Thirty tribes were studied, over two thousand five hundred photographs taken. His most indelible impression: the contrast between the rugged resistance of the natives to their harsh environment and the fragility of foreigners.

A racial difference this was not, for when the natives abandoned primitive for refined foods, they for the first time developed dental decay and became susceptible to infectious processes to which they were previously immune—malaria, dysentery, tick-borne diseases such as sleeping sickness, and others. The immunity when eating primitive foods extended to chronic diseases. An interview with the doctor in charge of a government hospital in Kenya revealed that in his several years of service among primitive people, he had seen no cases of appendicitis, gall bladder problems, cystitis, or duodenal ulcer.

In six tribes studied, no tooth ever attacked by decay was found, nor a single malformed dental arch. Several others had nearly 100 percent immunity to decay, and in thirteen tribes no irregular teeth were found. Where some members had moved to cities and adopted modern foods, extensive decay was found; children born of these individuals often showed narrowed dental arches with crowding of the teeth.

A wide range of diets was encountered, and differences between tribes were seen in physical stature and strength of typical individuals; stronger tribes dominated weaker neighbors. Among tribes studied were the following:

Nilotic tribes, including the Masai.   Herders of cattle and goats, the people lived on milk, meat, blood from their steers, plants, nuts, and fruits. Blood was whipped in a gourd and the clot cooked. The liquid remaining, especially important in the nutrition of children, pregnant and lactating women, and warriors, was used raw.

These cattle people were superbly developed physically, brave, and mentally sharp. Every Nilotic tribe observed dominated agricultural neighbors. This was not an undesirable trait or a sign of over-aggressiveness, for in the harsh African environment, as in all of nature, survival of the strong often was at the expense of the weak. The strength of the cattle people helped insure their survival.

Protection of their animals from predators called for greater skill and bravery by the Masai than required of other African tribes. One or two men or boys often guarded entire herds with only spears. Price called the skill of Masai in killing a lion with only a spear "one of the most superb of human achievements." Scenes of lions in full charge in films give indications of the courage involved; it is an absolutely frightening image.

Eighty-eight Masai were examined by Dr. Price; a total of ten cavities were found in four individuals.

Kikuyu tribes.   These neighbors of the Masai were primarily agricultural, eating mostly sweet potatoes, corn, beans, bananas, and millet. Smaller and much less rugged than the Masai, their teeth were quite good, but not up to the standard of cattle-herding tribes; 5.5 percent of teeth examined showed cavities. Dental arches were generally well formed.

For six months prior to marriage, young women used a special diet including extra animal source foods; these foods were also emphasized in pregnancy and lactation. Children were spaced at least three years apart; each pregnancy was preceded with special feeding. Such practices were typical of traditional cultures everywhere.

Other Agricultural People.   The chief foods were corn, beans, millet, sweet potatoes, bananas, and other grains. The people were smaller than herdsmen and tribes using large amounts of freshwater fish, and had been dominated by such tribes.

Other groups having in common a dietary made up chiefly of whole grains were examined at ports and missions. The individuals were not eating as their ancestors had. Some kept a few animals, and most used some milk and fish. Six to eight percent of the teeth in these groups had cavities.

Maragoli tribe.   Strong and well developed, these people ate quantities of fish, whole grains, sweet potatoes, and other plant foods. One tooth with a cavity was found in the nineteen individuals examined.

Muhima tribe.   These cattle-raising people lived on meat, milk, blood, and wild plant foods. They were tall, strong, and dominant, defending their families and animals with spears. This was one of six tribes Price found that had no teeth with any evidence of decay.

Sudan tribes, including the Neurs.   These herdsmen supplemented milk, blood, and meat with fish and shellfish from the Nile River. Among the Neurs, women were often over six feet tall, men over seven. No cavities were found in any people of this tribe.

They believed the seat of the soul was the liver and considered it their most important food. The growth of a person's character and body was said to depend upon feeding that soul by eating livers of animals.

* * *

Wherever natives had used large amounts of refined foods for some time, decay was rampant and tuberculosis prevalent; other chronic diseases appeared in time. The natives' immunity to infectious diseases typically striking foreigners disappeared; they too became susceptible. Dental arch abnormalities typically appeared in the next generation.

Modernized natives were aware of a problem. The question most asked by native boys at mission schools was why were they not so strong as boys growing up without contact with mission or government schools.

As elsewhere Price had visited, the contrast between traditional and modernized natives was stark. These words of a mining prospector, spoken after twenty years among the native people of Uganda, echo the sentiments of many people who observed traditional cultures before the foods of modern commerce arrived: "The heaven of my choice in which to spend all eternity would be to live in Uganda as the natives of Uganda lived before the coming of modern civilization."

Perhaps he romanticized. Yet, such reports were not uncommon, nor are they inconsistent with recent reports by contemporary anthropologists studying surviving hunter-gatherer cultures.

Tribes eating grains-based natural foods diets had well formed dental arches and resistance to infectious diseases, but their resistance to dental decay, physical development, and strength were inferior to tribes eating more animal source foods. The people strongest physically and often 100 percent resistant to dental disease were herdsmen-hunter-fishermen. In towns and ports where some groups ate a combination of refined and primitive foods, problems developed, but not to the extent occurring when native foods were abandoned entirely.

* * *

Primitive people everywhere discovered essentials of life, and following fundamental nutritional laws put them in harmony with nature. Modern civilization has chosen to ignore these fundamental truths. The sophistication of our technical knowledge has bred an arrogance precluding an appreciation of the primitives' superior skill in interpreting cause and effect. The wisdom of primitive societies in understanding laws of nature and living in harmony with these laws is a treasure humanity must not lose if we ever wish to regain our lost strength and resistance to disease.

Words like "primitives" and "savages" reveal our prejudices. Most writers have emphasized aspects of traditional cultures reinforcing these images. Western society has assumed that domination by white culture made it superior, that these non-white people had little to teach us. Representatives of western civilization exported religion and food to the rest of the world, refusing to realize they gave little for what they took. Immoral actions were accompanied by a lack of common sense; westerners failed to learn from cultures which, through destructive ignorance and malicious exploitation, were being forever destroyed.

Inability of many people in modern populations to reflect traditional moral values in their lives is a matter of concern. Links between morality and biology are intriguing and will later be explored. While concerning ourselves with primarily physical matters to this point, references to the characters and moral qualities of primitives Price met have been inescapable.

About this subject, Dr. F.M. Ashley-Montagu, a world-renowned anthropologist and author of various popular and scholarly books, wrote in the June, 1940 issue of *Scientific Monthly*, under the title "The Socio-Biology of Man:" "In spite of our advances, we spiritually and as human beings are not the equal of the average Aboriginal or Eskimo—we are very definitely their inferiors. We lisp noble ideals and noble sentiments—the Australians and the Eskimos practice them—they neither write books nor lecture about them."

Though many today would prefer otherwise, neither nutrition nor moral ideals are a matter of opinion. The price of society's decision to ignore natural laws governing these fundamental aspects of human life is the physical and spiritual bankruptcy threatening western society.

AUSTRALIA, THE TORRES STRAIT ISLANDS, AND NEW ZEALAND (1936)

Aborigines of Australia

Price wished to study cultures in as wide a range of physical conditions as possible. The Australian Aborigines lived in an extremely difficult environment; over one-half of Australia receives less than ten inches of rain per year. Poor soil and subsequent scanty plant and animal life in the interior regions made all the more remarkable the physical condition and culture of Aborigines there.

Their skill in tracking and trapping animals was renowned, and they were said to see animals moving over a mile away. Their social organization too was quite remarkable. The boys and girls were required to pass through a long and involved series of tests and trials (physical, mental, and moral) to enter adulthood. People knowing them well invariably stated Aborigines never stole and were completely trustworthy.

A spiritual people, they believed in an afterlife. The stars represented spirits of ancestors; spirits of great character made up constellations, and boys and girls learned their names. These were people who had conquered life's temptations and lived completely in the interest of others. Their religion was built upon this principle—as is Christianity.

In every isolated primitive group, Dr. Price saw physical excellence in all individuals. But the majority of Aborigines had been deprived of their homelands, placed on reservations, and used as laborers. The contrast between them and those left alone was more extreme than any place Price had seen. Whites enslaving Aborigines ate the same refined foods and their physical degeneration was equally marked.

Aborigines from both interior and coastal districts were studied. Special effort was made to examine children aged ten to sixteen after the permanent teeth had come in. Only then could the developing shape of the adult dental arch and pattern of the adult face be determined, allowing a full assessment of the effects of the individual's nutrition. A large number of skulls of Aborigines in museums at Sydney and Canberra were also examined.

Aborigines living primitively all had broad, beautifully proportioned faces, with wide and well-contoured dental arches. Museum skulls too were uniformly excellent.

Aborigines near the coast were larger than inland tribes, and skulls from near the coast were more massive. Coastal people ate quantities of fish, sea cow, a great variety of shellfish, sea plants, land plants, and fruits. Inland, food was scarcer; people ate roots, stems, leaves, berries, seeds, large and small animals of every variety (including rodents, insects, beetles, and grubs), various animal life from the rivers, birds, birds' eggs—nearly everything moving or growing.

All members examined in primitive groups from both coastal and inland places had excellent bodies, with almost no decay or abnormalities in the shape of the dental arch and face. Apparently this had been the case for thousands of years, for the primitive museum skulls were all perfect.

Those forced to eat refined foods showed in the next generation the same dental abnormalities present in white people. Tuberculosis and crippling arthritis became common, particularly among those with no access at all to native foods.

The story of the Aborigines is perhaps sadder than that of other primitive peoples decimated by contact with western civilization because the Aborigines were so completely exploited. They are a reminder that the white man was not welcome in primitive lands; guns were his introduction and the arbiters insuring his stay. Perhaps primitives in some places welcomed westerners at first, but ultimately they had no choice. Had they seen everything to come, they almost certainly would have resisted initial contacts more strongly.

But processes destroying traditional cultures were so insidious as to be perhaps unrecognizable in early stages. Who was to know that foods would be the difference between sickness and health, life and death; that the biological integrity of thousands of generations would be disrupted? What choices were available were not usually made wisely. When conditions deteriorated, it was in most cases impossible to return to traditional ways.

Some native people exposed to westernization chose to maintain traditional ways, entirely refusing to eat refined foods. These people maintained also their strength, health, and integrity. Perhaps they served as models for any of their fellows seeking help.

Torres Strait Islanders

The Torres Strait is the body of water between northernmost Australia and southernmost New Guinea. Many small, fertile islands supported populations of several hundred to a few thousand people when Weston Price visited. Government stores selling refined foods had in recent years been established on many islands. Adults had reached maturity eating only native foods before establishment of the stores, and very few other factors in the environment had changed.

Surrounding waters were rich with fish and shellfish. Plant foods were abundant and of such importance that Thursday Island, the location of the administrative center for the islands, was not originally inhabited because the soil was poor. The native diet consisted of a great deal of fish and shellfish of many kinds, tropical plants, seaweed, taros, bananas, papayas, and plums.

Natives living on native foods had almost no cavities. Almost all had broad, normal dental arches. They were a happy, peaceful, and contented people; there was almost no crime.

Thursday Island was the home of most whites in the Torres Strait; imported foods had been available for several decades. Native people lived mainly on the rest of the islands and acutely resented the intrusion of modern ways, particularly refined foods. Government stores were seen as a danger, and on several occasions the issue had nearly provoked violence.

The incidence of dental decay on a given island was directly proportional to how long a store had been present. Children born after parents began using refined foods often developed abnormal dental arches, as did a large majority of white children on Thursday Island.

The government physician for the Torres Strait islanders stated that in his thirteen years with them, among the native population of four thousand he had never seen a malignancy. He had operated on several dozen malignancies among the white population of about three hundred. Among natives, any conditions requiring surgery were extremely rare.

The general health and resistance to disease of traditional cultures is demonstrated in such interviews with physicians who spent years with the people. Though he focused primarily on dental health, Price's studies showed that a resistant individual develps neither dental nor other disease. He noted people suffering from tuberculosis and rheumatoid arthritis nearly always had extensive dental decay. Physicians interviewed consistently stated native people living on traditional diets remained nearly or entirely free of all disease. This was observed by early anthropologists, and confirmation has recently come in several research articles, to be discussed in chapter 4.

New Zealand Maori

The reputation of the Maori among anthropologists has, since the discovery of New Zealand, been that of the most physically well developed race in the world. An early study of 250 Maori skulls revealed only one tooth per two thousand with a cavity, and nearly 100 percent had normally formed dental arches. This was superior to even the Eskimos.

Maori have told a man at a telescope exactly when an eclipse of a satellite of Jupiter, supposedly invisible to the naked eye, was about to occur. No one from any other race has ever been reported to do so, but paintings in cave dwellings reveal that some prehistoric people saw stars we see only with telescopes.

Weston Price traveled eighteen hundred miles through twenty-five districts examining native Maori families and children in native schools in various stages of modernization; the cavities rate varied with the stage. In more isolated groups, 2 percent of the teeth had been attacked by decay, and in many districts 100 percent of the older generation had broad, normal dental arches. In modernized groups, from 40 to 100 percent of the younger people had abnormalities.

Tribal tradition placed much emphasis on shellfish, especially certain species, as was the case throughout the Pacific. Kelp and fern foot were eaten in quantity. The Maori relied primarily upon the sea for nourishment.

ANCIENT AND PRESENT-DAY PERU (1937)

Ancient Civilizations

Long before Spaniards pillaged the Mayan and Aztec civilizations of Mexico and South America, cultures flourished in Peru, existing in the high plains country of the Andes Mountains and the arid desert region extending from the Pacific Ocean to the Andes. This desert, forty to one hundred miles in width, runs one thousand inhospitable miles down the length of South America, and is marked by vast sand dunes with scarcely a sign of greenery.

But throughout are found complex foundations of fortresses and extended residential areas from past civilizations. Great aqueducts brought water from the mountains, enabling people to grow quantities of corn, beans, squash, and other plants in river bottoms where alluvial soil from the Andes had collected for ages past. These foods and seafoods nourished the cultures.

Fifteen million mummies were estimated to be in the succession of ancient burial mounds found along the entire coast. The foundation of these cultures was ultimately the sea animal life of the Pacific Ocean. Sweeping north from Antarctica, the Humboldt Current carries with it sources of food supporting a vast population of fish and shellfish.

The dead were wrapped in cloth by the early coastal races. Many articles were buried with them, including jars containing food and items the dead person used in life. Nets and tackle of fishermen were buried with many.

Thousands of specimens, well preserved because of the dryness of the climate, existed in Peruvian museums. Skulls of 1,276 ancient people were studied by Price; not one significant deformity of the dental arches was found. Each showed normal, broad arches capable of accommodating thirty-two teeth without crowding. Sea foods again provided raw materials for consistent reproduction in accordance with nature's laws.

Villages were visited where descendants of one of these ancient cultures lived. Isolated on the north coast of Peru, they were fisherfolk living traditional lives with no modern foods. Their physical development was excellent.

Cultural achievements of the ancient civilizations were considerable. Engineering feats remain unexplained. The great aqueducts of the coastal people, sophisticated and estimated capable of delivering sixty million cubic feet of water per day distances up to one hundred miles, were cut through boulders without hardened tools or blasting powder. Roads and suspension bridges built by the Incas crossed mountain divides fourteen to sixteen thousand feet above sea level, linking all parts of the empire to Macchu Piccu, their mountain fortress. A superb engineering achievement, the walls were built of white granite lifted from quarries in a river bank two thousand feet below.

The Tauhuanocan culture preceded the Incan and left magnificent monuments. One of the largest single stones ever moved and used in a building is found in one of their temples; it is thought to have been brought over two hundred miles through mountainous country. Many structures from this culture are found in the Andean Plateau from Bolivia to Equador, all characterized by intricately fitted, many-sided large stones, some of them twenty feet long. The fit is such that most crevices do not allow the passage of a knife point.

How were the stones cut and moved, and how were they and the white granite of Macchu Piccu raised? No one knows.

The Incan society was a highly organized and perhaps a successful socialistic state. Some sources report there was no hunger or crime, and that the ruling Incan carefully practiced laws his people were required to live by.

Foods in the high plateau country of the Incan and Tauhuanocan cultures were less diverse than at the coast. Plants and grains were used, including potatoes, corn, several varieties of beans, and quinua, a seed cereal. Llamas and alpacas were domesticated, and some wild game was available. A colony of guinea pigs was kept by each household for food; they are one of the few animals to make vitamin D in their bodies and provide a rich source.

When Price visited, dried fish eggs and kelp were regularly obtained through commerce with the coast and were universally available in high country markets; for centuries this had been so. The Indians said dried fish eggs were necessary to maintain fertility, and kelp to prevent the "big necks" whites often developed—the enlarged thyroid gland (goiter) which results when the body attempts to compensate for a deficiency of iodine.

Skulls from pre-Columbian burials in the mountains were studied. All were free of dental decay, with broad dental arches and well developed third molars.

Despite the severe climate of the mountains and the arid conditions of the coast, ancient Peruvians of both areas developed ways of eating and living leading to physical integrity and significant cultural achievements. The accumulated wisdom of their centuries of living in harmony with nature has been largely forgotten; subsequently, people in these lands today have developed diseases and structural physical problems inherent to the use of refined foods.

Andes Mountain and Amazon Jungle Indians

Andes Mountain Indians. In high mountain plateaus of southern Peru and Bolivia, many descendants of the ancient Tauhuanocan and Incan cultures still lived according to their ancestors' methods when Price visited. On market days, they brought down wares to trade and to socialize, giving him opportunities to examine several groups. Contact was arranged through local authorities.

The most isolated showed the lowest incidence of tooth decay and degenerative changes. No decayed teeth were found in one group of twenty-five; each individual had all teeth normal for his age.

Strength and endurance were characteristic of isolated groups. Loads in excess of two hundred pounds commonly were carried all day long, day after day. In freezing weather they slept with ponchos about their heads; legs and feet remained bare. Many lived at elevations upwards of twelve thousand feet.

While traditional mountain cultures in Switzerland and Georgian Russia used quantities of dairy products, Andes Indians achieved physical excellence without them, for dairy animals introduced have never adapted well to the climate. Llamas, wild deer, birds, and guinea pigs were their animal source foods.

Amazon Jungle Indians. The Amazon region of Peru begins in the eastern foothills of the Andes, where fertile soil, warm climate, and abundant rainfall results in fish-filled streams and forests rich with tropical vegetables, fruits, and wild animals—foods for the Amazon Jungle Indians. Price met and examined a group of thirty.

A proud, beautiful people with great strength, no teeth ever having decayed were found, and each individual had perfect dental arches. Another tribe of the same racial stock was in contact with a mission and had reduced the use of native foods in favor of refined foods available through the mission. Many had rampant tooth decay, and young children had dental arch deformities. They were becoming civilized.

* * *

Decay and missing teeth were expected. But Dr. Price's monumental study for the first time thoroughly and convincingly linked many problems to inadequate nutrition. Among these problems were changes in the shape of the dental arches, head, and face; infertility, miscarriages, difficult labor, and birth defects; susceptibility to acute diseases; and prevalence of tuberculosis, arthritis, cancer, and other chronic diseases.His discovery of characteristic animal source nutrients in the diets of all groups enjoying immunity from these problems further adds to the revolutionary impact of his findings.

Five pages of Weston Price's photographs follow, a graphic conclusion to this survey of his work. The benefits of raw foods, as demonstrated in the work of Francis Pottenger, are the subject of the next chapter, and in the chapter following, the history of the human diet, the relationship between evolution and food, and current research about the health and foods of surviving primitive cultures are considered.

PHOTOGRAPHS FROM
NUTRITION AND PHYSICAL DEGENERATION

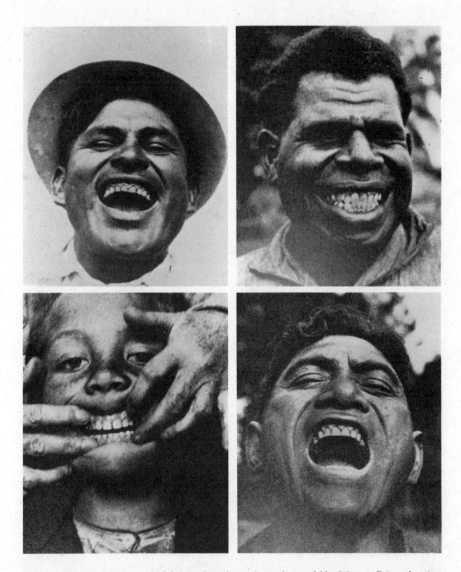

Figure 1. Photographs typical of those taken throughout the world by Weston Price of native people living on traditional foods. Uniformly broad dental arches were found everywhere—with all thirty-two teeth present, little or no decay, and no crowding of teeth.

    upper left—Peruvian coastal fisherman

    upper right—Great Barrier Reef (Torres Strait) fisherman

    lower left—Swiss girl (Loetschental Valley)

    lower right—New Zealand Maori fisherman

The photographs in this section were taken by Weston Price in the 1930's; most appear in his book, *Nutrition and Physical Degeneration*. These prints were made by Marcus Halevi and appear here courtesy of the Price-Pottenger Nutrition Foundation. Dr. Price's book may be ordered from the Foundation at P.O. Box 2614, La Mesa, CA 92041.

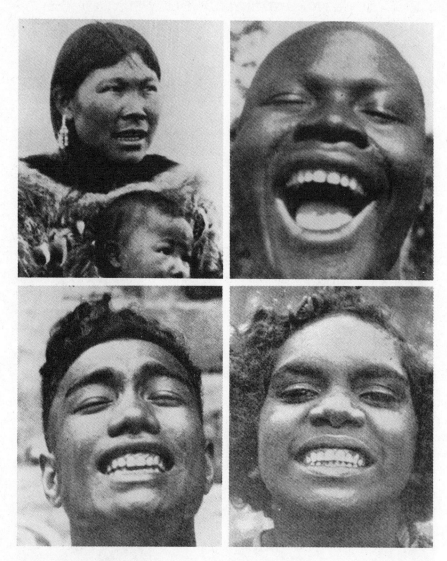

Figure 2. Further examples of the remarkable but quite natural physical development resulting wherever people ate according to the traditional wisdom of their culture.
    upper left—Eskimo woman and child
    upper right—African woman
    lower left—Aborigine man
    lower right—Aborigine woman

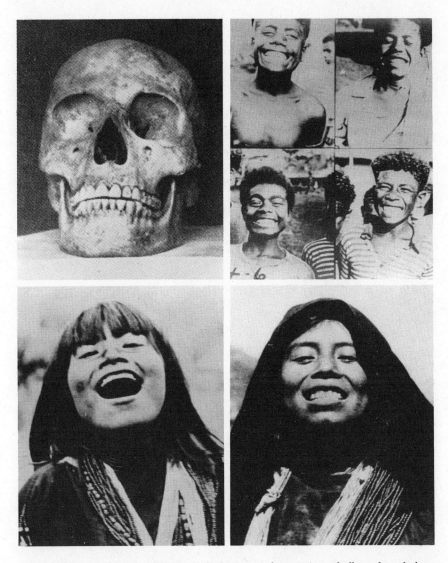

Figure 3. Archeological evidence studied in several countries—skulls and teeth from ancient cultures—showed in generation after generation that tribal patterns repeated themselves with no significant changes.

upper left—This ancient Indian skull was among the skeletal remains Price studied in North America, Australia, and Peru. In Peru, he examined 1,276 successive skulls without finding one with the narrowed dental arches of most modern people.

upper right—Melanesian boys. These four boys lived on four different islands and were not related. Each had nutrition adequate for the development of the physical pattern typical of Melanesian males; thus their similar appearance.

lower left—Peruvian jungle Indian girl

lower right—Peruvian jungle Indian woman

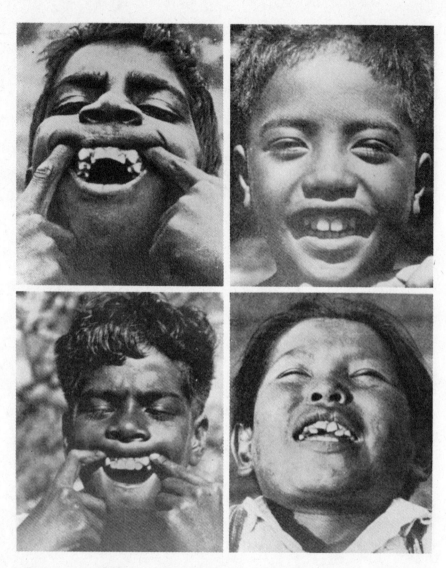

Figure 4. Typical changes occurring in the first generation born after the introduction of refined foods—narrowing of the dental arches with subsequent crowding of teeth. These problems occurred in addition to the agonizing dental decay which both the parents and the children experienced.

    upper left—Aborigine boy
    upper right—Polynesian boy
    lower left—Torres Strait Islands boy
    lower right—Eskimo boy

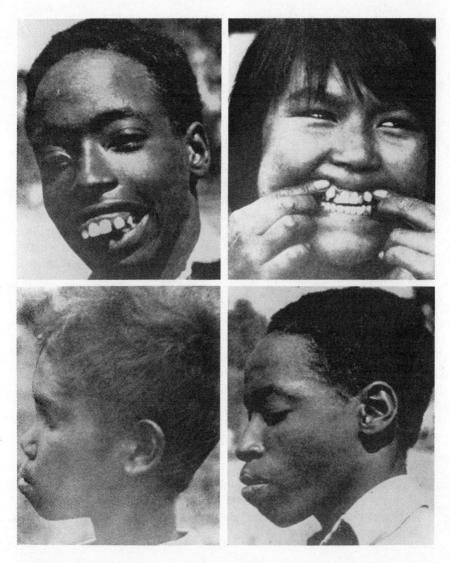

Figure 5. Further examples of degenerative changes typically seen in children born of parents eating refined foods.

upper left—African boy with extreme protrusion of the upper teeth and shortening of the lower jaw.

upper right—Eskimo girl with crowding of the upper dental arch which has caused the bicuspids to protrude. This is often seen in cultures eating refined foods. Contrast this with the young people in Figures 1 through 3.

lower left—Aborigine boy. Changes in the shape of the face and dental arch have caused the lower jaw to be thrust forward. Price virtually never saw such changes in people eating native, natural foods.

lower right—African boy; the same thrusting forward of the chin in a boy on the other side of the world. The cause is the same.

3

Benefits of Raw Foods

Archeological evidence indicates humans used fire at least four hundred thousand years ago; splintered and charred bones of large mammals Peking man hunted littered his caves. He probably used fire to help get at the marrow, and he may have roasted some meat.

Cooked food is more quickly chewed than raw; the change from an entirely raw to a partially cooked diet freed some time formerly spent eating—time now spent cooking. Cooking has always been both social and practical, combined with elements of ceremony, habit, convenience, and pleasure.

A home heated by wood gathers people near fire for hours in cold months. In caves and later primitive shelters, cooking and sharing meals about the warmth of fire was an everyday routine, as has been so in all cultures since.

And yet in every traditional culture examined, anthropologists find that customs dictate certain foods be eaten raw. Reasons invariably relate to preventing disease, insuring fertility, or promoting optimal growth in children.

Francis Pottenger was a physician and researcher whose work provided almost certain proof that raw foods contain unique nutrients vital to human beings. He conducted a now classic series of controlled experiments which involved over nine hundred cats for over ten years. He kept detailed records of his thousands of patients for over thirty years, discovering correlations between the cat experiments, his contemporary Weston Price's discoveries, and his clinical work treating people with chronic and acute diseases.

Dr. Francis M. Pottenger

Son of the physician who founded the once famous Pottenger Sanatorium for treatment of tuberculosis in Monrovia, California, Pottenger completed his residency at Los Angeles County Hospital in 1930 and became a full-time assistant at the sanatorium. From 1932 to 1942, he also conducted what became known as the Pottenger Cat Study.

In 1940, he founded the Francis M. Pottenger, Jr. Hospital at Monrovia. Until closing in 1960, the hospital specialized in treating nontubercular
34

diseases of the respiratory system, especially asthma. Pottenger maintained his private practice until his death in 1967.

A regular and prolific contributor to the medical and scientific literature, Dr. Pottenger served as president of several professional organizations, including the Los Angeles County Medical Association, the American Academy of Applied Nutrition, and the American Therapeutic Society. He was a member of a long list of other professional organizations.

Pottenger's Cats and Raw Foods: The Ten-Year Study

Extracts from adrenal glands of cows and steers were part of treatment patients received at the tuberculosis sanatorium, which manufactured the extracts from fresh glands shipped from Denver and Los Angeles. No laboratory assays capable of determining hormone content of biological extracts existed in the 1930's. To determine potency, cats which had had their adrenal glands removed were kept alive with extract; the amount required to maintain animals adequately determined the level of that batch's potency.

Despite careful surgical techniques and a diet of raw milk, cod liver oil, and meat scraps from the sanatorium kitchen, many cats died after the surgery to remove their adrenal glands. There was no obvious explanation, but the cats showed signs of nutritional deficiencies. Many had problems reproducing, and many kittens born in the laboratory pens had skeletal malformations and internal malfunctions.

Pottenger had a keen interest in nutrition; a high-protein natural foods diet was an important part of treatment at the sanatorium. Liver, tripe, brains, sweetbreads, and heart were fed to patients; scraps, all cooked, were fed to cats. When the cat population grew because Pottenger's neighbors donated so many, he began securing raw meat scraps for some cats.

These cats were, before long, in plainly better health than cats remaining on cooked meat. Their operative mortality markedly decreased, they reproduced more easily, and their kittens were healthier.

This inspired Pottenger to embark on a series of controlled experiments. Because pathological problems in cats eating cooked meats were similar to those in his patients, he believed a controlled feeding experiment with animals would isolate variables of importance in human nutrition as well.

The experiments met the most rigorous scientific standards of his day. His outstanding credentials earned Dr. Pottenger the support of prominent physicians. Alvin G. Foord, M.D., Professor of Pathology at the University of Southern California and pathologist at the Huntington

Memorial Hospital in Pasadena, co-supervised with Pottenger all pathological and chemical findings of the study.

The study is over forty years old. The technology of science has grown
more sophisticated, as the search for causes of disease has moved to the
intracellular level. But because of the strength of his insights, Pottenger's
inquiries and observations provide demonstrations about fundamentals
of nutrition and disease.

Two areas of inquiry in particular address questions modern science
has largely ignored. First, what is the nutritive value of heat-labile elements—nutrients destroyed by heat and available only in raw and undercooked foods? Second, what determines the difference in nutritional
value between one animal and another, one egg and another, one glass
of milk and another? The ten-year study answers these questions.

Raw Meat Versus Cooked Meat.   Effects of a raw meat diet fed one
group of cats, versus those of a cooked meat diet fed another, were
measured in the initial experiment, begun in 1932. The raw meat diet
consisted of raw meat, including bones and organs such as liver, heart,
brains, kidneys, and sweetbreads; raw milk; and cod liver oil. The cooked
meat diet was exactly the same except meats were cooked. In both diets,
raw milk was "market grade"—milk available commercially. A high
grade raw milk from cows kept at pasture or fed fresh-cut greens was
later used in select experiments.

Cats were kept in large outdoor pens, and successive generations were
followed. The raw meat group reproduced easily, and as each generation
developed there was for each sex striking uniformity in size and skeletal
development. A broad face with wide dental arches and no crowding of
teeth was the rule. Fur was uniform, with good sheen and little shedding.
Inflammation and diseases of the gums were rare.

These animals were resistant to infections, fleas, and other parasites.
They were friendly, even-tempered, and well coordinated—when
dropped from up to six feet or thrown, they always landed on all four
feet. Miscarriages were rare, and litters averaged five kittens. Cause of
death was generally old age, or occasionally fighting among males. Autopsies invariably revealed normal internal organs.

The cooked meat group showed many contrasts to the raw meat group,
contrasts which grew with successive generations. Litter-mates varied
greatly in size and skeletal structure, particularly dental and facial pattern. Often by the third generation bones became so soft as to be actually
rubbery. Vision problems, infections of internal organs and bones, arthritis, heart problems, underactivity of the thyroid gland, inflammation
of the joints and nervous system, skin lesions, allergies, intestinal parasites and vermin, and a host of other pathologies were common. Coor-
dination was poor; when tossed a short distance, the cats had trouble

landing on all four feet. Pneumonia and lung abscesses were the most usual causes of death in adults, pneumonia and diarrhea, in kittens.

At autopsy, analysis of the bones of cooked meat animals determined calcium and phosphorous content for second and third generation kittens to be one-third to one-half that of raw meat kittens. A marked difference between the two groups was also found in the average calcium to phosphorous ratio (2.08 to one for raw meat kittens versus 2.63 to one for cooked meat kittens).

Many cooked meat females were irritable and aggressive, while males were often docile and unaggressive, with little interest in females but keen interest in other males (an interest never seen in raw meat-fed males). Abnormal sexual activities also were seen between females in the cooked meat group. At autopsy, females often showed small ovaries with a congested uterus; males often showed testes which had failed to develop the ability to produce sperm.

Cats born outside the Pottenger Sanatorium, donated to the study, and placed on the cooked meat diet were called first generation deficient cats. Kittens born of them and fed the cooked meat diet were called second generation deficient cats. Kittens born of second generation deficient cats and fed the cooked meat diet were called third generation deficient cats.

The miscarriage rate among first generation deficient females was about 25 percent, among second generation deficient females, about 70 percent. Many cats died in labor; deliveries were difficult; many kittens were born dead or too frail to nurse. The kittens born of cooked meat mothers weighed an average nineteen grams less than those of raw meat mothers.

No fourth generation deficient kittens were ever born in the ten years of the study. Third generation deficient kittens always died before reaching six months of age, terminating the strain.

Raw Milk Versus Pasteurized Milk. Four groups of cats were used. All received for one-third of the diet raw meat, including organs, and cod liver oil. The other two-thirds was either raw milk, pasteurized milk, evaporated milk, or sweetened condensed milk. The raw milk/raw meat diet produced many generations of healthy cats, while the various heat-processed milk/raw meat diets produced successively sicker cats unable to reproduce by the third generation; the inclusion of one-third raw meat in the cooked milk diets did not prevent severe problems.

The most severe degeneration occurred in cats fed sweetened condensed milk; they became extremely irritable and nervous and developed heavy fat deposits and marked skeletal deformities. Cats fed evaporated milk were nearly as damaged. Those fed pasteurized milk showed lesser damage, similar to that seen in cooked meat animals of the prior experiment, i.e., skeletal changes, decreased reproductive capacity, and infectious and degenerative diseases (problems which were among those seen in the sweetened condensed and evaporated milk groups).

In a variation of this experiment, the effects of raw milk from cows fed fresh greens versus those of raw milk from cows fed dry feed were compared. Cats fed cooked meat and raw milk from fresh feed cows did significantly better than cats fed cooked meat and raw milk from dry feed cows. The latter produced deficient kittens and had difficulty nursing. Deficiencies were much less marked for animals fed cooked meat and also fed raw milk from fresh feed cows.

Fresh Greens Versus Dried Greens.   Guinea pigs were used to compare the effects directly. A group of animals was fed grains, cod liver oil, and field-dried alfalfa. Deficiency symptoms appeared—loss of hair, diarrhea, pneumonia, paralysis, and high infant mortality. Fresh cut greens were then introduced (grass cut after sundown, sacked, and delivered before sunrise). The animals gained weight, infant deaths decreased, loss of hair decreased, and no new cases of paralysis developed.

Some guinea pigs that had developed severe symptoms initially and not fully recovered were then allowed to feed on grass and weeds growing outside the pens. Within a few weeks, all diarrhea and loss of hair stopped, and their hair was soft, shiny, and velvety; the animals appeared even healthier than those kept inside the pens on fresh-cut greens. Seeking an explanation, Pottenger discovered the temperature inside sacks of cut grass used for feed was from five to thirty degrees warmer than the outside air. The grass had become somewhat cooked in the sacks, and heat-labile nutrients apparently had been altered.

* * *

Pottenger was not the first to maintain experimental animals for extended periods on natural foods. From 1902 until 1935, Dr. Robert McCarrison, a British physician in the Indian Medical Service and founder of the Nutrition Research Laboratories at Coonoor, India, studied goiter and other health problems of the Indian people. He did extensive experiments with large populations of laboratory animals, and in 1933 published a report containing statistics about several studies.

In conjunction with those studies, McCarrison kept a control colony of about one thousand white rats for over three years. The animals were killed and autopsied when two years old. In over fifteen hundred autopsies, no sign of disease was ever found. In the three years, there was no illness, no death from natural causes, and no infantile mortality. The animals were fed whole wheat flour cakes of unleavened bread lightly smeared with raw butter, sprouts, raw carrots and cabbage, raw milk, and raw meat and bones once a week. All foods were fresh; the animals lived in large, airy, clean rooms, and were exposed to the sun daily.

Parallels Between Pottenger's and Price's Work

While the experiments of Drs. McCarrison and Pottenger show the value of raw foods in keeping animals remarkably healthy, one might wonder about relevance to human needs. Cats are carnivores, humans omnivores; and while animals' natural diet is raw, humans have cooked some foods for hundreds of thousands of years. But humans, cats, and guinea pigs are all mammals. And while the human diet is omnivorous, foods of animal origin (some customarily eaten raw) have always formed a substantial and essential part.

Problems in cats eating cooked foods provided parallels with human populations Weston Price studied; the cats developed the same diseases as humans eating refined foods. The deficient generations of cats developed the same dental malformations that children of people eating modernized foods developed, including narrowing of dental arches with attendant crowding of teeth, underbites and overbites, and protruding and crooked teeth. The shape of the cat's skull and even the entire skeleton became abnormal in severe cases, with concomitant marked behavioral changes.

Price observed these same physical and behavioral changes in both primitive and modern cultures eating refined foods; he noted changes in character, morals, and behavior that accompanied the adoption by a culture of refined foods. In traditional cultures, strength of character and relative freedom from moral problems of modern cultures were characteristic. Studies of populations of prisons, reformatories, and homes for the retarded revealed that a large majority (often approaching 100 percent) had marked abnormalities of the dental arch, often with accompanying changes in the shape of the skull.

This was not coincidence; thinking is a biological process, and abnormal changes in the shape of the skull from one generation to the next can contribute to changes in brain functions and thus in behavior. The behavioral changes in deficient cats—nervousness, irritability, increased aggressiveness of females and passivity of males, with concomitant homosexual behavior—were due to changes in nutrition. This was the only variable in Pottenger's carefully controlled experiments. As with physical degenerative changes, parallels with human populations cannot help but suggest themselves.

Human beings do not have the same nutritional requirements as cats, but whatever else each needs, both may need a significant amount of certain high quality raw foods to reproduce and function efficiently.

* * *

Beginning with Albert Einstein, theoretical physicists have sought a single grand theory uniting the theories of relativity, electro-magnetism, and gravity. Details remain elusive, but many believe an encompassing explanation for the physical phenomena of the universe will indeed be found.

Such a theory, however, will not explain the biology of the degenerative physical and mental changes which have accompanied the abandonment of humanity's traditional foods, and the adoption of the refined foods of modern industrial society. To explain our modern predicament—and hopefully guide us out of it—we need a unified biological theory, based on an understanding of humanity's roots and attempting to work in harmony with forces inexorably shaping us. Physics seeks an understanding of physical forces affecting the universe; human health requires an understanding of biological forces in foods that affect human evolution.

Pottenger's work shows nutrients in foods easily affected by heat have effects on health and reproduction. The nutritive value of raw milk was shown dependent on the feed of the cow. The nutritive value of foods of animal origin, as measured by the food's effect on the health of an experimental animal, was shown to depend directly on the diet of the animal of origin.

Raw Foods and Calcium Metabolism

Pottenger maintained in-patient facilities and an out-patient practice for over thirty years, giving him an opportunity to study effects of his nutritional programs on many patients. He observed problems with calcium metabolism in a majority. Poor development of the teeth is the first and most obvious sign. Later arthritis appears; nearly all older people in America today show symptoms.

Other problems commonly connected with faulty calcium metabolism include back problems and other skeletal disorders, including spondylitis; gall stones and kidney stones; atherosclerosis, often leading to coronary heart attacks; hardening of the arteries of the brain, often leading to strokes; cataracts; and bursitis. Deposition of calcium in abnormal places is their common denominator.

Though many people develop these problems eating diets deficient in calcium, so too do others with diets rich in calcium. A diet rich in calcium (including calcium supplements and vitamin supplements to aid in the assimilation of calcium) does not prevent or reverse these problems unless the diet contains adequate fresh, raw foods.

Pottenger found clues about calcium problems in X-ray studies documenting changes in the skeletal system of his patients (the dangers of X-rays were little understood in his time). One study compared skeletal structures and bone age (the development of the growth center of bones in relation to the standard for a child of that age) in 150 children drinking four different types of milk—breast milk, raw certified milk, pasteurized milk, and canned milk.

The only group with consistently excellent development of the bones and skeleton and with normal bone age was the group drinking raw certified milk. Nearly all of the children drinking pasteurized milk or canned milk developed either very fine, small bones, disturbances in calcification of bones, or marked weaknesses in joints and ligaments. Bone age in a majority of these children was below normal.

Among children fed breast milk, development of bones was dependent on the diet and state of health of the mother. Children of mothers using high quality foods, including raw certified milk, had well developed bones with normal bone age. Children of mothers using diets including the cooked milks had bones with delayed development of growth centers and poor calcification, and weak joints. Breast milk is superior to raw certified milk only if the diet of the mother is of proper quality.

Other cases and studies of Dr. Pottenger demonstrated the value of raw milk and other raw foods and problems that occur when the diet lacks raw foods, which came to play an increasingly larger role in his approach to disease.

Raw Foods and Chronic Diseases

Dr. Josef Romig told Weston Price of how modernized Eskimos and Indians with tuberculosis usually recovered when returned to their native villages and native diets. Native Eskimo and northern Indian diets were similar to the diet Pottenger successfully used for patients with tuberculosis and other diseases. Liberal amounts of liver, heart, sweetbreads, kidney, brain, tripe, meat, fish, fertile eggs, and raw milk were used; organs were emphasized. These animal source foods were from animals kept at pasture or fed fresh greens.

Much of this diet was served raw, including organs, in a variety of recipes. Food was cooked as lightly as was palatable for the patient. Raw vegetable salads with sprouts were served twice daily. Breads made from sprouted whole grains were baked at low temperatures, minimizing destruction of nutrients. Bone meal and marrow were also prepared at low temperatures. Small quantities of fruit and sesame seeds were used, and the use of vegetable oils was minimized. This type of diet, carefully individualized for each patient, is a reasonable approach to chronic disease.

Raw Foods and the Digestive System

The digestive system adapts well to raw foods introduced at a rate appropriate for the individual. An acute inflammation in the digestive tract—gastritis, ulcers, colitis, certain types of diarrhea, among others—may easily be irritated by raw vegetables or fruits, which should in such cases be slowly introduced only when the acute problem has resolved and healing has begun.

But for most people, becoming accustomed to more raw foods involves more mental than physical obstacles. While popular wisdom holds cooking makes foods more digestible, this is true only of grains. The human digestive system is fully capable of digesting a wide variety of foods raw. Many foods may be more easily chewed when cooked, but for the fully functioning human digestive tract, all but the grains are most easily digested raw or lightly cooked. This is particularly true of animal proteins.

Raw food consists mostly of hydrophylic colloids. Hydrophylic means water-loving, and a colloid is a suspension of solid particles in a gel-like fluid. Eaten uncooked, these colloids absorb large quantities of digestive juices, forming a gelatinous mass which maintains the mucosa of the stomach and digestive tract in a healthy state.

The heat of cooking precipitates out colloids, making them hydrophobic (water-hating); the hydration capacity of the colloids is decreased, and they become less able to absorb digestive juices. Colloidal cellulose and pectins in plants can withstand greater temperatures without being precipitated than can proteins; this is why cooking has a less pronounced effect on the digestability of plants than on that of animal source foods.

In the ten year cat study, cooked food cats were consistently found at autopsy to have much longer intestines than raw food cats. Intestines of the former had many distensions and general lack of tone; the length was often up to twice that of raw food cats. The argument has been made that the length of the human digestive tract demonstrates humans are best suited for a vegetarian diet; remains of the digestion of animal flesh may putrefy when stagnant in the rather long human intestines. We may speculate that the eating of overrefined and overcooked foods contributes to that length; problems due to flesh too long in the intestines may be due to intestines that are *too long*. The low fiber content of refined foods contributes to this problem.

Safety, Convention, and Tastes

Evolution, anthropology, animal experiments, and clinical experience aside, the usefulness of information about raw foods justifiably hinges on questions of safety, convention, and personal taste.

The amount of raw vegetables in the diet should be increased rather slowly, allowing the body to adapt gradually. The mind too requires time to grow used to new and changing ways. While safety and convention are not major issues for plant foods, they are for animal source foods.

Consider a steak ordered rare, in many restaurants served nearly raw in the middle. The meat has passed through an inspection system of sorts. The steer was fed hormones, antibiotics, and grains containing residues of a variety of chemical poisons; varying amounts of each are in the meat, be it well done or raw. Government inspection guarantees that the meat contains no harmful organisms; it is accepted as safe. But mistakes, oversights, and occasionally corruption occur in the inspection system. And most animals are raised today in a manner which raises questions about their health and desirability as food for human beings.

Meat and organs from pasture-fed, naturally raised cattle must also be inspected. Such meat is more desirable than the usual commercial varieties. Though available in many areas now, meat of this quality in much of the country is hard to find.

One can order meat rare, even very rare; in the latter case, it may be served nearly raw. Very rare meat is socially acceptable; raw meat is not. This obviously has nothing to do with safety. Taste as well as convention is served; a charcoal-grilled very rare steak has more flavor than raw meat.

Health benefits make it desirable to become accustomed to lightly cooked meat, if one eats meat. Tastes change slowly; one may gradually become accustomed to rare and even raw meats. Occasionally individuals highly motivated by a desire to recover from serious problems, or prevent them, succeed in making these changes more abruptly.

Sushi has become popular—raw fish has been accepted in America. Many species may safely be eaten raw. Raw shellfish taste best to the non-connoisseur when hunger is sufficient; for the initiated, nothing compares. Most fish may be lightly cooked to the point of flaking apart, which is undercooked by most standards; most people prefer it cooked more. Restaurants generally overcook all fish; by ordering it undercooked, one may avoid having it served overcooked.

There are two considerations about the safety of raw animal source foods: the health of the source animal and the health of the individual eating the food. Both healthy people and healthy animals are highly resistant to disease. And by definition, healthy animals do not carry disease.

Brucellosis, or undulant fever, may be contracted by eating the meat or drinking the raw milk of infected animals. Modern commercial meat and dairy animals are susceptible to this disease—their health is poor as a result of overcrowded quarters, a lack of fresh grass and exercise, and overuse of chemicals in their management. Animals are best kept partly at pasture and in uncrowded conditions. If allowed to exercise and inspected regularly, they produce milk and meat which is healthy and safe.

Occurrence of brucellosis in cows was correlated with trace mineral deficiencies in an article of Pottenger's ("Brucella Infections," *The Merck*

Report, July, 1949). Minerals present in tissues of healthy cows were found on spectrographic analysis missing in tissues of cows with brucella infections. Cows fed the trace minerals manganese, cobalt, copper, and iodine were immune when exposed to the disease in other animals.

In subsequent work with over eighteen hundred patients with brucellosis, Pottenger found that supplements of these minerals (together with his dietary program) consistently resulted in significant improvements in blood picture, visible symptoms, and the patient's sense of well-being. The previous diet of nearly every patient indicated a state of malnutrition long before symptoms of brucellosis first came to attention.

The corollary of increased susceptibility of weakened individuals to the spread of disease from animals is that healthy individuals are resistant to such spread. This is why primitive Africans were resistant to organisms causing so much disease among whites in Africa, and it is why traditional people everywhere ate animal life without fear of infection. The animals were by and large healthy, but the first line of defense was superior resistance. That this resistance was in part the result of eating the animal life—much of it lightly cooked, some of it raw—completed the circle of cause and effect.

One can eat in a somewhat unconventional manner—if done with flair—and still be accepted by one's friends. Some interesting conversation may result. Compromise is required, in social situations as well as with one's own taste buds. Raw and lightly cooked foods simply cannot be forced; as with all food, they must be enjoyed if lasting habits are to be developed. While one may strive to try new things, let the first consideration be the selection and preparation of natural foods that are enjoyed. Upon this base may be built a long lifetime of refinements.

In a later chapter, several diets placing a widely differing emphasis on raw foods will be reviewed; some make no mention of the issue, others stress the importance of raw foods, and one stresses a need to cook most foods. All are to varying degrees successful; we will see that the most successful have a deep understanding of the value of raw food nutrients. But first, we turn to times when raw foods dominated the pre-human and human diet. Physical splendor was assumed; mental acumen was necessary for survival. Comparing and contrasting what is known of the diet and health of humans throughout evolution with contemporary hunter-gatherers and modern people is the subject of the next chapter.

4

Evolution
Food
and Health

From Ancient Ancestors
to
Contemporary Hunter-Gatherers

*T*he history and evolution of the human diet is a subject rich in controversy and rife with opinion and conjecture. But evidence exists, and
anthropologists are generally in accord, about roughly what our ancestors ate, if not precisely when they ate what. Agreement also exists on
the health of present-day primitive people eating diets similar to early
man's. An examination of the evidence, inferences, and conclusions of
anthropologists and medical researchers sheds light on why contemporary traditional cultures enjoy excellent health.

Evolution and Diet

Modern human beings, anatomically and genetically our equivalent, had
evolved by about forty thousand years ago. The agricultural revolution—
the cultivation of plants and the domestication of animals—of the past
ten thousand years is thought to have had little effect upon our genes.
One exception is that, in some parts of the world, people have evolved
the ability to digest milk as adults. More recent changes (masses of people
leaving the countryside to live in cities, modern commercial agriculture,
the refinement of much of our food) have not had the time required to
cause changes in our genes.

Thus we are genetically equipped to eat foods our hunter-fisher-gatherer ancestors ate—the pre-agricultural revolution diet. Many of us are
descendants of ancestors who settled into agricultural life less than two
thousand years ago; for others, agricultural roots go further back. Agriculture markedly affected human diets, with a shift to more vegetable
foods (grains especially) and a decline in animal consumption. The effect
on the size of humans was profound—European big-game hunters of
thirty thousand years ago were an average of six inches taller than their

farmer descendants. A similar change occurred in the Americas among Indians shifting to a more agricultural way of life in the period just before Europeans arrived.

Over the past two hundred years, larger amounts of animal source foods in western diets have resulted in an increase in average height to close to that of our big-game hunting ancestors. But more recently, diseases afflicting neither the hunter-gatherers nor the agriculturists have become major health problems. Writing in the January 31, 1985 issue of *The New England Journal of Medicine* under the title "Paleolithic Nutrition," Boyd Eaton, M.D., and Melvin Konner, Ph.D., reported that heart disease, high blood pressure, diabetes, chronic intestinal disease, and most types of cancer have been reported by medical authorities to be virtually unknown in hunter-gatherer cultures surviving today—the Hadza of Tanzania, the Kung and Kade San (Bushmen) of the Kalahari, the Philippine Tasaday, the Aché of Paraguay, the Australian Aborigines of Arnhem Land, and the Arctic aboriginal Eskimos, among others.

The publication of such information in this particular professional journal, long a bastion of conservative medical opinion, is an important milestone. For many years, other medical journals and professional publications have carried articles linking diet, health, and specific diseases, yet the medical establishment in this country has steadfastly ignored the evidence. With the appearance of "Paleolithic Nutrition" and related articles in *The New England Journal of Medicine*, perhaps more American physicians will become aware of the intimate connection between diet and disease.

Investigations published in Canadian and American journals over the past thirty years have shown young people in primitive cultures to be free of the early symptomless indications of these chronic conditions that have been found in young Americans. This was shown in autopsies of both hunter-gatherer youths killed in hunting accidents and young Americans killed in the Korean war. And examinations of people over the age of sixty in these primitive cultures found them relatively free of these diseases.

Present day traditional agricultural cultures in Georgian Russia and the region of the Vilcabamba Valley in Ecuador have also been demonstrated to be largely free of chronic diseases. Investigators have commented for years on the rarity of chronic diseases in America around the beginning of this century. Paul Dudley White, President Eisenhower's personal physician during the years the former president suffered his two heart attacks, wrote in 1943 in his textbook *Heart Disease:* "...when I graduated from medical school in 1911, I had never heard of coronary thrombosis, which is one of the chief threats to life in the United States and Canada today....it is now responsible for more than 50 percent of all deaths."

Archeologists consider cavities in the teeth of skeletons evidence of a people who lived under a fairly well developed agriculture; Price was not the first or only investigator to show hunter-fisher-gatherers to be nearly or completely immune to dental decay. But although our hunter forefathers were larger, stronger, and more resistant to dental disease than our agricultural forefathers, both types of culture were, for the most part, apparently free of modern degenerative diseases.

The refinement of grains, the production and consumption of sugar, and the decline in quality of foods from both plant and animal sources have contributed to the emergence of chronic disease as a major threat. Around 1900, new methods for milling flour were introduced which completely stripped the very perishable wheat germ from the grain. By 1910, these methods were in general use, and many people lost their major source of vitamin E and an important source of several other nutrients, including the B-vitamins and several minerals. Refined flour became a staple in foods, as did sugar, vegetable oils, and additives. Trends since then have been toward the use of more refined foods. Domestic animals have been injected with chemicals, drugs, and hormones, as the mechanization of agriculture has transformed them into meat and milk machines.

We turn now to the evolution and changing diet of ancestors of the human species, and of pre-agricultural humans who roamed the earth as hunter-gatherers for hundreds of thousands of years before the agricultural revolution began to end their way of life.

* * *

Early ancestral relatives of humans lived in trees probably more than five million years ago, eating fruit, eggs, and nestlings. Changing climatic patterns in Africa near the equator are thought to have driven these creatures down from trees in times of drought to forage for food in grasslands. Certain direct ancestors of humans, classified in the genus *Homo*, and other creatures of the genus *Australopithecus*, appear in fossil records of two to nearly four million years ago. *Australopithecines* were similar to our ancestors in many ways; both are thought to have descended from the same ancestral line, and both walked with feet nearly identical to those of modern man. Though the head has undergone drastic changes, particularly in the size of the brain, they walked upright. We know this from the position of the foramen magnum, the hole in the base of the skull through which the spinal cord passes en route to the brain.

Australopithecus was first named by anatomist Raymond Dart when skeletal remains of the creature were discovered in 1924. For many years, it was thought to be the direct ancestor of humans. Recent discoveries, however, indicated *Australopithecus* was a vegetarian cousin of the *Homo* line leading to man. The jaw and teeth are heavier, more suited to chewing and grinding roots. The teeth of *Homo* species of the same period are smaller and lighter, more suited for tearing and chewing meat. While *Homo* developed, *Australopithecines* became extinct between one-half and one million years ago.

Between one-and-a-half and two million years ago, *Homo erectus* appeared—the first human. Meat consumption increased during this time—animal bones litter his caves, he had tools for hunting and cleaning animals, and he lived in areas well populated with large game. He spread far from central Africa, where he most likely originated—a classical find of his species is Peking man, about four hundred thousand years old, and the first we know with certainty who used fire.

Further changes led to Neanderthal man, the first of *Homo sapiens* (*Homo sapiens neanderthalensis*). First appearing about eighty thousand years ago, he ate a diet estimated to have been perhaps 50% meat. But as Cro-Magnon man and other modern humans (*Homo sapien sapiens*) appeared some forty thousand years ago, they improved weapons and communications skills, and groups of men became more efficient at hunting big game. Meat assumed an even more dominant role in human nutrition.

This trend was reversed in the period shortly before the beginnings of agriculture. Need for fresh hunting grounds had spread humans all over the globe, and by the eve of the agricultural revolution, we numbered some three million. Together with changes in animal populations and climate, this population growth may be the reason why hunting for large animals became less important for many cultures. A new pattern emerged, as fish, shellfish, and small game assumed increasing importance. Tools for processing plant foods became more common at this time, some ten to twenty thousand years ago. Trace mineral analysis of strontium levels in bones has shown vegetable consumption was increasing as meat consumption decreased.

Contemporary Hunter-Gatherers

A mixed diet is typical of the estimated three hundred thousand contemporary hunter-fisher-gatherers. Animal source food constituted an average of 35 percent (by weight) of the diet in several cultures studied, the remainder coming from plant sources. The range for animal source food was from 20 to 80 percent. A similar range was found among cultures Weston Price studied, though some used even more animal source food much of the year.

One contemporary tribe carefully studied in the 1970's is the Kung. Only about two hundred still carry on their ancient way of life in the Kalahari Desert of Botswana. Like all remaining hunter-gatherers, they occupy a marginal area modern civilization has not yet claimed. Yet they have existed there for at least ten thousand years.

The Kung are one of the groups medical teams studied in concluding that contemporary hunter-gatherers do not develop the diseases of civilization. About 10 percent of the Kung are over sixty years old, approximately the percentage found in America. They live quite a leisurely life; men hunt two or three days a week, and women spend an equal amount of time gathering plant foods that constitute about two-thirds of the diet. Much time is spent socializing, visiting, sharing food, and teaching children. Some anthropologists have called hunter-gatherers the original affluent societies; many definitely do not lead the hard and short lives of popular conception.

Richard Leakey writes in *Origins*, his marvelous account of human evolution, that the sharing of food formed the strongest bonds among early hunter-gatherer humans living in small groups. Many anthropologists believe this socialization distinctly led to our development into complex social beings. Vegetarian cousins of early man, the *Australopithecines*, were solitary feeders who did not share food with companions; they became extinct. The sharing of meat specifically formed social bonds around which the life of early humans revolved, and helped make possible our subsequent evolution.

Among the Kung, killing and sharing meat is surrounded by great excitement and almost a sense of mysticism. Customs dictate how and with whom animals will be shared, and this is done with a great deal of fanfare and ritual not attending the sharing of plant foods. Dr. Leakey offers no explanation of why meat rather than some other food is the center of such ceremony and sense of importance.

Consideration of historical evidence and recent research reviewed earlier suggests meat was placed on a pedestal simply because the human animal recognized the essentiality and central place of animal source food in the diet. In other cultures fish played this role; in yet others, dairy products came to the fore. Hunter-gatherer societies were marvelously efficient; if they had not been, early pre-humans would not have proceeded to three million subsequent years of evolution. The traditions, rituals, and mysticism of the Kung surrounding the capture, sharing, and eating of meat are logical. Meat may supply only one-third of the bulk of their food, but they recognize it as essential and behave accordingly.

Analysis of hunter-gatherer diets shows an average fiber content of forty-six grams, eight to ten times that of the modern diet. The calcium content of sixteen hundred milligrams is at least twice as great; this figure is calculated from plant foods and animal flesh consumed, and does not reflect bones eaten (parts certainly were). The sodium intake was only one-sixth that of ours, while protein intake was at least twice today's average. Trace mineral content was high.

Less fat is consumed on a hunter-fisher-gatherer diet. Concentrated vegetable oils are unknown. Wild grazing animals contain little fat; fifteen African herbivores assayed had an average fat content of 3.9 percent. Today's beef cattle are from 25 to 50 percent fat or more; other domestic food animals are usually even fattier.

The composition of fats in a hunter-fisher-gatherer diet is different from that of fats eaten by most people today. As we'll see in later chapters, the fatty acids in vegetable oils are precursors of different prostaglandins than are the fatty acids found in free-ranging animals and in saltwater fish; evidence indicates the latter fatty acids are more desirable. Primitive diets are low in the fatty acids richly supplied in vegetable oils, but high in those richly supplied in fish oils.

Grazing wild animals were another primitive source of beneficial fatty acids; their fat has over five times more unsaturated fatty acids per gram than the fat of domestic animals (which have more saturated fatty acids), and four percent of them are eicosapentaenoic acid (EPA). Analysis of modern domestic beef showed only trace amounts of EPA. We'll look further at EPA in examining recent information about fish oils in chapter 7.

Implications For Post-Agricultural Revolution Diets

These analyses of ancestral and contemporary primitive diets present a comparison of traditional with modern foods. Whether weighted more toward vegetables or more toward meat and fish, ancestral diets included more fiber, less vegetable fat and saturated animal fat, and more polyunsaturated animal fat (especially EPA) than modern diets.

And while post-agricultural revolution diets changed considerably, maintenance of many elements of hunter-gatherer diets was until recently characteristic. Fresh meat from free-ranging domestic animals was a staple, used regularly nearly everywhere. Such meat has certain qualities of wild game. Raw milk and dairy products from such animals have similar qualities; they too were regularly used until recent years. Fish remained a staple for coastal and river people, as did fresh raw vegetables and fruits for rural people everywhere. So too did whole grains prior to modern milling techniques.

Agricultural cultures everywhere ate these foods for thousands of years; their people were healthy and largely resistant to diseases prevalent today. Whether one ate more in the manner of the hunter-fisher-gatherer, or more in that of the agriculturist, one had available a wide spectrum of foods that built healthy bodies.

As we look into the long lives of people in Vilcabamba, Hunza, and Georgian Russia in the next chapter, we will realize that their foods have much in common with those discussed in this chapter. The subtleties of some of the differences will be explained as well; the long-lived people provide many examples of how the traditional foods of early agriculturists differed from those of hunter-gatherers on the one hand and modernized cultures on the other. Nutrition is never as simple as may sometimes appear, but if we keep in mind that Weston Price showed the full spectrum of human disease to be ultimately caused by less than optimal nutrition, we will see subtle influences causing profound effects.

5

*Long-Lived People
of
Vilcabamba
Hunza
and Georgian Russia*

*R*eports of many people remaining vigorous into extreme old age are the stuff of popular legends, and Vilcabamba, Hunza, and Georgian Russia have generated their share. Isolated and remote, Vilcabamba is a village of several hundred people in the Vilcabamba Valley in the Andes Mountains of southern Ecuador. Hunza too is remote and mountainous, an ancient kingdom of some forty thousand people living near the borders of China and Afghanistan in the high valleys of the Himalayas in Pakistani-controlled Kashmir. Georgian Russia covers a much larger area, and it too is mountainous. One of the three Soviet republics of the Caucasus region, it has a population of some five million.

Many people in these places state ages well over one hundred years. In the 1971 census, the village of Vilcabamba listed nine in a population of 819; how many other centenarians lived on small farmsteads in surrounding mountains and hamlets is unknown. But Ecuador is Catholic; church baptismal records have been carefully made and preserved for centuries. These records verify many centenarians, several of whom were over 120 in 1975.

Georgia reported 1,844 centenarians, or thirty-nine per one hundred thousand people; for some, birth records exist. In comparison, centenarians number three per one hundred thousand in America. Many old people in Hunza claim to be over one hundred, but there is no written form for the language and no recording of births.

Verifying Ages and Health Status

Controversy invariably surrounds extraordinary claims of longevity, and verifying the ages of people in these regions is difficult. Examining reports of evidence for people in and around Vilcabamba, however, makes clear that stated ages are largely true. Alleged experts on life extension have discredited all reports of great longevity because a supposedly common practice in Georgian Russia had a man take his grandfather's name, and with it his age, to avoid compulsory military service. This may indeed have occurred, and some Hunzas and Georgians may well have exaggerated their ages to investigators. But these are not reasons to discredit all claims of great longevity among these people.

Church baptismal records in Vilcabamba provide believable evidence. Several medical investigators have taken pains to verify the ages of old-sters in Georgia and Vilcabamba, and have stated that with reasonable certainty a number of these people were over 120 years old, and many others were well over one hundred. The church records show several people in the mountains near Vilcabamba who died in the 1920's and 1930's were over 150 years old. This is consistent with reports from Soviet gerontologists that Russia's oldest man recently died at the age of ap-proximately 168.

Attempts to verify the stated ages involved several independent meth-ods which were matched one against another. Documents of dates of birth, such as church baptismal records, were considered most reliable. Passports, old letters, and even woodwork carved in homes to record births all proved useful.

Each oldster was questioned about his age at marriage, the time until children were born, and the present age of children. Memories of events of historical or local importance were recorded. Calculations of the per-son's age made from this data correlated well for 704 centenarians in Georgia whose ages were known from birth records; for 95 percent, the calculated age exactly matched the age on the birth record. For the rest, the error averaged 5 percent, and in no case was the error more than ten years.

Verification was more difficult in Hunza because the absence of written records made it impossible to confirm exact ages. But as in Vilcabamba and Georgia, investigators agree the physical vigor in extreme old age, rather than the age itself, most impresses visitors. The old people lived in the mountains and were farmers, and often had been hunters or herdsmen (a few men over ninety still were). Everyday life had since early childhood involved much walking and other exercise, and they continued to walk and work, usually until shortly before death.

Dr. David Davies, a gerontologist at University College in London, did a thorough job of documenting the ages of a number of centenarians in Vilcabamba. He made four trips to the Vilcabamba Valley and the sur-rounding mountains between 1971 and 1973. In *The Centenarians of the Andes* (1975), he describes these trips.

He spent a great deal of time in churches searching baptismal records. The priests would not let these books out of sight; the books never left the church premises. The earlier were made of parchment, with a skin covering; some dated back to 1655. Dry climate and care had preserved them in highly legible condition.

Baptismal records of people still living dated to 1847; one individual was 126 at the time of the investigation. Records were found for several others over 120. Death certificates were found for four people who lived to 150 and died in the 1920's and 1930's in the mountains near the Vilcabamba Valley. The records were kept by Jesuits, who in those years controlled the export of Peruvian bark found in the area, at great profit. As a source of quinine, it was then the chief medicinal for malarial fevers. Davies points out that the Jesuits certainly would not have wanted to attract visitors, and one can think of no reason why they would have falsified the documents.

Civil registers were kept separately beginning around 1900 in state offices in villages; these too recorded births and deaths. Deaths of the old people, births of their children, and wedding dates were recorded. These dates of death matched those in the church records. Other dates were used to corroborate life history methods of estimating age. These data were checked for correlation with the documentation and stated ages of individuals.

Children and grandchildren were also interviewed to corroborate further ages of centenarians, as were other oldsters of about the same age. Interviews were held separately to prevent possible prompting. Memories of the old people are described as remarkable, and the various methods consistently verified ages listed in baptismal records. Dr. Davies' reasonable conclusion: "Thus we have been entirely satisfied that the ages of these centenarians are authentic."

He further reported these people were lucid, agile, and active in old age, and did not get cancer, heart disease, diabetes, high blood pressure, or other diseases afflicting people in modern cultures. These diseases were common in towns just fifty miles away. Even in the village of Vilcabamba and other villages in the valley, chronic diseases had begun appearing with the introduction of refined foods. When centenarians who had moved down from the mountains to be near younger relatives were exposed to these foods, they were less healthy; in some, symptoms of diabetes appeared.

Centenarians nearly always had spent their lives on their small mountainside farms outside the villages. When remaining there, they experienced eventually a time when health declined and aging occurred rapidly. Typically within a few months death came.

"Every Day Is a Gift When You Are Over 100," which appeared in *National Geographic* in January of 1973, is an account of long-lived people by Dr. Alexander Leaf, a physician and teacher at Harvard Univeristy who spent parts of two years traveling in the three regions. The woman who spoke the words of the title was named Khfaf Lasuria, a resident of the Abkhazia region of Georgian Russia. Leaf concluded after a lengthy interview that she was over 130 years old.

She recalled events of her life for Leaf in great detail. She had retired from her work as a tea-leaf picker two years before; when over one hundred in the 1940's, she had held the record as the collective farm's fastest picker. Still independent, she took care of herself, regularly taking a bus alone to a distant village to visit relatives, keeping a garden, and caring for her chickens and pigs.

She greeted the doctor with a toast of vodka; she drank a small glass each morning, and a glass of wine before lunch. Each household in Abkhazia had its own vineyard and made its own wine. The wine was dry and drunk fresh, and was a source of enzymes, minerals, and other nutrients. Many old people drank two or three glasses a day. On festive occasions, many Abkhazians drank considerable grape vodka (also homemade), and wine. But the older people often abstained from vodka and their wine glasses were smaller.

Mrs. Lasuria smoked about a pack of cigarettes a day, and she inhaled; she began smoking in 1910. A small number of old people of these three regions smoke, but many reportedly do not inhale.

Leaf was surprised to find a handful of overweight centenarians in Georgia, but they too worked and walked vigorously in the mountains. Exercise is almost certainly one key to longevity. A Russian gerontologist studied over fifteen thousand people over eighty in Georgia and found that over 70 percent walked regularly in the mountains and over 60 percent still worked. Oldsters who failed to maintain useful roles tended to die sooner.

A Georgian cardiologist and gerontologist, Dr. David Kakiashvili, tested the hearts and lungs of many of the old Georgians with modern investigative techniques. He found many had silent cardiovascular diseases that had never caused symptoms. All had exercise-induced superior cardiopulmonary function which he believed was protecting them. Dr. Miguel Salvador, a well-known and respected Ecuadoran cardiologist, extensively studied 338 elderly Vilcabambans and found only one with a weak heart.

In several studies of the Abkhasians by other Georgian gerontologists, dating back to 1932, only the slightest signs of heart conditions were ever found, these in some of the very old. No reported cases of cancer occurred in a nine-year study of 123 people over one hundred years old; the vast majority were also found to have good neurological and psychological stability. A study of the vision of another group aged over ninety found 40 percent of the men and 30 percent of the women able to thread a needle without glasses; hearing was good in 40 percent of the group.

Further evidence of an absence of chronic diseases in Vilcabamba was provided by Dr. Jorge Santiana, a cancer specialist and associate of Dr.

Salvador. Santiana too visited Vilcabamba and examined many of the elderly. He found only one growth—benign.

And yet, Davies discovered two problems in the health of Vilcabambans. First, mortality in infancy and early childhood was high. This he discovered in examining church baptismal records; 40 percent died of epidemics and viruses before the age of three. And second, the vast majority of older people, including most centenarians, lost most or all of their teeth at a fairly early age. The gums were firm; individuals could chew foods easily, but were without many teeth during later years. This was in contrast with Georgians, whose teeth generally remained excellent into extreme old age. We'll later return to these problems.

Most old people in Georgia were married. The study of fifteen thousand Georgians over eighty revealed that, with rare exceptions, only married people attained extreme age. Many couples had been married upwards of seventy and eighty years. Among centenarians, 91 percent of the women had two or more children; 68 percent had four or more. Only 2.5 percent were childless. Among both men and women, a strong interest in the opposite sex was considered normal into old age; an active sex life well into the nineties was not unusual.

In contrast, Dr. Davies found in Vilcabamba that most women over one hundred had never married. The life of married women there was considerably harder; they were overworked, treated as sexual objects, and exhausted by middle age. Of fifty married women interviewed, all but one over the age of twenty-five had between four and fourteen children, many more than the women in Georgia. Vilcabambans are Roman Catholic.

People in these cultures expected long lives; young people interviewed spoke of living to one hundred. Old people enjoyed high social status and were esteemed for wisdom and experience. Multi-generation, extended family households were universal, and the word of the oldsters was generally regarded as law. Even people well over one hundred continued tending animals, gardening, caring for children, working in the fields on a limited basis, and tending domestic chores.

While common elements are present among long-lived people, a long and healthy life is an individual matter. In dietary matters as in other habits, each person within the framework of what was available set his own patterns. Individual diets undoubtedly had an influence on individual longevity.

Foods used in the three regions have much in common, but there is conflicting and somewhat confusing evidence. We'll now examine the diet in each place to provide a basis for contrasts, comparisons, and conclusions.

Georgian Russia

Soviet gerontologists studied dietary habits of one thousand people over the age of eighty, including more than one hundred centenarians. About 70 percent of the calories were of vegetable kingdom origin, and the remainder were derived from meat, milk products, and eggs. This proportion is nearly identical to the average found in contemporary hunter-gatherer cultures, and corresponds with estimates for the diet of hunter-gatherer cultures existing at the time of the beginnings of the agricultural revolution.

Caloric intake of these Georgians was estimated at seventeen to nineteen hundred calories per day, high for people over eighty years old; this is explained by their physical activity. Soured raw milk, usually from goats, and raw milk cheeses were used at nearly all meals. The cheeses are low in fat, and daily fat intake was only forty to sixty grams (about 25 percent of the total calories were from fat). Eggs were commonly used; most people kept chickens, goats, and sometimes pigs and sheep. These animals were eaten regularly, and there were many meat courses on festive occasions. Protein intake averaged seventy to ninety grams per day (an amount found in twelve ounces of lean meat).

Vegetable gardens were kept by most people. Fruits were common, but were not a large part of the diet. Grain staples included whole grain bread baked in outdoor ovens and unflavored cornmeal-mush patties eaten with sauces spiced with hot red pepper. Homemade butter and homemade wine were used daily, and many people enjoyed small amounts of homemade grape vodka.

Vilcabamba

The village of Vilcabamba lies thirty miles southwest of Loja, a small town some five hundred mountainous miles south of Quito, the capital of Equador. *Vilca* means "sacred" and *bamba* means "valley" in the language of Quechua Indians once inhabiting the Vilcabamba valley. Legend has it the valley was the original paradise of Adam and Eve; myths and romantic stories abound. Visitors say a very special atmosphere surrounds the place.

The valley is nearly at the equator, and the altitude at the village is a little over five thousand feet. The temperature is steady year around, usually about sixty-eight degrees at midday. Chief crops of the valley and adjacent mountain slopes are wheat, barley, yucca root, corn, and some grapes. Coffee and sugar cane are grown for export. A wide variety of green vegetables, legumes, celery, cauliflower, and cabbages are grown.

Most of the old live on small mountain farms and grow vegetables, grains, and fruits. Most keep chickens, a goat or two, and perhaps a cow and other animals. Soured milk products are used, though less than in Georgia. By some reports, the Vilcabambans eat little animal protein—an average of twelve grams a day according to an Ecuadoran medical team that studied the elderly. But Dr. Davies' details typical meals with centenarians which included raw or lightly boiled eggs, cottage cheese made fresh from cows' or goats' milk, and occasionally fresh meat. Many centenarian families had more meat because one member was a herdsman.Both eggs and cheese were commonly used, though less so than in Georgia. Vilcabamba was poor; people could not keep as many animals as the Georgians.

Davies tells of his stay with one centenarian family. At dawn, the old man hiked fifteen minutes up a steep mountainside to his fields, bringing back fresh corn, while his wife gathered eggs around the house. These foods would typically be lightly boiled and eaten with homemade brown bread, boiled beans, homemade raw cottage cheese, and perhaps yucca, wild potatoes, fruits, or green vegetables. Meat was eaten if an animal had been killed recently.

Few English-speaking people have visited Vilcabamba. Little original information about the diet has been written; most accounts are repetition of the few original reports, particularly that of the Ecuadoran medical team. Dr. Davies' book indicates more eggs, milk products, and meat are used by old people than has been reported in several popular books by individuals who have never visited Vilcabamba. Davies spent time in the mountains visiting centenarians, learning they all kept chickens and dairy animals. Vilcabamban villagers, more accessible to other investigators, did not keep as many animals. The Ecuadoran medical team did not single out centenarians in their studies of the elderly; their data, based on a sampling of older people in the village, did not reflect specifically the average diet of centenarians.

The details of the diets of centenarians as a group and of individual centenarians might provide invaluable clues about longevity. Like the Ecuadoran team's study, the study in Georgia of one thousand people over the age of eighty grouped all data and presented averages; no search was made for differences between diets of centenarians and those of the rest of the elderly.

A detailed examination of foods and lifestyles of individual centenarians (including analysis for fat-soluble nutrients, and vitamin and mineral content) would add another dimension to our understanding of these people. Other considerations would include the quality of the soil and the health and diet of animals used for milk, meat, and eggs.

Two other men reportedly over 125 years old both lived on the coast of Equador and had been fishermen, as was the case for the majority of that country's isolated individual centenarians. Davies did not investigate them because he felt isolated remarkable individuals might live to a great age simply because of great stamina. His interest was in examining environments where large numbers of centenarians lived, looking for influences upon the aging process. But Davies writes that in his previous studies of surviving primitive cultures (he has led expeditions studying several primitive societies and has authored several books about his work) he often found individuals living to a great age near the coast.

This is a significant clue in understanding longevity because the quality of animal life of the sea is similar to that of the dairy products, eggs, and meat produced in the mountains of Vilcabamba, Georgian Russia, and Hunza. Protective nutrients richly supplied in fish, free-ranging animals, and milk products and eggs from such animals are common elements in diets of coastal and mountain centenarians throughout the world. We will investigate these nutrients further in the next two chapters.

Vilcabambans had only limited amounts of animal source foods; the amounts were not quite adequate. More were available to Georgians, and fishermen centenarians certainly were richly supplied. Only the Vilcabambans suffered from loss of teeth, likely because their diet lacked adequate fat-soluble protective nutrients found only in animal source foods. But foods available are of the highest quality, and are sufficient both to protect them from most problems and to give many of them great longevity.

These issues are complex. Recently published information about similarities in the structure and composition of fats in fish and grazing animals was a vital clue. While many claim Vilcabambans live so long because they consume little food of animal origin, evidence indicates they live so long in spite of it. What they do consume is of the highest quality; they would simply be better off with more.

Witness the Georgian centenarians. The very old eventually lose some teeth, but Davies and other investigators report most have very good teeth. Infants and young children suffer very little mortality. The diet is rich in meat and dairy foods of the highest quality and in nutrients found in substantial quantities only in these foods and in fish. These nutrients are known to control mineral metabolism (thus the effect on dental health), benefit the immune system, and have a host of other profound effects.

High mortality among the young in Vilcabamba also may be explained in part by these same considerations; many simply do not have sufficient strength to resist disease. Apparently nutrition which is adequate in most ways for adults is not adequate for the very young. Imagine a population living in a way conducive to good health and longevity, and eating optimal foods, but without quite enough of certain foods and associated nutrients. Some problems must appear somewhere, though the people as a whole may be healthy and many might live to be very old. Is it not logical and even expected that nature would find a way to limit the population and prevent further scarcity? Nature's way is to take the weakest of the young, both in human and in wildlife populations.

Birth control was practiced by virtually all traditional cultures Weston Price studied. These cultures were conscious of the need to space children at least three years apart and accomplished this through customs and tribal laws. Further to insure healthy children, women ate special foods before and during pregnancy and while nursing. Young children too ate special foods.

Any such customs regarding the spacing of children among Vilcabambans were lost when they became Roman Catholics upon the arrival of the Spanish; the practice of any form of birth control was forbidden. Very large families inevitably resulted, with no planned spacing of children. Frequent deaths among infants and young children resulted.

Among elderly Vilcabambans, even with loss of teeth, the gums and jaws remained strong. The misery accompanying the decay and extensive loss of teeth that marked the introduction of refined foods in the cultures Price studied was conspicuously absent; teeth simply fell out in middle and later years. The people had the strength and resilience to adapt to this loss.

Vilcabambans ate more meat and milk products when available, for example if one family member was a herdsman. Their consumption of animal source foods was limited by scarcity rather than choice.

Several elements of Vilcabamban life are disconcerting, including the high death rate among the young and the dental problem. Davies observed the men often did not treat the women very well and tended to drink excessively quite often. Married women spoke of being unhappy with their lot in life, as did some very old women who had never married. Many people smoked (in Georgia it was only a few). The balance and happiness found in the people of Georgia were seldom seen among the Vilcabambans, except among the mountain farmers.

Hunza

Hunza is isolated. The nearest air travel is to Gilgit, Pakistan, and even then only in good weather, through a narrow mountain gorge. Several days' travel over difficult mountain roads is then required to reach Hunza. Permission to visit, granted by the Pakistani government and the ruler of Hunza, is difficult to obtain. Those who have visited have been unable to document ages of old people, for there is neither a written language nor birth records. Western visitors have given conflicting reports.

Sir Robert McCarrison, a British physician who worked in India for nearly thirty years as earlier described, spent most of his time from 1904 to 1911 in Hunza. He later wrote in *Studies in Deficiency Diseases* that the people were "...unsurpassed in perfection of physique and in freedom from disease in general....the span of life is extraordinarily long....during the seven years I spent in their midst....I never saw a case of asthenic dyspepsia, of gastric or duodenal ulcer, or appendicitis, of mucous colitis, or cancer." The Hunzas and the Hunza diet inspired McCarrison's animal feeding experiments.

The book *Hunza, Lost Kingdom of the Himalayas,* by John Clark, was published in 1956, detailing his twenty months in Hunza in 1950-51. An American geologist who first spent time in the Far East as an Army engineer during World War II, Clark returned on his own to see what he could do to help what he described as a small, poverty-stricken Asian country. He had training in anatomy, first aid, and public health, plus twenty years of field experience in first aid while working as a geologist in remote areas.

At the Mir's urging he set up a medical dispensary upon his arrival. He describes the people as desperately poor, sometimes malnourished, and much in need of medical help for a variety of problems, including malaria, dysentery, worms, trachoma, impetigo, goiter, dental decay, rickets, and tuberculosis. He saw many of these problems daily during his entire time in Hunza, often treating fifty to sixty people a day, using antibiotics, sulfa drugs, and anti-malarials he had brought into the country. Eventually he was forced by the Pakistani government to leave; his plans for helping the Hunzas to improve their way of life and escape poverty had been rejected.

The book *Hunza Land: The Fabulous Health and Youth Wonderland of the World*, by Renee Taylor, was published in the early 1960's. A film, "Hunza....The Valley of Eternal Youth," based on her travels in Hunza, was made. Taylor wrote several other books about Hunza, stating there was little or no sickness of any kind, no need for doctors, and that Hunza is "the land of just enough." She stayed at the Royal Palace and quotes the Mir extensively. She wrote that many of the people were over one hundred years old, and that virtually everyone was healthy and happy. No documentation was offered about the health status of any of the people.

Dr. Leaf wrote of Hunza that he had an impression of many extremely fit and vigorous old people moving about the very mountainous countryside. A picture of a man said to be the oldest in Hunza and claiming to be 110 is shown; Leaf regarded the age as approximate. He describes a dietary survey taken by a Pakistani nutritionist. Fifty-five Hunza men were found to have an average daily caloric intake of less than two thousand calories, with fifty grams of protein and thirty-six grams of fat; meat and dairy products were estimated to supply only 1.5 percent of daily calories. Leaf apparently did little field work or interviewing in Hunza, and his only comment on the Hunzas' health or longevity is to report that the Mir, from his personal knowledge of the state's history, verified ages of many of the elderly.

The above accounts are in accord that the Hunza diet is sparse in animal source foods; few families could afford more than one or two animals. The country is in the high Himalayas and villages and farms are built largely on steep valley hillsides; usable land is crowded. Clark wrote there was no winter pasture, and summer pasture was much overgrazed; the land would maintain few animals.

The chapatti is the mainstay of the diet, made from wheat, barley, buckwheat, or millet flour freshly ground from whole grain, kneaded, and baked over an open fire. Sprouted seeds are used, and fresh vegetables; the people all farm small plots of land. Apricots, mulberries, grapes, and walnuts are grown. Grapes are made into homemade wine. Apricot seeds are both eaten and made into an edible oil. When an animal is butchered, every possible edible portion is consumed. Clark wrote this would typically be only twice a year; then meat would be eaten for a week or so.

What milk is available is mostly from goats; milk and buttermilk are used sour. Some butter and cottage cheese are made. Those who care for animals in high summer pastures may eat much of these foods; most of the population has little.

Dr. McCarrison's account of Hunza is an objective medical report by a physician who knew the country well. McCarrison was one of the fathers of modern nutritional science; his experiments, research papers, and books have stood as classics in the field for over fifty years. To list the honors he received during his career would fill pages. His character, creative intelligence, and ability to record objectively the situation in turn of the century Hunza cannot seriously be questioned.

Reports since then are both scarce and conflicting. John Clark's book is a well written and carefully constructed account of his nearly two years of living among the people of Hunza. The holder of a doctorate in geology, he was a professor and research associate at Princeton University at the time of publication. His purpose in Hunza was both humanitarian and political; he wanted to teach the people technological expertise about farming, animal husbandry, and modern woodcrafting that would enable them to raise their standard of living and turn away from possible Communist influences. While he did not formally survey the health and longevity of the people, he did record in detail his observations and experiences.

Illnesses he reported were acute infectious processes and deficiency states, rather than chronic diseases. Prevailing problems reflected deficiencies of adequate nutrients of animal source, compounded in some cases by inadequate total caloric intake. The Hunzacuts go through a period each spring, just before fresh foods begin growing, when very little food is available.

The legend of Hunza was strong before Dr. Clark's time in the kingdom. He writes in his preface: "I wish also to express my regrets to those travelers whose impressions have been contradicted by my experience. On my first trip through Hunza, I acquired almost all the misconceptions they did: The Healthy Hunzas, the Democratic Court, The Land Where There Are No Poor, and the rest—and only long-continued living in Hunza revealed the actual situations. I take no pleasure in either debunking or confirming a statement, but it has been necessary clearly to state the truth as I experienced it."

There is no reason to doubt Clark. Taylor's and other later accounts were written by some of the few Westerners who were allowed into the country; their visits were brief. As guests of the Mir who stayed at his palace, they may have seen no more than the ruler wished. A film was made, this too perhaps influenced by official decisions about content. The creation of a myth may have been considered desirable. The myth has been further perpetuated by populizers of vegetarian and largely vegetarian diets.

Early and reliable reports such as McCarrison's established Hunza as a rather special and healthy place; hence it was that much easier later to create and perpetuate a popular legend. But, if McCarrison's account of 1904–11 Hunza, and Clark's account of 1950–51 Hunza, are both accurate, we are left to account for why things changed.

This is difficult. The capacity of the land may have been overextended; by the time of Clark's tenure in Hunza, every square inch was in use. But in a land that prospered for over two thousand years, why did problems develop in less than fifty? For whatever reasons, John Clark's book makes clear that by 1950, a small but significant percentage of the people of Hunza suffered from problems directly caused by inadequate nutrition; he reports treating over five thousand people during his time in the country.

Conclusions About Long-Lived People

Conflicting reports generate controversy, and while possible explanations exist, only a personal investigation in the three places could hope to resolve the issues. But we are left with reasonable proof that people in Vilcabamba and Georgian Russia live to be very much older than most authorities state is possible, and that they do so with great vigor. This may be the case in Hunza as well. An extremely active, emotionally rewarding life and a special kind of natural foods diet appear to be the influences most responsible.

Georgians have demonstrated the most resistance to health problems, whereas Vilcabambans and Hunzas suffer from problems uncommon in Georgian Russia. The Georgians alone obtain sufficient amounts of protective nutrients, richly supplied in their meat and dairy foods.

The Traditional American Diet

Foods that rural pre-industrial America relied upon were similar to those of Georgian Russia. One hundred years ago, over half our people lived on farms. They made bread from whole grains, grew vegetables and stored and preserved the surplus, raised beef cattle without chemicals and hormones, kept chickens, pigs, and dairy animals at pasture, fished in creeks and rivers, and hunted for wild game. Some people living near the coast fished daily; others combined elements of farming and fishing life. People spent their days outdoors and working.

The milk and cheeses were raw, the garden free of pesticides, the grains whole, the animals lean, free of hormones, and fed their natural diets. The diet of our farm people was roughly the diet of Georgian Russians and of traditional people everywhere who cultivated plants and kept animals for food.

These people were largely free of the diseases of civilization—hypertension, heart disease, arthritis, colitis, obesity, diabetes, cancer, and stroke, to name the more common. Well into the twentieth century, these diseases had nowhere near the prevalence in America they have today.

The average age of death in 1900 was forty-five to fifty years of age. But one-third of all babies died in infancy or early childhood, keeping the average down. Sanitation in cities was poor, and the nutrition of people in cities did not compare with that of people on farms. Antibiotics and advances in public health knowledge, combined with resultant improvements in sanitation, have drastically reduced death among the young. Average life expectancy is thus up to seventy-five years, but the average forty year-old today can expect to live only four years longer than the average forty year-old could expect to live in 1900. Health and quality of life of the elderly have declined; the very prevalence of chronic diseases implies extended suffering that in the past occurred on a much more limited scale.

One hundred years ago, many deaths at very young ages caused the average life expectancy to be only forty-five to fifty years, despite the fact that many people lived to be sixty, seventy, eighty, and older. A somewhat larger percentage of people today live to those ages; the claim is made that this is why there is a rising incidence of chronic diseases. But the moderate increase in the percentage of people living longer today has been nowhere nearly enough to account for the increases of several hundred percent which have occurred in the incidence of each of the diseases mentioned above. Each now afflicts many people before they reach fifty or even forty. While unusual or even rare among the population as a whole one hundred years ago, most of these diseases were then nearly or literally unheard of at age forty or fifty.

Protective nutrients are found in the traditional diets Weston Price studied, in the raw foods diets of Pottenger's experiments and clinical work, in ancestral and contemporary hunter-gatherer diets, and in the diets of the long-lived people. These nutrients and other characteristics of successful diets are the subject of the next chapter. When present, these nutrients exert extremely beneficial effects; their relative deficiency in modern diets may well prove to be the ultimate cause of the growing epidemic of modern degenerative diseases.

6

Protective Characteristics of Traditional Diets

*D*iets of traditional groups immune to dental and degenerative disease had several characteristics in common (these people will be referred to as immune groups). Nearly all foods were whole, unrefined, and unconcentrated. The only modification was cooking, often minimal; many were eaten raw. Major exceptions to this whole-foods generality were the use of butter and cheese in the Loetschental Valley of Switzerland and of seal oil and other concentrated animal and fish oils by Eskimos.

The foods of each immune group had been used by the group for centuries or longer and were indigenous to the group's region. No imported foods were used. Customs dictated the importance of eating certain foods at specified times in life. Specific foods were known to prevent specific problems. Certain special foods believed to insure the birth of normal, healthy offspring were particularly valued and were included in the pre-conception diet of both parents.

None of the diets contained large amounts of fruit, which was used when available, though in limited quantities. Even where large quantities of fruit were available, fish and shellfish, animals, and vegetables were preferred.

Immune groups used none of many foods commonly used today. The obvious include sugar, white flour, canned goods, and other supermarket standards. Less obvious are vegetable oils and fruit juices, both commonly used by health-conscious people. Nor did they use significant amounts of honey, the only sweetener sometimes available. Alcohol was used moderately if at all, in raw fermented beverages rich in enzymes and minerals. They took no vitamin pills.

Fish and shellfish were used in quantity by immune groups near the sea, supplemented by sea mammals or land animals or both. Freshwater fish, animals, and sometimes milk and cheese were the most important protein foods for inland groups. Seaweed was used by every immune group living near the sea. Inland groups traded for it or, in the case of certain African tribes, used special iodine-rich freshwater plants. Green vegetables and plants, in many groups gathered wild, were staples for all. Most used at least some fruit. Organs of animals or fish or both were considered vital.

Given these common characteristics, we will now consider specific fat-soluble nutrients, fiber, minerals, and raw food proteins and enzymes. These biochemical and structural elements, abundant in primitive diets and lacking in modern, help explain why the foods of traditional people largely protected them from disease.

Fat-Soluble Nutrients in Foods of Animal Origin

Foods rich in fat-soluble vitamins and the essential fatty acid eicosapen-taenoic acid formed substantial parts of traditional diets. These foods fall into three categories:
  1) Sea foods, especially fatty fish such as salmon.
  2) Animal and fish organs, especially liver.
  3) Dairy products from animals feeding on fresh green pasturage, particularly cheese and butter, which concentrate fat-soluble nutrients.

Vitamin D is richly supplied in these foods. Vitamin D is a complex of several vitamins; one, Vitamin D_3, is produced in humans by action of ultraviolet light on skin. Vitamin D_3 helps regulate the absorption and utilization of calcium and other minerals, and other members of the D-complex appear to play similar but complementary roles.

Sunlight does not stimulate production of these other members of the D-complex; they are supplied in the above foods. This may be a reason these foods proved essential for building immunity to dental and degenerative disease, for these other members of the D-complex may play crucial roles in maintaining health. Indeed, why would they be present in animals' bodies if each did not serve a function?

Price found when patients with active decay eliminated refined foods and ate sufficient protective foods, the decay process often ceased. This was the case in young people of the Loetschental Valley who experienced decay only while outside the valley. The decay ceased without fillings, and photographs in his book detail this. Present-day dentists occasionally observe cavities that have ceased to be active; this relates to dietary changes.

Price's chemical analyses of dairy products from all over Europe and America showed the fat-soluble vitamin content much higher in those made from milk from animals fed fresh green pasturage. It was highest when grass was growing most rapidly. Dairy products from animals not eating fresh grass did not contain significant amounts. In Pottenger's experiments, milk from cows fed fresh greens had a significantly healthier effect on animals than milk from cows fed hay, perhaps because of the presence of EPA in the former.

Fish fats are rich in EPA. Wild grazing animals have small but significant amounts, yet domestic beef fattened on grains contains almost undetectable amounts. EPA is similar in structure to a fatty acid found in domestic animals, arachadonic acid, and to one found in vegetable oils, linoleic acid. All are precursors of different prostaglandins, each of which has subtly different effects.

Desirable prostaglandins are formed from EPA; some seem responsible for keeping arteries optimally dilated and platelets from clotting abnormally (platelets are small particles in the blood which aid in clotting). Other prostaglandins made from EPA seem to enhance the functioning of the immune system, and many other effects are being studied by medical researchers. Evidence indicates high EPA consumption is one reason Eskimos and other primitive people (consumers of large amounts of fish and wild game) rarely suffer from heart disease and other chronic and acute diseases.

*   *   *

An assumption was made above in stating that dairy products from animals feeding on fresh pasturage contain EPA. Analysis of wild African grazing animals found significant amounts of EPA, and we may assume milk from such animals contains EPA. Analysis of domestic beef found almost no EPA; such animals are fattened on grains and fed little or no fresh grass the last few months of life, likely explaining the lack of EPA in their fat (for reasons later to be explained). We may assume fat in animals fed a diet similar to that of wild animals—fresh pasturage— contains significant amounts of EPA; so too would cheese and butter made from milk from animals so fed. However, to the author's knowledge no analyses of such foods for EPA content have yet been made. Price did his work before EPA was identified and understood.

The health of people in the Loetschental Valley lends credence to the assumption. This immune group alone ate little meat or fish, instead using large amounts of cheese and butter made from milk from animals kept at pasture. Protective nutrients supplied by animals and fish in other immune groups were likely supplied by these dairy foods.

Sea foods, organ meats, or raw dairy products of the proper quality are, in the author's experience, essential for full recovery from chronic disease and maintenance of optimal health. Experiences of traditional cultures when these foods were displaced by refined foods indicate they are essential also to insure normal development, birth, and growth of the foetus and child. Considerations of the proportions and kinds of these foods best suited for individual tastes and needs will be discussed in later chapters.

Fiber

Most people benefit from more fiber, for typical diets are low in fiber. Meat and foods made from refined flour have little; sugar, fats and oils, and alcohol, none. Foods high in fiber—whole grain foods and vegetables—may greatly benefit the digestive tract.

Diets high in fiber nearly always end constipation. Individuals with chronic stomach or intestinal problems must use vegetables and fruits cautiously, however; especially eaten raw, they may initially worsen symptoms. Well-cooked vegetables and whole grains rarely aggravate such problems.

The traditional diets were high in fiber. Plants, roots, and fruits were widely used, and in some places, whole grains. In northern Canada, Alaska, and the Outer Hebrides, few land vegetables were available, but much seaweed was used. Seaweed holds considerable water in passing through the digestive tract, forming a gel which increases the bulk of the stools and the speed at which they move through the bowels.

People eating traditional diets led active lives. Because their caloric needs were greater than those of most Americans, they ate more food and thus more fiber. This also provided greater amounts of essential nutrients.

Higher cancer rates occur in countries with high fat, high meat, low fiber diets, such as America, where the typical diet is mostly meat, fats, and refined carbohydrates. Lower cancer rates, especially colon cancer, occur in countries with high fiber diets, as in rural areas of Africa, where native people eat mostly natural foods. But low cancer rates, to the point of near absence, occurred among certain cultures with diets high in fiber and also rich in animal and fish fats, as shown by Price. That this remains the case among contemporary hunter-gatherers will be demonstrated in the next chapter.

The explanation lies partly in a consideration of the quality of the animals consumed. Animals eaten by traditional cultures are healthy, low in fat, and free of hormones, antibiotics, and pesticide residues. Fish has similar qualities, though heavy metals now contaminate some species and chemical residues, others, the latter particularly in some coastal waters.

Cooking affects the digestibility of protein; raw or lightly cooked protein is more easily digested, particularly by an individual with a healthy digestive tract. Such foods hold more water in their passage through the digestive system than do overcooked proteins, decreasing the fiber needed for adequate bowel function. A diet containing raw or lightly cooked fish and meat, raw dairy products, and raw vegetables and fruits may provide adequate fiber. This is the primitive diet, and it promotes excellent bowel health. Most of us eat little raw protein; whole grains may provide the additional bulk needed for efficient and comfortable elimination.

Minerals

Minerals originate and reside in the soil or the sea. In a forest, minerals leave the soil as vegetation and are returned by animal droppings, carcasses, and decaying vegetation. The cycle continues.

Modern agriculture has broken that cycle. A few elements without which the land would not produce crops are replaced—nitrogen, potassium, and phosphorous. Others, including trace minerals, are not. Since life first emerged from the sea and gained a foothold on the barren masses of the primitive continents, a delicate balance of natural forces has worked in harmony to evolve life's rich diversity. Chemical agriculture ignores that equilibrium. These natural forces provided foods required for optimal health and strength. Whether modern commercially produced foods can accomplish this is questionable.

Evidence about the role of trace mineral deficiencies in the development of diseases has emerged in recent years. Such deficiencies may be directly traced to agricultural methods which produce food for people and feed for animals yielding meat and dairy products. Modern agriculture does not return to the soil what is taken out. Refining processes further strip grains of minerals and other nutrients.

Price analyzed foods of immune groups for mineral and vitamin content. In every case, the foods supplied at least four times our minimum daily requirement for each nutrient tested. Calcium intake ranged up to seven times as much; phosphorous intake, from five to eight times as much. Magnesium intake for several groups was more than twenty times as much, iron and iodine intake, up to fifty times as much. Intake of both fat-soluble and water-soluble vitamins was in every case at least ten times our minimum daily requirements.

Mineral supplements benefit many people; often health problems are accompanied by deficiencies of calcium and magnesium and of trace minerals. But excesses occur if overdoses are taken, and increased intakes of some minerals can cause deficiencies of others. Supplementary zinc, for example, can drive down body levels of copper.

The use of special foods to provide nutrients is preferable to the use of pills. Whereas mineral and vitamin pills are assembled in laboratories, natural foods have been assembled in nature's laboratory over the course of evolution. The best way to get minerals is in foods; the full balance of accompanying nutrients is then supplied simultaneously.

Research and clinical experience indicate that a deficiency of minerals in modern diets contributes to health problems. High incidence of osteoporosis among the elderly is an example; it is due in part to calcium deficiency. Liberal amounts of minerals in foods of immune groups resulted from environments in which ecological balances were respectfully allowed to maintain and replenish themselves. Perhaps because humans took little, they were given a great deal.

We have since taken a great deal, from forests, plains, and seas. Only a fraction of our wilderness and wildlife heritage remains. Unless we live with the land, rather than on it, and maintain it rather than rape it, what capacity the planet has left to supply traditional foods will be lost. The ability to resist disease, and much of the biological strength human beings have evolved over thousands of years, will be lost with it.

Raw Food Proteins and Enzymes

Raw food's values are little understood by either the public or food scientists. It is difficult to measure the effects of enzymes and other raw-food nutrients that are easily destroyed or changed. Food industry products are rarely raw foods; the industry has little interest in researching the benefits of raw foods.

Enzymes are in every living cell; catalysts, they speed up the biochemical processes of life. Enzymes in the body are denatured—broken down, destroyed—if the body's temperature exceeds about 107 to 108 degrees. Death may occur if the body's core heats beyond this; life depends on enzymes.

Enzymes are a type of protein, and proteins consist of chains of amino acids linked by chemical bonds. The body can make many of the amino acids it requires; the eight it cannot produce are called essential and must be consumed. Textbooks of physiology and biochemistry state dietary proteins are broken down in the small intestine into constituent amino acids that are absorbed into the bloodstream. Scientists and medical students are thus taught that enzymes in foods have no nutritional value beyond that of their constituent amino acids. Since all proteins (and thus all enzymes) supposedly are broken down and reach the bloodstream as amino acids, standard teaching holds that enzymes in raw foods have no unique or special effects. The possibility that enzymes and other proteins in foods may be absorbed intact, or in large fragments having significant biological effects, has long been dismissed as the province of faddists seeing mystical properties in raw foods.

But in recent years evidence has been published by W. A. Hemmings (of the University College of North Wales) and other researchers indicating that a significant portion of dietary protein is absorbed intact, in large fragments of many linked amino acids. Studies were done by feeding radioisotope-labeled animal protein to rats and measuring the radioactivity levels in different parts of the animal's body. The researchers stated about half of the ingested protein freely passed as intact protein and large identifiable fragments into the bloodstream. These proteins went to tissues throughout the animal's body and were broken down over a period of days or weeks. The researchers believe a similar process occurs in humans, indicating different raw foods each have unique and potentially significant biological effects.

Such evidence supports the experience of healers who for thousands of years have stressed raw foods are essential to the healing process and the maintenance of health.

Over forty years ago, Francis Pottenger proved raw foods were required to maintain the health of cats. He applied elements of this knowledge to the care of his patients with tuberculosis and other chronic diseases, with excellent and well documented results. Unfortunately, while his work was initially well received by the medical profession, it has in the ensuing years been largely ignored.

Every primitive culture Weston Price studied ate many foods raw; tradition often dictated which. The milk, cheese, and butter of Swiss villagers and African herdsmen were seldom heated. Organs everywhere were often eaten raw or lightly cooked. Eskimos of Arctic regions, where no plants were available much of the year, ate some fish raw. This practice prevented scurvy; the vitamin C in meat and fish is destroyed by cooking. Much meat was eaten raw, lightly cooked, or smoked. Salmon eggs were important for coastal people; uncooked eggs were dried in fall for use in winter.

In the South Pacific, islanders and coastal Australian Aborigines ate much fish and shellfish raw. When shellfish were cooked, native people arranged them circularly about a small fire, with the animals' valve ends toward the flames. Just enough heat was used to open the valves, saving much work.

Dried raw seaweed was used by coastal people everywhere. Many vegetables and other plant foods were used raw, especially young greens. Fruits were nearly always eaten raw.

Using Protective Nutrients

Biologically we are hardly different from these people. The long journey through time preparing them to face the environment has similarly prepared us. When protective nutrients were lost from diets, health problems followed, as is the case today.

Consuming enough of these nutrients is a step toward building strength and resistance to disease. Certain foods are more appropriate than others, depending on one's ancestry and tastes. Most modern people have little interest in raw meat, for example. The point in detailing traditional use of specific parts of animals, often raw, is not to suggest that one emulate this, though one might. Rather, the concern is finding adequate sources of nutrients primitive wisdom teaches are important.

Another consideration relates to the high quality of foods used in traditional cultures. Animals used for food and dairy were lean, healthy, and free of pesticide residues, antibiotics, and added hormones—as were fish. Vegetables, grains, and fruits grew on living soils rich in elements natural to soil and free of pesticides.

Health can be dramatically improved without eating such foods. But optimal health requires foods of the highest quality.

Raw and lightly cooked foods may be eaten in quantity if enjoyed; they should not be forced. Eating animal source foods raw is controversial, and when from contaminated animals is dangerous.

A reasonable approach might utilize raw eggs (some of the B-vitamin biotin is lost by binding with the protein avidin in raw eggs, but the amount is minor and insignificant) and certified raw milk where available in eggnog; rare beef; and raw fish to taste. Some enjoy rare steak and hamburger essentially uncooked in the center; others use certified raw milk and butter and eat raw milk cheeses. In years past, millions used raw dairy products. While some danger exists, the safety of raw beef, fish, and dairy products depends largely on the health of the source animals. In the author's opinion, danger resulting from a lack of essential nutrients found in raw foods is far greater than that associated with eating the foods raw if they are derived from healthy animals and have been inspected and approved by appropriate government agencies.

If animal source foods are used raw or lightly cooked, sources ideally should be similar in quality to animal source foods of traditional cultures. Today, fish comes closest. Meat and milk should be government certified.

Vegetables, especially salad greens and sprouts, are best raw, though cooked vegetables add variety and, in colder weather, warmth. Raw food vegetarians may enjoy quite good health, particularly if the diet includes raw dairy products. Quantities of raw vegetables eaten for caloric needs supply large amounts of enzymes. Those eating no animal source foods often develop problems involving mineral metabolism and vitamin B_{12} deficiencies, or both. But until then many strict vegetarians feel good, and such exclusively vegetarian diets often initially help people suffering from chronic diseases. However, the addition of animal source foods of proper quality enhances results.

Foods of the highest quality are more expensive and may be difficult to find. The financial reward is considerable, however, if one succeeds in building health to the point where visits to a physician are no longer a regular affair. This is a reasonable goal. Intangible rewards are even greater; nothing equals the feeling of a smoothly functioning body.

Fish is the food most readily available that provides nutrients richly supplied in ancient, primitive, and traditional diets. An in depth examination of nutrients in fish, and contemporary medical research into the effects of fish on human health, are the subjects of the next chapter.

7

Fish
Fat-Soluble Nutrients
and Health

*T*raditional people used much fish (here meaning both scalefish and shellfish) wherever available and fishing cultures were among the most physically well developed and disease resistant found. In considering the possible reasons, we might ask the following questions:

What do experts in biochemistry and physiology know of effects of nutrients in fish?

Is there evidence that nutrients unique to fish are of special benefit? If so, what are these nutrients? How much fish need be eaten for optimal benefits?

Have published studies by physicians and other researchers shown fish to prevent or reverse particular diseases?

The answers provide a further understanding of why traditional people enjoyed splendid physical development and excellent health.

Essential Fatty Acids and EPA

Essential fatty acids have collectively been referred to as Vitamin F. Fatty acids consist of chains of carbon atoms bonded to other elements. Unsaturated means that some of the chemical bonds in the carbon chain are unstable; oxygen may form bonds with the carbon atoms adjacent to these unstable bonds and cause rancidity. A highly unsaturated oil can stay liquid at room or even colder temperatures, while saturated fatty acids such as those found in butter or meat are solid at room temperature.

Many recent articles in *The New England Journal of Medicine*, *The Lancet* (England's most widely read medical journal), and other professional journals have been about physiological effects of fish consumption and fatty acids in fish oils. Several focused on eicosapentaenoic acid, known as EPA, found in high concentrations in certain fish.

EPA is a long-chain, highly unsaturated fatty acid that can be used in metabolism to make prostaglandins, as can several other fatty acids including linoleic, alpha-linolenic, gamma-linolenic, and arachidonic acids.

Prostaglandins are hormone-like substances exerting control over events throughout the body, for example the production and release of chemicals by blood platelets and cells lining the walls of blood vessels. These chemicals control the tendency of the platelets to form a clot, thus influencing the chances of a thrombus (clot) forming, lodging in the coronary arteries, and causing a coronary thrombosis (heart attack).

Linoleic and alpha-linolenic acids are essential fatty acids; the body cannot make them and they must be supplied in the diet. Though experimental animals freely convert alpha-linolenic acid to EPA, some researchers believe EPA too should be considered essential for humans because we have at most a limited ability to make EPA, and it has unique and beneficial effects.

Many prostaglandins made from either EPA, linoleic acid, or arachidonic acid affect the same bodily functions, often in different ways; for many functions, the body can utilize prostaglandins made from any of the three. But recent medical research shows the prostaglandins made from EPA have different and often healthier effects than those made from arachidonic acid, probably in part because western diets contain overabundant amounts of arachidonic acid. What seems to be required for optimal function is properly balanced production of prostaglandins made in the body, on the one hand, from arachidonic acid, and on the other, from linoleic acid, alpha-linolenic acid, and EPA. Those made from arachidonic acid are known as the "omega-2" prostaglandins; those made from linoleic acid are known as the "omega-1" prostaglandins; and those made from alpha-linolenic acid and EPA are known as the "omega-3" prostaglandins. The chart on the next page details the metabolic pathways of the fatty acid precursors of these three series of prostaglandins.

EPA is concentrated in the fat of marine (saltwater) fish and shellfish, especially the cold-water varieties. Concentrations of a closely related fatty acid, docosahexaenoic acid (DHA), occur in the same sources. DHA is also concentrated in the brain and in retinal cells of the eyes of mammals, including humans; the significance of this will be demonstrated in experiments discussed later in this chapter.

Chloroplasts—the green cells in plants—contain small amounts of alpha-linolenic acid; most animals readily convert it to EPA. Humans are thought to accomplish this conversion under the right circumstances, the EPA then being utilized for synthesis of particularly beneficial prostaglandins. This pathway is favored in metabolism over those utilizing arachidonic and linoleic acids, indicating some advantage the body gains from production of the prostaglandin series derived from EPA. All of the prostaglandin pathways are inhibited by many influences, including deficiencies of magnesium, zinc, iron, vitamin B6, or other nutrients; excessive alcohol; cortisone-like drugs; increased adrenaline associated with stress; aging; and the presence in the body of unnatural fatty acids such as those found in margarine and hydrogenated vegetable oils.

The meat of grain-fed animals is fatty and contains almost no EPA; arachidonic and linoleic acids are dominant. Linoleic acid is dominant in seed oils such as safflower, sesame, corn, sunflower, and peanut oils. The presence in the cells of the human body beyond certain minimal amounts of either of these fatty acids results in their utilization for the production of prostaglandins. Such conditions are thought to block the conversion of alpha-linolenic acid to EPA. Most chronic diseases, including arthritis, arteriosclerosis, and cancer, are associated with excessive arachidonic acid and prostaglandins derived from it.

Grazing animals, wild or domestic, eat little arachidonic or linoleic acid. Fresh greens supply alpha-linolenic acid in chloroplasts, and it is converted to EPA. This pathway is favored because their chloroplast-rich diet is devoid of grains, which contain linoleic acid. Most domestic animals are grass-fed for part of their lives, but are fattened on grains for several months before slaughter; it is likely that this is why their fat contains only barely detectable amounts of EPA.

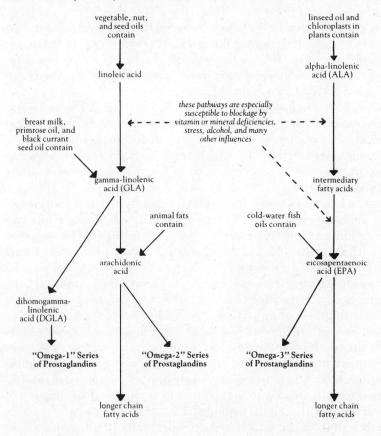

Foods, Fatty Acids, and Prostanglandins

Some strict vegetarians eat many fresh raw greens and sprouts. Such people may be very healthy, though most eventually show symptoms of deficiencies. These subtle aspects of fatty acid metabolism help explain their relatively good health—their bodies may make EPA from alpha-linolenic acid.

Minimizing sources of excessive linoleic and arachidonic acids, while emphasizing sources of EPA, DHA, and alpha-linolenic acid, favors the metabolic pathways producing EPA. Sources of linoleic and arachidonic acids include most nut and seed oils, and fatty meats and dairy products from grain-fed animals. Sources of EPA, DHA, and alpha-linolenic acid include fish and shellfish, meat and dairy products from grass-fed animals, and green vegetables. The small amounts of linoleic and arachidonic acids the body requires are supplied by such a diet.

The More Fish, the Less Heart Disease: A Twenty-Year Study

The article "The Inverse Relation Between Fish Consumption and Twenty-Year Mortality From Coronary Heart Disease" appeared in *The New England Journal of Medicine* (May 9, 1985). The results of a twenty-year study of 852 middle-aged men in the town of Zutphen, the Netherlands, were detailed by a team of Dutch researchers.

Men free of known heart disease were selected in 1960. Dietary histories were obtained from the participants and their wives, with special attention to fish consumption. Twenty percent of the men ate no fish in 1960. Among the rest, the intake varied from a fraction of an ounce to eleven ounces per day. The average for all the men was three-quarters of an ounce per day.

The research team followed these men for twenty years; seventy-eight died of coronary heart disease. Statistical analysis was done on all data. The conclusion: an "inverse dose-response relation" existed between the amount of fish a man ate and his chances of dying of coronary heart disease. The more fish consumed, the less risk of heart attack; this relationship held true from trace amounts up to the maximal intake.

The men eating an average of at least one ounce of fish per day were compared with those eating no fish; their death rate from coronaries was more than 50 percent lower. Statistical analysis proved these results independent of all other factors for coronary heart disease; fish consumption was a protective factor, independent of all variables. The influence of EPA on clotting tendencies is likely one reason for these results.

The men were divided into groups by the amount of fish consumed. Those with the highest intake averaged 2.5 ounces of fish per day, two-thirds of it lean (cod and plaice) and one-third fatty (herring and mackerel), providing about .4 grams of EPA per day, mostly from the fatty fish. However, the consumption of lean fish also proved to protect against heart disease, and the more consumed, the greater the protection. Nutrients in addition to EPA seem to be involved.

While more fish gave greater protection, the men averaging only an ounce a day of any fish—one or two modest portions a week—had less than half the death rate from heart disease than those eating no fish. The regular inclusion of some fish in the diet seems prudent; indeed, eating large amounts of fish and shellfish may be one of the most beneficial changes one could make in the diet. Primitive Greenland Eskimos, shown in several studies to have an extremely low incidence of coronary heart disease when living on their native diet, eat upwards of fourteen ounces of fatty fish per day, providing at least seven grams of EPA.

Fish Oils Dramatically Lower High Blood Fats

The article "Reduction of Plasma Lipids, Lipoproteins, and Apoproteins by Dietary Fish Oils in Patients With Hypertriglyceridemia" appeared in the same issue of *The New England Journal of Medicine*. Hypertriglyceridemia refers to the presence of excessively high triglycerides in the blood. Triglycerides are normal fats found in the blood; they are a type of plasma lipid. Excessive amounts have been correlated with heart disease and circulatory disorders.

Twenty patients were placed on three successive controlled diets differing only in the kind of fat included. The first diet was low in fat and cholesterol, and contained no fish oil. The second contained fish oil (in fish and in supplements) amounting to 20 to 30 percent of the daily calories. The third used an equal amount of polyunsaturated vegetable oils.

In every patient, blood triglyceride and cholesterol levels fell while on the diet rich in fish oils. In four weeks triglycerides fell an average of 64 per cent for the patients with moderate elevation of triglycerides, and they fell an average of 79 per cent for the patients with severe elevation; the new levels were, on the average, less than one-third the old. Cholesterol levels fell 27 percent for the moderately elevated group and 45 percent for the severely elevated group.

The reductions were from the levels measured while the patients were on the low-fat, low-cholesterol diet prior to the fish oil-rich diet. Many then still had milky-appearing blood plasma, a characteristic of fatty blood. Within days on the fish oil-rich diet, this disappeared.

When the patients were taken off the fish oil-rich diet and placed on the diet rich in polyunsaturated vegetable oils, they experienced alarming developments. Among those who had moderately elevated blood fats prior to the fish oil-rich diet, levels of triglycerides and cholesterol rose considerably, but remained below previous levels. Vegetable oils are known to reduce these blood fats; they proved less effective than fish oils.

The vegetable oils caused more striking effects in the patients who had severely elevated blood fats prior to the fish oil-rich diet. These people had experienced large reductions in triglycerides and cholesterol while on the fish oil-rich diet. Within three to four days on the diet rich in vegetable oils, all had increases in triglyceride levels. After ten to fourteen days, levels had on the average tripled and blood cholesterol had increased by an average of over 30 percent. Because abdominal pain and liver tenderness was developing in many of these patients, and because of the severely elevated blood fats, the vegetable oil-rich diet was discontinued at that point. The plan had been to continue it for four weeks, the same length of time the fish oil-rich diet was used.

A return to the fish oil-rich diet was followed by the disappearance of the abdominal pain and liver tenderness. The blood fats dropped to the previous levels, and eventually even lower as the diet was continued.

These dramatic results demonstrate the danger of believing advertisements implying alleged health benefits of polyunsaturated vegetable oils. Because early studies determined that in most individuals these oils caused reductions in some blood fats, the public was led to believe large quantities were beneficial. More recent studies have shown these oils do not reduce the blood fats thought to do the most harm when elevated, i.e., the very low density lipoproteins (VLDL) and associated triglycerides. These fractions of the blood fats are most affected by fish oils.

Polyunsaturated vegetable oils are suspected of being cancer-causing agents and of speeding up biochemical processes involved in aging. Some fatty acids vegetable oils supply in large quantities are essential nutrients, but the fish oil-rich diet supplied adequate amounts without the inclusion of vegetable oils. Limiting dietary polyunsaturated vegetable oils aids the body's ability to convert the alpha-linolenic acid in plant chloroplasts to EPA, and thus increases production of more favorable prostaglandins. Olive oil contains about one-tenth the polyunsaturated fatty acids found in most vegetable oils; moderate use is recommended as a substitute.

The fish oil-rich diet in this study supplied from twenty to thirty grams of EPA per day (nearly twice that of even Eskimo diets); two ounces of fatty fish such as mackerel or salmon supply about one gram of EPA. Both the twenty-year study and the fish oil study point toward high fish consumption; a diet rich in marine fish and shellfish would seem to be ideal.

Fishermen and Farmers in Japan: A Comparison

Further insight into the amount of fish one might eat for optimal protection against coronary heart disease, as well as other disorders involving abnormal clotting of the blood, is provided in a study by a group of Japanese researchers (*The Lancet*, November 22, 1980). The main source of dietary protein in Japan is fish, and the Japanese have a low incidence of heart disease. Believing EPA may be a major reason, the researchers carried out platelet aggregation studies to look for differences between the people of a fishing village and those of a farming village.

In the fishing village, the average daily intake of fish among the people studied was nine ounces per person, supplying 2.5 grams of EPA. In the farming village, the average was three ounces, supplying .9 grams of EPA. In the fishing village, the people had significantly higher blood levels of EPA.

In the platelet aggregation studies, the platelets of the people in the fishing village showed significantly less tendency to adhere and form a clot. In consistence with EPA's role as a precursor of prostaglandins which cause decreased platelet aggregation, the tendency of platelets to clot is directly related to the level of EPA in the blood.

The difference in platelet aggregation between the fishermen and the farmers was apparently due to the greater fish consumption and subsequently higher blood levels of EPA of the fishermen. The farmers ate as much fish as the group of men who were the biggest fish eaters in the twenty-year Netherlands study—an average of three ounces a day. The fishermen ate three times as much, approaching the consumption of Greenland Eskimos.

While the Netherlands group (eating an average of three ounces of fish daily) had over 50 percent less coronary heart disease than those eating no fish, they were not immune; some had heart attacks. Decreased platelet aggregation among fishermen eating nine ounces of fish a day, compared with farmers eating three ounces a day, suggests optimal levels of fish intake are closer to nine ounces per day than to three.

The Effects of a Mackerel Diet on Blood Platelets

Mackerel nearly exclusively constituted the diet of seven volunteers studied by West German researchers; the daily intake was from eighteen to twenty-nine ounces. Blood studies were conducted, with particular attention to platelets.

A platelet is formed when certain bone marrow blood cells called megakaryocytes fragment. Each platelet has a membrane surrounding it, and this membrane is a storehouse for fats. The researchers found that the composition of these fats, while on the mackerel diet, became similar to the composition of fats in mackerel; within a few days of beginning the diet, the membranes became rich in EPA.

The tendency of the blood to clot thus changes when eating large amounts of foods rich in EPA; changes occur in the structure of the cells responsible for clotting. Recall the old saying: "You are what you eat."

Concern has been expressed that EPA-rich diets may cause problems related to an inability of the blood to clot, and subsequently prolonged bleeding time. Eskimos on their native diets do have longer bleeding times than most Americans. But their blood does clot well and their wounds heal well. Our EPA-lacking diet appears to have shortened bleeding time; the Eskimos' is apparently normal.

Fish Oils in Vision and Intellectual Function

Sharpness of vision and brain development are related to blood levels of EPA and DHA; these fatty acids are essential for good vision. DHA is a normal constituent of the cells of the retina, and the amount present is dependent upon the amount in the diet. Animal tests at Oregon Health Sciences University in Portland indicate deficiencies reduce the ability of retinal cells to be stimulated, with consequent reduction in sharpness of vision.

In other studies at the Oregon Regional Primate Center, the development of vision during gestation and early life was impaired when female monkeys were fed a diet deficient in EPA, DHA, and linolenic acid for two months prior to and during their pregnancies. The infant monkeys were then fed the deficient diet; when twelve weeks old, their vision was only half the strength of monkeys fed a normal diet. The cells of the retina and brain of animals with deficient vision were analyzed; the fat content showed very low levels of EPA and DHA, explaining the loss of sharp vision.

The ability of Maori to see the moons of Jupiter with the naked eye was apparently related to the rich supply of EPA, DHA, and alpha-linolenic acid supplied in their foods.

EPA and DHA, especially DHA, are also found in high concentrations in the cerebral cortex of the normal human brain. Deficiencies may impair the functioning of the brain—learning, reasoning, and overall intellectual powers. Rats fed a diet deficient in these fatty acids were unable to learn to run a maze as well as rats fed a control diet.

The wisdom of primitive diets is demonstrated by this research; every traditional culture Weston Price studied emphasized foods rich in EPA, DHA, and alpha-linolenic acid. Seafoods, organs, and in some cultures dairy products from pasture-fed animals were particularly emphasized for mothers-to-be (prior to and during pregnancy, and later during lactation) and young children. Recent research has indicated the human brain acquires about half its fat composition before birth, and most of the rest during the first year after.

The primitives did all that research tells us people should do to insure the optimal development of the next generation. Regretfully, the caging and sacrificing of innocent animals has been necessary in order that western people may learn, after much disease and suffering, the lessons traditional cultures have understood for thousands of years.

Fatty Acids and Linseed Oil

Chloroplasts in green plants contain alpha-linolenic acid, which mammals can convert to EPA, as has been discussed; some researchers suggest that an individual consuming enough foods rich in alpha-linolenic acid, such as linseed oil, may form sufficient EPA to benefit from its effects. Use of linseed oil (also called flaxseed oil) as a food supplement and as a salad oil is thus sometimes recommended by nutritionists and physicians.

While grazing animals convert alpha-linolenic acid to EPA, the extent to which the human body can do so is not clear. One research team in the Clinical Chemistry Department of Aalborg Hospital in Denmark gave a volunteer one tablespoon of codliver oil three times a day for one week. Cod liver oil is about 10 percent EPA. A ten-fold increase in the EPA content of the blood fats occurred within the week. Linseed oil was given to the same person two months later, in the same dose; after one week the individual showed only insignificant increases in EPA.

The human body nevertheless may well make the conversion of alpha-linolenic acid to EPA under certain circumstances. The proportion of different kinds of fatty acids in the diet has a major influence; had the individual been on a diet very low in arachidonic and linoleic acids—unlikely, since they predominate in most modern foods—he may have formed measurably more EPA from the linseed oil.

Fat-Soluble Nutrients in Dairy Products

The butter and cheese made from milk the cows gave in June was particularly prized by the Swiss people of the Loetschental Valley. This summer butter and cheese was higher in fat-soluble nutrients than samples analyzed from other times of the year.

Weston Price tested over ten thousand samples of butter and cheese over the course of many years. Consistently he found the content of fat-soluble vitamins was highest during the months when grass grew most rapidly. For much of North America, there are two such periods, one in late spring, and the other in late summer. In more northern areas, the two periods occur more closely together than in southern areas, around mid-summer. But for every area, a graph of the fat-soluble vitamin content of the dairy products of the area (plotted against the time of year) echoed a graph of that area's rate of plant growth (plotted against the time of year).

Statistics for mortality from heart disease and pneumonia for all districts in the United States and Canada were then plotted. Price found the rise and fall in mortality from these two diseases followed regular yearly cycles in each section of the country. These cycles were exactly opposite the curve for the vitamin content of the dairy products and the curve for the rate of plant growth for that section of the country. In more northern districts, where the twin peaks of the vitamin curve (and also the twin peaks of the plant growth curve) tended to blend together into one mid-summer peak, mortality rates tended to bottom in mid-summer. In more southern districts, where distinct peaks occurred (one for late spring, and one for late summer) in both vitamin and plant growth curves, there were two low points on the mortality curve—one in late spring, and one in late summer.

The incidence of children's diseases in Ontario was analyzed, including chicken pox, measles, nephritis, scarlet fever, and others. For each disease, a graph of the number of cases was opposite the graph of vitamin levels in the dairy products of Ontario (both graphs were plotted against the time of year).

This is evidence of profound natural forces at work. All life depends upon the sun. Is it strange the green life springing from the sun's rays, the fresh greens making higher life forms possible, should prove so vital?

Fresh Greens in the Diet

A basic and effective diet for chronic disease, always adapted for the individual, might include fresh raw and cooked vegetables, especially greens and sprouts; fish; liver from naturally raised animals; perhaps some grains, fruit, and certified raw milk if desired; olive oil and vinegar; and butter.

Fresh greens are vital and may be used in large amounts if this proves suitable for the individual. Sprouts are the vegetable foods most abundant in vitamins, minerals, and enzymes. These fresh, raw, organically grown young plants are available in many markets and may be grown in any home.

Though some alpha-linolenic acid in greens and linseed oil appears at times to be converted to EPA, such conversion fails to provide optimal amounts. Traditional diets and recent research on fish oils point toward fish as a central food for optimal health and prevention and reversal of chronic diseases.

Cod Liver Oil

As children, many people took cod liver oil during the years this old remedy was given almost universally as protection against colds, flus, and other infectious diseases. Cod liver oil is a reasonable way to increase EPA intake; one would need to eat ten ounces of fatty fish daily to supply five grams of EPA, and an optimal intake is likely at least that.

One tablespoon of cod liver oil, the maximum usually used as a daily supplement, provides 1.4 grams of EPA, 1.3 grams of DHA, 14,000 I.U. of vitamin A, and 1,400 I.U. of vitamin D. A concentrated and potent food supplement, cod liver oil should be used sparingly.

Preparations of concentrated EPA and DHA are available. Those most potent, as of this writing, are capsules containing 225 milligrams of EPA and 150 of DHA. For the individual eating little fish, such a supplement in addition to one tablespoon of cod liver oil per day is a reasonable way to increase the intake of EPA and DHA.

Emulsified cod liver oil is favored by many people with an aversion to the taste of fish oils. The taste is innocuous, with only a faint hint of a fish-oil taste and smell. Since it is only one-third cod liver oil, up to three tablespoons per day may be recommended. Many people unwilling to take full-strength cod liver oil will take the emulsified version.

Fish oils are highly subject to rancidity. The use of six-ounce bottles minimizes contact of the oil with oxygen, and refrigeration further slows oxidation. Vitamin E, a natural anti-oxidant, may be taken as a supplement to minimize the effects any small amounts of rancid oil may have.

The biochemical structure of the prostaglandins was discovered in the 1970's, leading to discoveries that particularly beneficial prostaglandins are made in the body from unsaturated fatty acids richly supplied in fish oils. Scientists are unraveling many mysteries, but as yet have fully elucidated only a fraction of the ways the body responds to foods.

More will be discovered about fish and other natural foods, EPA and other subtle nutrients. The immune-stimulating effects of EPA may be linked to absence of cancer in primitive people. Causes and explanations will be found as science dissects and analyzes.

Beyond that, a synthesis must eventually be reached. As he strove to transcend individual parts and comprehend the whole, Weston Price grasped for the totality of the interaction between biological cause and effect and the human condition when he wrote, simply: "Life in all its fullness is Mother Nature obeyed."

Each piece of the whole that is understood provides additional information useful in building health and eliminating disease. In the next chapter, we review some widely differing, well-known diets, each of which has proved helpful to many individuals. We will then go on to a synthesis, incorporating our several sources of knowledge of traditional foods into a plan one may use to create his own best traditional diet.

8

A Review of
Several Well-Known Diets

*S*cores of dietary regimes have become popular. Many contain elements and principles of use in understanding the effects of food on health. These include the Pritikin diet, two high-protein weight loss diets (the Atkins diet and the Scarsdale diet), the Gerson diet, raw foods diets (which may incorporate fasting), and the macrobiotic diet of Michio Kushi.

Each contains elements of traditional diets. All recommend mostly fresh, unrefined foods. Each has helped many people but has drawbacks; a common one is restrictiveness. Inflexibility is another; individual problems occuring in response to certain foods may cause difficulty in finding appropriate dietary adjustments. A lack of flexibility may even be a problem as health improves, for a diet should change as an individual changes. A program initially bringing marked improvement may later fail to maintain health.

While these regimes have been of great value to many individuals, none incorporates fully the principles behind traditional human diets—principles necessary for designing nutritional programs in accord with our deepest physiological and psychological needs. But an integration of strengths from each into knowledge of traditional human foods yields a better understanding of the relationship between food and human health.

The Pritikin Diet

Nathan Pritikin established an in-patient diet and exercise rehabilitation center in Santa Barbara in 1976. His program grew popular; one of his books, *The Pritikin Program for Diet and Exercise,* has sold over two million copies.

The diet severely restricts all fats, vegetable and animal alike, especially cholesterol (though technically not a fat, cholesterol is often classed with fats). Fresh raw and cooked vegetables and whole grains are emphasized; animal protein is restricted to four ounces daily.

Impressive results may be achieved, particularly in people with heart disease and high blood pressure. Because the diet is low in fat, cholesterol and triglyceride levels decrease. An exercise program of extensive walking, and later jogging, aids in the improvement and even disappearance of symptoms in some individuals.

The fatty fish and fish-oil diets described earlier are more successful in lowering triglycerides and cholesterol. Differences between fats in fish and those in commercial animals (and subsequent effects on metabolism) are not recognized in the Pritikin diet, nor are differences between cholesterol-rich food from healthy animals (fish and pasture-fed farm animals) and cholesterol-rich food from fatty, conventionally raised animals.

For several years this author worked in a large New York medical practice with individuals on the Pritikin diet for heart and circulatory problems. Larger amounts of high-quality animal foods, especially fish, shellfish, and liver, enabled people on the diet to follow the routine more consistently, and yielded greater improvements than seen in individuals following the standard Pritikin regime.

Because of his success, Pritikin wrote that his diet is "the world's healthiest diet...the most significant breakthrough in man's age-old quest for rejuvenation," and that "for centuries the hardiest, most long-lived peoples in the world have thrived on these foods." He followed his diet for over twenty-five years, apparently reversing the course of his heart disease and controlling the leukemia which eventually led to his hospitalization and subsequent death.

For centuries, the hardiest, most long-lived peoples in the world have indeed thrived on fresh vegetables and whole grains—among other foods. But the strongest of these cultures used substantial portions of the highest quality animal source foods. Cancer, heart disease, and other degenerative diseases were extremely rare.

Pritikin's work is significant and important, demonstrating the power of a program which emphasized giving up bad habits and adopting a more natural lifestyle. But selective use of circumstantial evidence is misleading, and the program does not consider evidence from anthropology, human evolution, and recent medical research in recommending a diet. Frequent references are made to the African Bantu people, who eat a low animal protein, low fat, high fiber diet and enjoy resistance to diseases of the cardiovascular and digestive systems. Yet no reference is made to other traditional cultures eating large amounts of animal protein and enjoying similar resistance. Many natural foods diets produce health relative to that seen in modernized cultures.

That Pritikin's program has been of benefit to many individuals is undeniable. But the same program helping initially may not maintain an individual's health. Changes away from the routine leading to chronic illness (i.e., sugar, refined flour, alcohol, fatty meats, commercial dairy products, smoking, and little or no exercise) and toward natural foods and regular exercise bring improvement and feelings of well-being.

But building lasting health and resistance to degenerative processes is more complex; there is danger in oversimplification. The magnitude of what has been fragmented and mostly lost—the wisdom of our ancestors—is such that only by being open to learn from all available sources can one hope to put the pieces back together.

High-Protein Weight Loss Diets

Several weight loss diets similar in their emphasis on protein foods have become popular. Two of the most well-known appeared in books that were best-sellers, *Dr. Atkins' Diet Revolution*, and *The Complete Scarsdale Medical Diet*.

Atkins' diet eliminates nearly all carbohydrates in early stages, forcing the burning of fats for energy and producing ketones. Ketones are not completely burned when metabolized, and are subsequently excreted; this may aid in weight loss. Their presence suppresses hunger; individuals eating mostly protein and fats (meats, eggs, fish, dairy products, fatty sauces), as the diet suggests, experience little hunger and yet may lose a great deal of weight. Salads and some fruits are also allowed.

The Scarsdale diet also causes ketosis (the presence of ketones on the breath and in the urine) and thus operates on much the same principle, although an average of 35 percent of calories are derived from carbohydrates. Weight loss results from low caloric and low fat intake; the strict part of the diet (suggested for use no more than two weeks at a time) averages one thousand calories a day, 20 percent from fats. The use of lean meat, fish, skim milk, and low-fat cheeses restricts fat and calories.

These diets superficially resemble diets of cultures Weston Price studied. Elimination of refined carbohydrates (sugar, white flour, and most alcohol) and restriction of even whole foods containing carbohydrates (whole grains, foods made from whole grains, and fruits) causes the dieter to eat more foods of animal origin and more vegetables. Most people with weight problems have eaten diets high in refined carbohydrates, so such changes are beneficial. Many succeed in losing weight, adjusting to the new diet, and staying with it.

The quality of the animal source foods used is nevertheless an important issue. The Atkins diet in particular stresses the use of fatty foods; the book presents evidence that refined carbohydrates rather than animal fats are the villains in the American diet. There is truth in this, but fats in modern commercial animals and milk products are very different in quantity and kind from those in animals living under more natural conditions.

These diets may successfully achieve goals of weight loss and decrease risk for diseases associated with overweight. This is no small accomplishment for the overweight person who has found it impossible to remain on other weight loss regimes. Having accomplished this, the individual wishing to optimize his health must then take further steps.

The Gerson Diet

Max Gerson was a physician who began practice in the mid-1920's in Bielefeld, Germany. He studied under Professor Ottfried Foerster, a renowned neurosurgeon of the day. Gerson's specialty was diseases of the nervous system.

Because Gerson cured his own migraines with a natural foods diet, he began treating his migraine patients similarly; they did well. One reported his skin tuberculosis or lupus (cutaneous lupus erythematosus) cleared up as well. Gerson found this hard to believe, for lupus was supposedly incurable. Laboratory reports and slides proved the lesions were indeed healing, and he began treating other lupus patients. They too recovered.

Because Gerson was a specialist in nerve diseases, the medical community claimed he could not treat skin diseases and attempted to revoke his license. The case went to court, and the judge asked the physicians charging Gerson if they cured lupus. They replied lupus was incurable. The judge responded, "Well, then, why don't you let this doctor do it?," and dismissed the case. Gerson went home, removed his shingle saying "Internal and Nervous Diseases," and put one up saying "General Practitioner."

He began treating tuberculosis, meningitis, and other diseases with his natural foods diet. The wife of Albert Schweitzer, in very serious condition with tuberculosis, in 1928 went to Gerson. She recovered fully under his care. Years later, her husband, at the age of seventy-five, recovered from diabetes under Dr. Gerson's care; he lived to be ninety. On the cover of Gerson's book we find Dr. Schweitzer's words: "I see in Dr. Max Gerson one of the most eminent geniuses in medical history."

In 1929, Gerson began treating cancer, often with favorable results. The dietary regime then consisted initially of fresh vegetables and fruits (many raw) and freshly prepared juices. During the course of treatment, buttermilk, pot cheese, yogurt, and egg yolks, all raw, were added. A mineral supplement was used, and frequent enemas.

As he developed his therapy in Germany and then in America after escaping and emigrating here in the late 1930's, other aspects were added, including fresh green leaf juice, fresh raw calve's liver juice, injections of raw liver extract, iodine, desiccated thyroid gland, potassium supplements, and coffee in the enemas. The details of the therapy and theory are presented in his book, *A Cancer Therapy, Results of Fifty Cases*, published in 1958. Dr. Gerson died in 1959.

His book presents proof, with complete medical records, X-rays, and diagnoses of terminal cancer by accepted, established medical authorities, that a significant number of Gerson's patients (previously diagnosed terminal) recovered from cancer. All fifty of the cases reported were alive and free of all signs of cancer at the time of publication. Most had first become Gerson's patients in the 1940's and early 1950's.

For over twenty years, Gerson submitted reports of his work to medical journals. The medical establishment steadfastly blocked publication, even attempting unsuccessfully for years to revoke his license for practicing "unorthodox medicine." In more recent years, the cancer orthodoxy has maligned Gerson's work as unproven and dangerous, grouping it with that of others who have dared suggest better ways to treat cancer patients than surgery, radiation, and chemotherapy.

An account of Gerson's story is told by journalist S.J. Haught in his book *Has Dr. Max Gerson A True Cancer Cure?* (First published in 1962, the book is now titled *Cancer? Think Curable—A Cancer Therapy*.) Mr. Haught's original intention was to expose Gerson as a fraud; his story was to be called "The Unveiling of a Quack." He was converted to Gerson's side by the evidence.

In the years since his death, many people have applied Gerson's therapy. His daughter has established a clinic in Mexico faithful to the therapy and has attempted, with some success, to incorporate recent developments in natural therapy. But no one using Gerson's therapy or any other has consistently achieved his results.

One of the foremost reasons may be that in Gerson's time, chemotherapy for cancer patients was in its infancy, and most people seeking his help had not been exposed to toxic chemotherapeutic agents. Because these agents depress the immune system, poison the liver, and leave the body weakened, he found that after chemotherapy people did not respond well to his dietary regime. Today, most cancer patients seeking nutritional therapy have already had chemotherapy, although many seek to improve their nutrition while on chemotherapy.

Also enhancing Gerson's results was the superior food available in his day. More people had been raised on fresh, high quality foods superior to those generally available today, and this may have enhanced their ability to recover from cancer. The foods available for use in the therapy were similarly superior.

The most intangible element in any therapy is the influence of the physician on the patient. This therapy is difficult both psychologically and physically, requiring a strict dietary regime, months of hard work, and attention to detail. An inspirational and even charismatic physician-healer can make an immense difference in results, simply by virtue of his ability to inspire the patient and the family to follow his program with care. By all accounts, Dr. Gerson was such a man.

Several aspects of the Gerson diet are of special interest in light of our knowledge of traditional diets. Fresh raw calve's liver juice and fresh raw green leaf juice are the central foods; both supply nutrients richly provided in traditional diets.

Gerson wrote liver juice is the most powerful weapon we have against cancer; the therapy calls for three preparations daily, each made from eight ounces of liver. Juice concentrates essential nutrients, allowing more to be consumed than if whole liver were eaten. For most patients, drinking raw juice is more tolerable than eating raw liver. He stressed that liver must be fresh, raw, and taken from animals raised without the use of hormones, antibiotics, or pesticides.

Injections of crude liver extract and vitamin B$_{12}$ were used. Gerson noted leukemias in particular required greater doses of liver juice, liver extract, and vitamin B$_{12}$.

Research by Dr. Albert Szent-Gyorgyi gives indications of the importance of nutrients found in liver for successful cancer therapy. Szent-Gyorgyi received the Nobel Prize in 1937 for medicine and physiology for his isolation and identification of vitamin C. He also discovered the function of bioflavonoids, and his work on contractile proteins is a foundation of muscle biochemistry and physiology. He reported in 1972 that his experiments had demonstrated that the growth of inoculated cancer in mice was strongly inhibited by extracts of liver. Other researchers have reported similar findings.

Fresh raw green leaf juice is the other dietary mainstay of the therapy. As with liver, the use of juice allows the patient to take in far more nutrients than possible with solid foods alone.

Salads, lightly cooked vegetables, fruit and fruit juices, and some whole grain foods were used, also buttermilk, pot cheese, yogurt, and egg yolks. Other foods of animal origin Gerson considered essential were thyroid and pancreas.Thyroid tablets were used to stimulate metabolism, for he found nearly every cancer patient had an underactive thyroid gland. Pancreas tablets taken with meals aided digestion.

Consistencies in Gerson's work, Weston Price's, and Francis Pottenger's are evident. Cancer remains the most difficult clinical problem patient and physician must face. The Gerson therapy is no panacea, but many physicians and other healers successfully use parts of Gerson's regime; many elements of the Gerson therapy are of benefit in cancer and other chronic diseases. An understanding of Dr. Gerson's work provides an essential piece of the puzzle that must be solved to treat effectively and prevent these diseases.

Raw Foods Diets and Fasting

Some diets advocate exclusive use of raw foods. The program known as natural hygiene was described in books by Herbert Shelton, who for many years maintained a health spa in San Antonio. The diet is strictly vegetarian—no animal foods are included (this is known as a vegan diet). Sprouts, fruits, and raw vegetable juices are emphasized.

The regime is similar to the raw foods regime of the Hippocrates Institute in Boston, a facility where people may go for raw foods therapy. Both regimes are frequently combined with therapeutic fasting as an approach to the treatment of chronic diseases.

A strength of these programs is that raw vegetables (especially sprouts and greens) and their juices are extremely beneficial foods. An exclusively raw diet eliminates harmful foods. Individuals often experience improvements, and may even apparently recover from serious chronic diseases.

Improvement or recovery may be tenuous, however. Deficiency symptoms may appear, and there is usually difficulty staying on the strict regime. Tremendous cravings often occur—the body knows something is lacking. The gaunt, hollow appearance of individuals who have followed a vegan raw foods diet over long periods of time speaks of a need for missing nutrients.

One example is that of a four-year-old girl whose mother had been a strict raw foods vegan since the sixth month of her pregnancy with the child. The child never had any food of animal origin, eating only raw vegetables, sprouts, nuts, seeds, and fruits. Markedly undersized for her age and with tiny bones, the pains she experienced in her legs suggested rickets. She was chronically tired, with little energy for playing or learning.

Deficiencies of essential fatty acids, vitamin D, calcium, vitamin B_{12}, and perhaps protein were suspected. Her mother was persuaded to include certified raw milk and eggs in the child's diet, though she would not include cod liver oil or fish. Within a month, though, the child had gained weight and had more energy, and the pains in her legs had disappeared. Within a few months her fatigue was gone and, though still small, she had grown considerably.

Her case is typical of children on vegan raw food diets for extended periods. While the mother had not encountered major problems of her own, the diet lacked nutrients required for the growth and optimal development of her child.

Fasting. Many people who advocate a raw foods diet recommend periods of fasting, sometimes for a week or two or even more. While a fast helps cleanse the body, nutrients must soon be provided. The elimination of harmful foods allows the body a rest, and extended periods of fasting may achieve good results. But consistent recovery from chronic disease, with much less discomfort to the patient, may be achieved when proper foods are introduced. A brief fast is optional.

Individuals not undernourished may fast for several or more days with considerable benefit and no great discomfort. But most chronically ill patients need not necessarily fast to recover their health.

The individual experiencing an acute gastrointestinal problem is an exception. When recent internal bleeding has occurred, fasting under a physician's supervision until the bleeding has stopped is usually the best course. This may take up to a few days. The proper foods, carefully prepared, may then be introduced.

A brief fast is almost without exception the best natural way to deal with acute illness. The acutely ill have no appetite; food is taken only at the urging of family members or out of boredom and habit. A sick child, like a sick animal, will not touch food. The natural response to the onset of illness is loss of appetite; when no food is taken, the body can most efficiently marshall its energy to fight illness, rather than being forced to channel energy into digestive processes. Stored reserves are more than adequate for energy. Recovery from colds, flus, and other acute illnesses is most rapid when a fast is initiated at the first sign. Rest is in order, and feeding usually should not begin until the temperature is normal and a strong appetite has returned.

Antibiotics are overused, but they may be life saving in acute problems. Herbal medicines are of benefit in most situations. Fasting is but one way to treat acute illness, and is at times best combined with other methods. When in doubt, seek a competent physician.

Social Aspects of Raw Foods Diets.   Most Caucasian Americans are descendants of people from northern and central Europe and Russia; a smaller number are of southern European and Middle Eastern origin. Foods have been cooked in northern regions since early explorations by prehistoric hunters. In southern Europe, the Middle East, and African regions where ancestors of Black Americans originated, cooking played a smaller but still significant role in the traditional preparation of foods.

To eat an entirely raw foods diet ignores this heritage. Socially, this puts an individual on a fringe; eating is a social event and the strictly raw foods person finds himself quite limited socially.

The Macrobiotic Diet

Macro is Greek for "long" or "great," bios for "life." The term macrobiotics was used by Hippocrates to describe healthy, long-lived people. Other classical writers too used the term, which came to mean living and eating in a simple and natural manner.

By the early 1900's, refined foods were widely used in many Japanese cities. Yukikazu Sakurazawa became ill eating these foods; he recovered eating brown rice, miso soup, vegetables, and other traditional Japanese foods. He later developed a philosophy of living and healing based on his understanding of traditional foods and teachings. While living in Paris in the 1920's, he adopted the pen name George Ohsawa and called his teachings macrobiotics.

For thirty-five years, his pupil Michio Kushi has been the leader of the worldwide macrobiotics movement. The author of books on the subject, he has done a great deal to popularize the use of whole and natural foods.

Macrobiotics as taught by Mr. Kushi and his followers is a way of life emphasizing a need to live in harmony with both nature and one's fellow man. The core is the macrobiotic diet, individualized for each person according to age, sex, climate and geography, activity level, and personal needs. A principle of the diet is that whole grains should be the major portion of everyone's diet. Claims are made that the macrobiotic diet has been followed by ordinary people throughout history, that early humans and their forebears were more herbivores than omnivores, and that whole grains were the principal food in all previous civilizations and cancer-free societies.

The standard macrobiotic diet consists of cooked whole grains (about 50 to 60 percent of daily food by volume); fresh vegetables, mostly cooked (25 to 30 percent of daily food); soup, featuring sea vegetables and fermented soy products (5 to 10 percent of daily food); beans (5 to 10 percent of daily food); and small amounts of fruit, fish, and desserts prepared with natural sweeteners. Vegetables and fruits used should be those indigenous to the region where one lives. Tropical varieties are avoided, as are all dairy products, eggs, and meats.

This type of diet has indeed been followed in many parts of the world at times, particularly in the Far East where population growth in geographical areas with limited resources necessitated the use of more grains and less food of animal origin. Traditional cultures with choices, however, always have used more animal source foods than the tiny percentage macrobiotics advocates. The notion that whole grains formed the basis of the diet of all cancer-free societies is entirely contrary to information from scores of anthropologists, nutritionists, and medical researchers who have investigated this subject since the turn of the century. Both whole grains and animal source foods of the proper quality have proven capable of forming a major part of the diet of cancer-free societies.

Macrobiotics as taught by Kushi and others can be a healthy regime when thoroughly understood and carefully followed. Individuals have recovered from chronic diseases on macrobiotic diets. One well-known case is that of Anthony Sattilaro, a physician who recovered from advanced bone cancer on a macrobiotic regime, as detailed in his book, *Recalled By Life*.

Limitations and Case Histories. Macrobiotics also has limitations. In one case, a fifty-seven-year-old man came to the author with a recent diagnosis of lung cancer, a spot the size of a quarter on his lung. He did not want conventional therapy and began a nutritional program integrating elements of the Gerson therapy with other aspects of traditional healing diets. The tumor remained stable for nearly a year, to the surprise of his family doctor, who continued to monitor his condition. This was an oat cell carcinoma, a type of lung cancer with a poor prognosis—few patients live more than a few months after diagnosis.

Growing impatient with the rigors of his therapy and the tumor's continued presence, he learned about macrobiotics. After consulting with a macrobiotic nutritional counselor, he stopped the therapy and began a strict macrobiotic regime. At that point, X-rays showed his tumor stable, and still the size of a quarter. He reasoned that if macrobiotics failed, he would quickly return to what he had been doing.

His condition deteriorated within weeks, his lungs filling with fluid; he required hospitalization. His tumor had begun growing rapidly and a few days later he died.

Another case was that of a twenty-three-year-old woman who had eaten macrobiotically for several years. She had a gradual onset of marked and occasionally severe abdominal and pelvic pain over the course of forty-eight hours. She consulted both a macrobiotic nutritional counselor and a medical doctor. The former modified her diet somewhat. Her symptoms became worse, and her medical doctor recommended hospitalization if she did not improve shortly.

Appendicitis was suspected, but physical findings and symptoms were more suggestive of an ovarian cyst. She had continued eating, though she had no appetite. Fasting and enemas were immediately instituted; unless improving by morning, or at any sign of her condition's worsening, she was to be hospitalized.

Her symptoms by morning had improved. They had largely disappeared within seventy-two hours of instituting the fast, and she began eating small amounts. Since then she has used considerably more raw vegetables and fish than called for in the standard macrobiotic diet. No further problems requiring treatment have occurred.

Small children eating macrobiotic diets with their parents commonly show failure to thrive (slow growth, underweight, and lethargy) due to deficiencies of fat-soluble vitamins (especially vitamin D), vitamin B_{12}, essential fatty acids, calcium, and perhaps other nutrients. These children suffer from a lack of raw food and animal source nutrients; dietary adjustments invariably lead to marked improvement within weeks.

Some individuals do well following macrobiotics while others do poorly. The amount of fish included in the diet has an influence—the more the better. In his recovery from bone cancer, Dr. Sattilaro regularly used modest amounts of fish. Vegetarian macrobiotic regimes including little or no fish most often lead to problems. Careful use of recommended amounts of beans, sea vegetables, and other special foods, each required for balance in the macrobiotic diet, enables other individuals to maintain health with apparently minimal use of animal source foods.

A craving for sweets is common among people eating a macrobiotic type of diet. Naturally sweetened desserts are regularly used, and followers often report eating additional sweets. In contrast, loss of the taste for sweets is often a side effect of a diet which includes substantial portions of animal source food.

An expressed concern of the macrobiotic movement is world peace; Michio Kushi has written of the desirability of one world government. Whole grains as the staple food for mankind is seen as an important means of promoting this end, for more people may then be fed and more equal distribution of wealth achieved. Food plays a role in personality; people eating a grains-based diet may exhibit more passive and less aggressive tendencies than those eating a diet based in animal source foods.

Food plays a pronounced role in shaping biological and cultural evolution. Government and industry leaders determining national policies seem unaware of this, as are most people. Macrobiotic leaders, however, are aware that the acceptance of a macrobiotic diet by large segments of the western world's population would have sociological as well as physiological effects. Perhaps it would be a step toward a less aggressive society and a more unified world, even toward one world government— but what kind of world, and at what cost? The quantity versus the quality of life is at issue.

In the nuclear age, survival of the human species as we know it depends on controlling aggressive tendencies; the same aggressive traits which carried us through evolution now threaten to destroy us. But loss of our biological strength has resulted in an epidemic of disease, physical and mental abnormalities, and lost reproductive capacity that has caused far more suffering than any war yet fought. This suffering is directly due to changes in diet. The macrobiotic goal of reduced aggressive tendencies is laudable, but only by producing and eating sufficient amounts of traditional animal source foods can we regain our biological strength and have both quantity and quality of life.

Changes taking place in the American diet have been mirrored by changes in national health. The interrelationships are obvious when one considers the implications of our study of our evolutionary ancestors, primitive cultures existing in the earlier part of this century, contemporary hunter-gatherers and long-lived people, and current medical research on nutrition. Each of the diets considered in this chapter in some way utilizes beneficial aspects of traditional foods. The next logical step— the creation and implementation of one's own diet for optimal health— is a complex process that may appear deceptively simple. We begin that process in the next chapter with a consideration of the elements of change, balance, and proportions in relation to food.

9

Creating a
Traditional Diet
For
Health and Longevity

*T*his chapter is designed to aid in selecting foods for a balanced traditional diet suited to individual tastes, personality, and genetic background. These are guidelines for experimenting with diet. By studying reactions to foods, one may create an optimal nutritional program. Once again, when medical problems are present or suspected, see a competent physician.

Effects of specific foods upon different conditions will be discussed in the next chapter. Particularly if any of these or other serious conditions exist, the services of a knowledgeable and understanding physician may be invaluable.

The Dynamic State of An Optimal Diet

The body's needs constantly change. To maintain balance, a sense of which foods are most needed *now* is required. Foods eaten at the last meal, and in the last day or two, strongly affect this sense. But there are longer cycles during which a need to emphasize certain foods may be felt. Some cycles relate to seasonal availability of foods; others are internal, and may last for a few days, months, or even years.

Several signals may be monitored as a guide in food selections. Difficult bowel movements, with hard stools and straining, signal a need for more fiber, best supplied in raw vegetable salads and whole grains. Exercise—daily walks, jogging, running, or other aerobic exercise—also aids regularity by stimulating both the intestines themselves and the consumption of more food. One reason traditional people consumed large quantities of vitamins, minerals, and other nutrients was that they ate so much. An active life necessitates this; one may eat a lot and still stay slim.

Appearance of excessive mucous in the respiratory system—sinus or nasal congestion, post-nasal drip, or early symptoms of a cold—is often a sign the body is reacting poorly to dairy products. Even raw milk products often cause these symptoms when from grain-fed animals.

Abnormal redness on the skin—pimples, rashes, small blemishes—is often a sign of eating sugar and sweets. Honey and other sweeteners, fruit juices, dried fruits, and even fresh fruit may cause this sign. The skin is an organ of elimination and often is the first part of the body to reveal an imbalance. The person eating no concentrated sweets for a time may have the quickest reaction when sweets are eaten—the body is well balanced and immediately eliminates excesses. Citrus fruit, pineapples, and tomatoes are also likely to cause these symptoms.

Certain fruits are quick to cause marked intestinal gas. Dried fruits, nuts and seeds, beans, and certain combinations of foods also often cause flatus, depending upon the amount eaten. Excessive gas, stomach or intestinal, is a sign the foods eaten have been improperly digested. When one eats well, digestion is smooth as silk.

Traditional Wisdom in Balancing Foods.   The traditional Chinese concept of yin and yang helps understand the desirability of a dynamic aspect in the diet, an aspect that aids in choosing foods wisely as one's needs constantly ebb and flow. In oriental philosophy, all of creation reflects a balance of yin and yang opposites. Yin is expansive, while yang is contractile. Other yin and yang opposites include hot and cold, dark and light, female and male. A person living in happiness and health is a harmonious balance of these yin and yang forces. The foods eaten are an important influence.

Some foods have more yin qualities, others more yang. Animal source foods are more yang, more strengthening. Grains are centered, a balance of yin and yang, while vegetables are slightly yin, more so if raw. Fruits are more yin. Concentrated sweets, drugs, and alcohol are extremely yin.

All aspects of life affect the sum of yin and yang—physical activity, climate, time spent outdoors, intellectual pursuits, personality, diet, sleep, the influence of friends. Health problems result from an imbalance of yin and yang forces—an excess of one or the other (or of both, for balance becomes difficult when excesses of both are present). An outbreak on the skin may be seen simply as excess yin (expansion). Diarrhea may be interpreted similarly. Constipation, on the other hand, reflects excess yang (contraction).

Foods thus manipulate the equilibrium of health. This oriental concept is useful both as a way of viewing medical problems and as an approach to understanding how personality may be consciously influenced through choice of foods and specific actions.

As an example, suppose a man wished both to grow healthier and stronger in character. How might he go about this? Yang is the stronger force; but strength must be tempered to be integral with a healthy and harmonious life. Animal source foods, especially organ meats, have a yang influence, so he may choose more of these foods. Drugs, chemicals, and excessive fats are yin, so he would seek foods free of them. To balance yang with yin influences, he would use vegetables. Among the grains, he may use buckwheat, the most yang—dense, highest in protein, requiring little cooking. He may avoid fruit juices and alcohol —extreme yin. Yet occasional strong drink in small quantities would not unbalance him. He would consciously shape the diet with strengthening, yang foods, counterpointed by yin foods of the proper quality.

Running strengthens when not done to excess; movement has a yang effect, especially rapid movement. So he might choose to run—sometimes long distances, but at times shorter and fast. When tired, he would rest, and grow stronger. And since cold is a yang force, he would welcome cold weather—the outdoors in winter, a cool room to sleep in, the balancing warmth of fire, and wood to cut and split.

Strength of character is built from way of life. Profound positive changes in personalities of both children and adults often accompany dietary changes and disciplined efforts to shape activities. Lifestyle changes in the directions indicated may have both a physically and a spiritually strengthening effect.

Signals the body gives may be translated into corresponding adjustments in the foods eaten. Food shapes the form of our lives, often without our awareness. Our option is to consciously use food to shape our lives in a manner of our choosing.

Proportions and Balance

Foods may be divided into the following groups:

1—*Animal Source Foods:* fish and shellfish; meat, organs, and bones; fowl; eggs; milk, yogurt, clabbered milk, kefir, cottage cheese, hard cheeses, and butter.

2—*Raw and Lightly Cooked Green Vegetables, Sprouts, and Sea Vegetables:* raw green vegetables include lettuces and other leafy greens palatable raw in salads; parsley; celery; and sprouts. Lightly cooked green vegetables include kale, broccoli, and others. Sea vegetables include dulse, kelp, and others.

3—*Other Vegetables, Whole Grains, Fruits, and Nuts and Seeds:* non-green vegetables; freshly cooked whole grains; sprouted breads; whole grain flour products such as breads and pastas; fresh and dried fruits; and nuts and seeds.

4—*Condiments and Alcoholic Beverages:* oils, vinegars, honey and other sweeteners, spices and seasonings, salt, pickled foods, beer, wine, and liquor—none strictly necessary but all at times desirable, and *in small amounts* doing little or no harm while enhancing flavors, providing variety, and making basic foods more interesting.

5—*Vitamin, Mineral, and Food Supplements:* additional vitamins and minerals useful in helping deal with environmental stresses and in correcting dietary deficiencies; and certain special foods in concentrated form useful in providing optimal nutrition.

6—*Everything Else:* refined and manufactured foods, particularly sugar and white flour. There is a fine line between such foods and those in group 4, and occasional use of small amounts of sugar and white flour has much the same effect as many foods in group 4.

Animal source foods of high quality and raw and lightly cooked green vegetables, especially sprouts, are the most primitive and basic foods, essential for prevention, healing, and recovery from disease. Non-green vegetables and freshly cooked whole grains may form a significant part of the diet, within individually determined limits; these are good foods, but overuse may limit use of more vital foods.

Fat-soluble nutrients essential to mineral metabolism and eicosapentaenoic acid (EPA) are found together only in fish, meat from grass-fed animals (especially the organs), and dairy products from grass-fed animals. These are of course foods Price found richly supplied in diets of immune groups. For raw food nutrients, fresh raw greens and sprouts should be emphasized, especially if little or no raw animal source food is used.

An example of a balanced regime would be one-third animal source food (fish and shellfish, meat, organs, eggs, raw milk and cheese); one-third raw greens and sprouts; and one-third whole grains, other vegetables, and fruits. Grain and cooked vegetable consumption increases in winter as raw vegetable consumption decreases. In late spring, summer, and early fall fruit might be used in quantity; consumption of grains may at such times decrease and even approach zero. Raw vegetable consumption too goes up in summer, when animal source foods are usually eaten less.

The author has spent weeks on the coast of Washington eating only salmon—over two pounds a day. During more vegetarian days, late one Kansas summer, little but musk melons and watermelons were eaten for two weeks. Cross-country drives have meant eating brown rice for days at a time, or perhaps raw greens and canned sardines. The earth provides a wide variety of foods that will sustain us.

The author has also fasted for up to seven days on spring water, though most uncomfortably. Literature about fasting describes how after a day or two hunger disappears, and as cleansing proceeds, one does not experience hunger pangs until fat reserves are depleted and true hunger returns. Alas, by the third day what felt like the excruciating pangs of advanced starvation had begun. Seven days was eternity; the fast was over nonetheless. That was ten years ago; brief fasts of one or two days have since provided sufficient cleansing.

These are examples of variance; obviously none exemplifies a balanced diet. Balance in diet is best achieved by seeing one's body and one's health in the long term. When principles are understood, nutrition may be approached in a creative way. People often complain they become tired of simple foods eaten daily and yearn for the variety of refined and prepared foods. But once one aquires a taste for whole and natural foods (and it is an aquisition for us who grew up on refined foods), they never are boring or tiring.

Experiences of Arctic explorer Vilhjalmur Stefansson illustrate this point. Despite adherence to medical advice of the early 1900's about prevention of scurvy, expeditions of early Arctic and Antarctic explorers suffered severely from the disease. Stefansson's expeditions were a notable exception. Rather than carrying fruits and vegetables, lime juice, and other provisions of a "balanced diet," he and his men lived much as Arctic Eskimos did, eating nothing but seal and a little polar bear for months, much of it raw and the rest lightly cooked. They got no scurvy. The little vitamin C in raw meat and fish, destroyed normally in cooking, provided adequate protection from the disease.

Stefansson found his men always became accustomed to the all meat diet and eventually enjoyed it. The first week was difficult; some men ate little or nothing. Gradually they ate more, until soon they were eating heartily, though with many complaints. Stefansson guessed if sometime during the first three months, they had suddenly been rescued from the seal and given a diet of varied foods, most would have sworn never to taste seal again. If it had been three or four months, a man may or may not have been willing to go back to seal again. But if the period had been six months or more, Stefansson claimed none were unwilling to go back to the all meat diet.

This is consistent with the experience of many people when introduced to simple natural foods diets. There may be considerable discomfort initially, followed by a period of grudging aquiescence. But if the individual stays with the diet for three to six months, he usually will never go back to refined foods.

Such diets are designed to be widely varied with a broad range of natural foods. And the emphasis in each is individually constructed, because a diet capable of preventing and reversing chronic diseases may be constructed in many different ways. Adequate amounts of fat-soluble nutrients of animal origin and sufficient raw foods must be included, and the bulk of the diet consists of vegetables, grains, and fish. Varying amounts of other animal source foods are recommended, depending on the availability of meats, eggs, and dairy foods of sufficient quality. Personal preferences, seasonal and geographical variability in the supply of foods, and restrictions necessitated by certain health problems may be easily accommodated within this broad framework.

Nutrition in Pregnancy

A remarkable discovery of Weston Price's was that in cultures where little or no dental decay was found, physical abnormalities of any kind in children were almost nonexistent. Wisdom about special foods and spacing the birth of children by at least three years are the two factors most responsible.

This traditional wisdom about spacing childbirth is sound. Many psychologists believe such spacing is ideal also for the emotional development of older siblings forced to compete at too early an age for the time and attention of the parents when siblings are born too soon after their own birth.

For at least six months before conception, an optimal nutritional program should emphasize foods from at least one of these three groups: 1—fish and shellfish; 2—liver and other organs; 3—certified raw milk and cheese from animals kept at pasture. Foods from groups 2 and 3 should be from naturally raised animals. Iodine-rich sea vegetables, such as dulse or kelp, and many fresh raw greens should also be used. These foods should for a woman enhance fertility and optimal development of the fetus. Their use as well by the prospective father before conception should insure maximum viability of sperm and minimize chances of birth defects. During pregnancy, a rich source of calcium is important, particularly during the latter third.

During pregnancy, exercise such as walking (or running for a woman accustomed to it) continued on a regular, daily basis enables a good volume of food to be eaten without exorbitant weight gain. Such volume and the inclusion of whole grains in the diet should insure freedom from the constipation that troubles many pregnancies. Avoidance of sugar, alcohol, white flour, and vegetable oils—empty calories—further insures consumption of adequate fiber.

Price's evidence that such a program produces maximally healthy and well developed babies is overwhelming. Women following such a program of diet and exercise have in the author's experience invariably had healthy pregnancies, births, and babies.

Many of the same foods emphasized immediately prior to conception and in pregnancy are especially important in treating disease through food. These and other considerations important in treating specific conditions are the subjects of the next chapter, as we continue to define how each individual may best select foods. Relationships and goals involved in a search for health are the subject of the subsequent and concluding chapter of part I. In part II, we will turn to a more detailed examination of the foods themselves, continuing to examine the differences between traditional and modern foods, and the effects of those differences on human strength, resistance to disease, and longevity.

10

Recovery Through Nutrition

Dietary Considerations
For
Specific Conditions

*A*lthough this chapter is about specific conditions, a specific diet for each will not be described. Different people with the same diagnosed condition have different nutritional requirements; sometimes these differences are marked. Detailed recommendations may be made only after individual assessment. Tastes and emotional states should never be overlooked; the finest plan is of no help if not followed. With this in mind, we'll discuss considerations most important in the following conditions.

Colds, Flus, Mononucleosis: When and How to Fast

Colds and flus disappear most rapidly when a fast is started at the first sign of symptoms. Everyone has individual characteristic signs marking the onset of colds and flus—for some, fatigue and a headachy feeling, or perhaps a loss of appetite, for others, a vague but growing soreness in the throat. The latter is often the first sign in those with no tonsils, which as a part of the immune system protect the throat from bacterial and viral invasion; their loss leaves one more susceptible to sore throats.

Typically, symptoms grow worse over the course of a day or two, as the illness becomes established. If a fast is instituted at the first sign, minor symptoms will usually begin to abate within twenty-four hours. The cold or flu can often be avoided by eating very carefully for the next few days.

The human body is remarkable; when allowed, corrective action comes naturally. The acutely ill feel no hunger because food in acute illness interferes with natural responses. But hunger may be strong when the earliest symptoms appear, for the illness is not yet established. Awareness and discipline aid greatly; too often we eat out of habit or boredom, or because of expectations of others. The temptation to eat before fully recovered may be strong, but doing so often brings back symptoms and blocks recovery.

106

After the fasting stage, the wisest diet is simply non-starchy vegetables and fish, chicken, or meat. The classic Jewish mother gives chicken soup; this wisdom originated when the chicken was fed and raised in the barnyard. Soup made of beef, chicken, or fish stock, and greens, carrots, and onions is excellent. When a virulent bug takes hold and can't be shaken off in a day or two, this diet is next best to fasting.

People often express disbelief about the effectiveness of a short fast. One patient called late one Thursday afternoon with flu symptoms. Her weekend travel plans were threatened; she felt ill and was feverish (101.5 degrees). She hoped to feel well enough to travel Friday afternoon. A fast was recommended, with only water, herbal teas, vitamin C, and cod liver oil.

"Nothing else," she was told. "Just rest. Don't eat tonight or tomorrow. No food, no juices. Take a warm water enema, body temperature, with a quart or so of water, once tonight and again in the morning. By noon tomorrow, the fever should break, and if your temperature is normal by late tomorrow afternoon and you feel up to it, take your trip. Do not eat tomorrow night either. Begin eating Saturday—but only vegetables, some soup, and fish, chicken, or meat. Do not overexert yourself. If symptoms reappear, fast again."

Despite her doubts, she followed directions. By morning, her temperature was close to normal; by evening she felt well enough to travel. She had aborted a bout with a cold or the flu.

Vitamin C is useful in such cases, but more than two to three grams a day may cause diarrhea. Regular use of this amount causes dependence, however. After taking over a gram a day for several days, stopping completely leaves one particularly susceptible to illness. This problem may be avoided by tapering off gradually over a period of several days.

Mononucleosis. Mononucleosis is an infectious viral disease marked by fatigue, high fever, sore throat, and swollen lymph glands. The diagnosis is made from characteristics of the blood cells seen microscopically. While people in their teens and twenties are usually the most susceptible, middle-aged people with mono may go undiagnosed for months if the possibility is not considered when symptoms are present.

Conventional medicine has no treatment for mono; since it is viral, antibiotics are ineffective, though they may be given if a concurrent bacterial infection is suspected. While effective against some bacterial infections, antibiotics may further weaken the patient and place an added strain on an already overburdened liver. The usual course is several weeks of bed rest followed by several more of gradual recovery.

Recovery from mononucleosis with carefully supervised natural treatment may be dramatic. Even when the disease is well established, an initial thirty-six to forty-eight hour fast usually brings the fever under one hundred degrees and reverses the course of any concurrent bacterial infection. By then the patient typically feels better and has some appetite; if so some food may be taken. With continued rest and careful eating only when the appetite is strong, patients are up and around and feeling fairly well, though still weakened, within a few days. Ninety percent recovery within one to two weeks and full recovery within two to four weeks has been the rule.

While not life threatening, mononucleosis can drag on for months and be most debilitating. Although unusual, some individuals suffer relapses, which may actually be flare-ups of a low grade but continuing presence of the disease. While no causal link has been established, patients with a history of recurrent mononucleosis have later developed Hodgkin's disease, a type of cancer of the lymph system. The chronically weakened immune system leaves an individual susceptible to the development of cancer. A healthy immune system eliminates the small number of cancer cells we all constantly develop spontaneously.

Infants and Babies.   In most cases, no food should be taken in acute illness until the temperature returns to normal; usually this takes from twelve to twenty-four hours. Even an infant may be safely fasted for a day or two if sufficient water is given. An acutely ill infant has no desire for food. Short tepid baths (water at seventy-five to eighty degrees for a few minutes) and small amounts of aspirin if the temperature is over 102 nearly always keeps a fever in infants under 104. If the problem seems serious or is accompanied by continuing diarrhea, if there is doubt about its nature, if the fever climbs over 105 degrees, or if it persists longer than twenty-four hours despite these measures, the infant should immediately be seen by a physician.

The breast-fed baby is profoundly affected by the diet of the mother; if ill, the mother's diet is almost invariably to blame. The above described dietary measures usually quickly eliminate illness in the baby.

* * *

With the exception of butter, milk products are not usually well tolerated while recovering from acute illness, and are best avoided. Salads and green vegetables should be favored over grains.

Acute illness is a warning sign of more serious things to come, and may for the most part be avoided by a healthy lifestyle and diet. The simple and straightforward measures discussed effectively deal with most occasional acute problems that do arise, in a safe and nontoxic way.

Allergies

Allergies too are early warning signs that foods are creating imbalances. The worst offenders are usually conventionally produced milk and cheese; removing them from the diet eliminates many allergies.

In young children, allergies most often manifest as coughs, colds, and recurrent middle ear infections, all of which usually clear up when conventionally produced milk and cheese are removed from the diet. An example is the case of a six-year-old boy whose marked hearing loss due to recurrent middle ear infections was causing him difficulties in school. Surgical implantation of drainage tubes was planned, but his parents decided to first try natural treatment.

Acute infections in both ears cleared within a week; within three his parents and his teacher noted a clear improvement in hearing. Subsequent audio testing showed his hearing to return gradually to normal over the next six months, and surgery was avoided. This little boy was a marvelous patient; within a week on the diet we planned together, he grew to love the foods. He once explained how he hadn't eaten any cake at a birthday party the day before because he was happy to be hearing better, and that was more important than cake.

Despite perversion by sugar, children's tastes often change rapidly; they tend to embrace good food when that is all there is to eat. Firm guidance is needed; they may refuse to eat in an attempt to pressure parents into giving them what they want. The alternative of good food or no food ends hunger strikes within a day or so.

Alternative allergy testing and treatment for both children and adults has become popular. Alternative refers to the clinical ecology approach which uses the newer allergy tests, such as cytotoxic testing, rather than the conventional scratch tests of traditional allergists. Some people swear by the results achieved; others have noted little improvement in their symptoms.

In cytotoxic tests, foods eaten often tend to test as being allergenic (positive); subsequent avoidance may cause improvement in symptoms. But mainstays of a traditional diet may test positive, including fish and green vegetables. And highly allergenic foods, such as conventional milk and cheese, may test negative if they are not being regularly used at the time. Such results may confuse patient and physician alike.

The tests are popular because of confusion about what constitutes proper diet; they attempt to provide a sophisticated solution for a simple but subtle problem. Yet the proper diet may be determined for an individual without these tests.

Many people test positive for pollens and other environmental factors. Both classical allergy shots and the intradermal injections of clinical ecology are designed to neutralize the effects of these allergens (substances triggering the allergic response), and many people get relief from these measures, particularly the latter. But adverse reactions to trees, grasses, flowers, dust, dogs, and cats are not normal and indicate the immune system is unbalanced and failing to function properly. The cause of the unbalance is almost always poor food selection. Offending foods often cause no overt response when eaten. Rather, chronic symptoms such as postnasal drip, congestion, itchy eyes, fatigue, or others are continually present, masking responses occurring when the food is eaten.

The individual then at times has a gross and obvious allergic response to pollens and other environmental factors. The response is real and is directly stimulated by the environmental factors, but it has developed because foods disturbing immune function have been regularly eaten. Conventional dairy foods are usually the worst offenders.

When traditional diets are followed, such problems clear up. Trees, flowers, and cats are not supposed to make people sick; when they do something is wrong.

Pottenger noted the development of allergies, and even of allergic bronchitis, in cats fed diets of cooked and refined foods. The naturally fed animals suffered no such aberrations. For human beings, allergies are caused by the modern diet. An understanding of how the body reacts to foods is an understanding of allergies.

Chronic Fatigue and Thyroid Problems

Chronic fatigue is a very common complaint. Some people feel tired throughout life and accept fatigue as normal. Others feel tired for up to several months prior to the diagnosis of a chronic disease.

If laboratory tests and a physical exam are normal, little attempt is usually made to treat fatigue. While it may be a sign of a serious but undetected problem, fatigue is often considered a vague complaint people must live with.

Chronic fatigue is a classic symptom of low thyroid function, or hypothyroidism. Laboratory tests for thyroid function often are normal in people with low thyroid function and some of the symptoms of hypothyroidism, which besides fatigue may include dry skin and hair, a tendency to gain weight easily, constipation, and sensitivity to cold weather. Seldom are all of these symptoms present; low thyroid function affects people differently.

The one common characteristic is a low basal body temperature, the underarm temperature upon first awakening in the morning (best taken at the same time daily before moving about or arising from bed). The most definitive readings in women are taken the first three days of the menstrual cycle.

The physician first describing this test, Broda Barnes, first trained as a physiologist, studying thyroid function in animals. In his thirty-five year career, he treated thousands of patients with natural thyroid tissue, using the basal body temperature test as one means of monitoring progress. He suggests 97.8 to 98.2 degrees as a normal range. Presence of symptoms associated with low thyroid function and a consistent basal temperature below 97.8 led him to treat with thyroid tissue. He associated low thyroid function with the development of chronic diseases and other conditions, including migraine, emotional and behavioral disorders, infectious diseases, skin problems, menstrual and fertility problems, hypertension, heart disease, arthritis, diabetes, cancer, and premature aging.

Hormones produced in the thyroid gland control the metabolic rate of every cell in the body. The thyroid thus affects pathological conditions as they arise and develop, and low thyroid function contributes to a developing chronic problem. Many clinicians have noted this relationship. Medical literature since early in this century shows many reports of beneficial effects of thyroid medication on a host of chronic conditions. Dr. Gerson noted his cancer patients almost invariably suffered from grossly low thyroid function and he included substantial amounts of thyroid tissue in his therapy.

Barnes kept records that revealed his patients taking thyroid had markedly lower incidences of chronic diseases, especially heart disease and cancer, than statistically expected. This is consistent with the experience of many physicians who find most patients with chronic diseases show some symptoms of low thyroid function and a low basal body temperature.

The lower end of the temperature range Barnes used is a bit high; the range of possible normals should be from 97.2 to 98.2. An individual in the 97.2 to 97.7 range may or may not have low thyroid function; many symptomless people fall in this range, but so do many people with overt symptoms. Those with basal temperatures below 97.2 nearly always show symptoms; people with chronic diseases usually are in this range.

As chronic conditions improve, symptoms of low thyroid function improve also, and basal temperature rises. Proper diet and adequate iodine intake aid thyroid function, as was elegantly demonstrated by Dr. Robert McCarrison. He showed the weight of the thyroid gland as a percentage of total body weight in white rats varied significantly when a natural foods diet rich in raw milk, vegetables, whole grain flour, and meat was changed to one of refined foods. Classic symptoms of hypothyroidism appeared when the animals were fed refined foods.

When prescribing thyroid, endocrinologists and internists usually call for a synthetic, rather than natural animal thyroid tissue. This allows a standardized dosage, not possible with precision when using the natural product because tissue from different animals varies slightly in potency. But people on synthetic thyroid may show conflicting symptoms of underactive and overactive thyroid function, and low basal temperatures. Several in the author's experience have had recurrent heart irregularities—irregular rhythms and palpitations—while on synthetic thyroid.

Such irregularities have not been noted in individuals on carefully regulated amounts of natural thyroid.

The thyroid gland is not an entity unto itself, and its effects on metabolism are best considered as one part of the overall picture. Low thyroid function is common, especially in middle-aged and older people. The first signs of improvement for many individuals making dietary changes are increased energy with less fatigue, and more frequent bowel movements. Improved glandular function, particularly of the thyroid gland, likely provides the stimulus for these changes.

Arthritis and Back Problems

Most people over the age of fifty (and many much younger) reveal at least some early symptoms of arthritis. With added years, the problem usually becomes worse; the bent posture, stiff hands, and slow gait of most elderly Americans is in stark contrast with the energy, activity, and strength noted among the very old in Georgian Russia, Vilcabamba, and Hunza.

No explanation for the development of arthritis has been put forth by conventional medicine. Deposits of calcium are found in affected joints, and involvement of an imbalance in calcium metabolism is accepted. These deposits occur early in osteoarthritis, the common arthritis of aging; in rheumatoid arthritis, they appear considerably later.

What causes these deposits of calcium in the arthritic process? Calcium serves a host of functions, and the absorbtion and utilization of dietary calcium is complex. Bones are a storehouse for calcium, and normal blood levels of calcium are maintained by an interplay of dietary calcium and calcium released from and taken into the bones.

Abnormal calcium deposits in the joints in arthritis are due in part to disturbances in calcium metabolism caused by poor diet. When dietary calcium is inadequate, the bones steadily lose calcium to maintain adequate levels in the blood. This leads to both osteoporosis (defined as an abnormal loss of calcium from the bones) and to abnormal deposits of calcium; often osteoarthritis and osteoporosis are present simultaneously, and clinicians often have difficulty distinguishing between them.

But arthritis also develops in people getting adequate dietary calcium. Eating refined carbohydrates, particularly sugar, causes disturbances in blood levels of calcium and phosphorous. Such disturbances are a major factor in the development of arthritis. Sweets of any kind aggravate symptoms of arthritis in most patients. Significant improvements in symptoms often lead to a "treat," a few cookies or similar sweets, soon followed by the reappearance of pain and other symptoms. This is no coincidence.

Commercial dairy products also aggravate arthritis. Pasteurization changes the way calcium is arranged in milk and disturbs its normal utilization. Often young and early middle-aged adults with back problems have been large drinkers of commercial milk. Evidence indicates the synthetic vitamin D_2 often added to milk also contributes to this type of calcium metabolism problem, which the author has never encountered in a raw milk drinker. Nor have any older people been encountered who developed arthritis while drinking raw milk. The evidence of Pottenger's cats is revealing; those fed pasteurized milk developed inferior skeletal structures and eventually mild arthritis, while those fed sweetened condensed milk developed gross skeletal abnormalities and debilitating arthritis.

The chronic bad back of a young adult is an early stage of the osteoarthritis of an older individual. Dental decay in children and young adults and periodontal disease in middle-aged and older adults all indicate disturbances in calcium metabolism. These problems respond well to traditional diets.

Fat-soluble nutrients controlling mineral metabolism have profound effects on these problems. Cod liver oil and fatty fish are excellent, readily available sources. If individuals chronically lack adequate dietary calcium, then cod liver oil and special foods rich in calcium, or calcium supplements, may have a rapidly beneficial effect within days, especially upon chronic back problems. Elimination of commercial dairy products and refined carbohydrates and inclusion in the diet of raw vegetables enhances results.

Fruit, particularly citrus fruits, and fruit juices aggravate arthritis. Nightshade vegetables—tomatoes, potatoes, green peppers, and eggplants—also usually aggravate the symptoms. Removal of all fruit, fruit juices, and nightshade vegetables from the diet is the best course for those serious about reversing an arthritic condition through careful nutrition. Later, small amounts of these foods may be tolerated.

Arthritis is often accepted as a part of growing old, perhaps until the pain becomes great. But pain is a great motivator, and people with osteoarthritis are often very successful patients. Literally every patient who has seriously attempted to follow the principles of nutrition outlined has experienced significant relief from arthritis.

The degree of improvement correlates with the care taken with the diet. Many people find they can control arthritis by eating with some degree of care, while continuing to eat some refined foods; arthritis is more easily controlled than other chronic diseases. Others following recommendations fully have experienced a complete reversal and no longer have symptoms. A return to refined foods invariably shortly results in a relapse of symptoms. This seems true of all chronic diseases.

Large portions of fresh raw and lightly steamed green vegetables are important in arthritis; they are rich in calcium and other minerals. Juice made from raw greens and carrots is helpful, especially if few other raw foods are eaten. Raw eggs blended into eggnog with raw milk (from grass-fed cows or goats if possible, though this is difficult to find) are excellent, as are fresh sunflower and buckwheat sprouts grown in flats or in the garden (they are occasionally available in health food stores). Fresh fish, especially fatty species such as salmon, may be eaten in whatever amount desired.

Heart and Circulatory Disorders

The most important single food for people with these problems is fatty cold-water species of fish such as salmon, preferably eaten at least several times a week. Equally, raw shellfish may be eaten in season as desired. People with these problems are usually warned to avoid shellfish and organ meats because of the high cholesterol content. However, the use of organ meats and of several dozen oysters or clams a week, when in season, has been the rule for various individuals the author has worked with during their recovery from heart disease. Recovery was adequate even in an individual who without fail consumed four to six ounces of liquor daily. Seafoods have not caused a rise in blood cholesterol.

Commercial varieties of dairy foods and meats should be avoided or minimized. But the fats in meat and dairy foods from grass-fed animals may well be beneficial and need not be avoided. Information presented earlier on fish, fats, and protective nutrients should serve as a guide in food selection for the person with a history of heart disease.

Calcium and the Heart. Abnormal deposits of calcium are present in both atherosclerosis (the buildup of plaque on arterial walls, particularly those of the coronary arteries) and arteriosclerosis (hardening of the arteries). In the former, calcium, cholesterol, and other fatty materials are involved; in the latter, the hardening is mainly calcification.

These two problems generally occur concurrently and are often associated with arthritis; imbalances in calcium metabolism affect all three. Abnormal calcium metabolism traceable to the diet appears the major contributing factor in the deposition of calcium in both joints and arterial walls.

These abnormal deposits occur in a host of problems. Arteriosclerosis may lead to senility and strokes when arteries to the brain are affected, and it contributes to the poor circulation to the extremities common in old age. Kidney stones and gallstones usually contain large amounts of calcium. In multiple sclerosis, calcium is precipitated into muscles, and in arthritis deposits occur on bone surfaces and in joints.

A loss of calcium from bones often leads to the spontaneous fractures of osteoporosis, especially of the hip in the elderly. Bones have become so weak in these cases that the break occurs under normal stresses of daily living. Losses of bone calcium leading to this take place over many years. Studies show radiologists are not unanimous on interpreting an X-ray as showing osteoporosis until at least 30 percent of the calcium in the bone has been lost. This means lesser losses are often not detected; we may assume many middle-aged and older people have undetected loss of calcium from the bones. This bone loss of calcium, rather than excessive dietary calcium, leads to the above problems involving calcium deposits.

People eating traditional diets consumed four to eight times the calcium official standards recommend today. Foods and food supplements rich in calcium should be used, especially by people with calcium related problems. On occasion, individuals have noted calcium supplements to cause constipation, a problem not usually caused by foods rich in cal-cium—raw milk, green vegetable juice, bone meal and bones, and egg shells. However, eating quantities of cheese does constipate many people.

Calcium deposition may relate also to hypertension, for a gradual deposition of calcium contributes to a hardening of the arteries. Resultant inelasticity of these vessels raises blood pressure.

Blood Pressure, Cholesterol Levels, and the Thyroid Gland. High blood pressure usually accompanies heart disease and is often involved in its development. Both high blood cholesterol and high blood pressure are classic signs of hypothyroidism, or low thyroid function. Extensive writings in medical literature in the earlier part of this century have detailed relationships between blood pressure, blood cholesterol, and the thyroid gland. Thyroid problems were then diagnosed symptomati-cally rather than through laboratory testing. Tests now used are often normal despite the presence of overt symptoms of low thyroid function, and articles in medical journals frequently point out the limitations of these tests.

Thus many Americans have both high blood pressure and high blood cholesterol that are caused in part by undiagnosed low thyroid function. Thyroid hormones control the rate at which cholesterol and other fats are metabolized; their relative lack thus leads to higher levels of blood cholesterol. How a lack of thyroid hormones contributes to high blood pressure is not as clear, but in the 1920's physicians involved in the new field of endocrinology proposed the concept of cellular infiltration.

Because fats in cells throughout the body (including those in cells lining the blood vessels) are not burned up at a normal rate when thyroid function is low, they accumulate along with other waste products of incomplete cellular metabolism. Liken this to a wood fire getting insuf-ficient oxygen—it smolders, and charcoal accumulates. The accumulation in cells lining blood vessel walls causes these cells to take on extra fluid and swell. As the vessels become less elastic, the blood pressure is slowly raised over the years. This is the concept of cellular infiltration, a physiologically sound theory to explain the observation that hypertension occurs in hypothyroidism.

Current standards for blood pressure and blood cholesterol reflect averages rather than what is healthy. Blood pressures among the elderly in Vilcabamba and Georgian Russia are in the range of 100 over 60 to 120 over 80. Americans are considered to be doing well if the blood pressure stays under 140 over 90. Cholesterol levels in these two traditional societies average under 120. Most Americans have levels over 200, many much higher.

Among people without marked blood pressure problems when beginning a traditional diet, blood pressure usually slowly falls into the 110 over 70, to 120 over 80 range (if not there to begin with). Those with markedly elevated pressure at the start (higher than 140 over 90) usually experience gradual reductions until no medication is needed (under 140 over 90). Further reductions occur if a careful program is continued and, if weight is a problem, it is reduced into a reasonable range.

Caffeine and the Heart. Caffeine often increases blood pressure, which may drop twenty or more points within a few weeks of abstaining from coffee even if no other changes are made. Caffeine also may cause palpitations (alarmingly strong and rapid heartbeats) and influence arrhythmias (irregularities in the rhythm of the heartbeat). Sugar too may bring on these symptoms.

An example is a gentleman who "converted," as he puts it, to eating mostly natural foods over the course of several years. Still, he maintained a fondness for sweets and coffee. He began mixing his regular drip coffee half and half with decaf; he drank twice as much. Once a week or so, he binged on rich desserts.

He began occasionally experiencing unnerving palpitations and arrhythmias during the night. Evaluation by a cardiologist revealed no serious problems, and he continued his regular program of jogging, tennis, and rowing; he was in quite good condition. The problem occurred only during the night.

Questioning revealed the problem occurred two or three nights a week, sometimes after binging on sweets and sometimes on nights he ate no sweets. He concluded that coffee rather than sweets caused the trouble. His cardiologist, knowing caffeine can produce the symptoms, advised he cut down or give up coffee.

He cut down to a cup or two a day, but the problem continued to occur. He seemed to think that such a small amount of coffee could not be responsible. He was persuaded to give up coffee entirely, which he nearly did (he still had a cup once or twice a week). The problem still occurred once a week or so, sometimes on the nights he had coffee, sometimes on other nights.

We discovered in time the symptoms often occurred on the nights he ate sweets. On nights he did drink coffee (with or without sweets), the symptoms might occur. Both coffee and sweets were capable of inducing his palpitations and his arrhythmia, though neither one did so every time; the occurrence of symptoms was apparently related to the dose. The combination of coffee and sweets was most likely to cause symptoms.

This case is typical of the potential effects of caffeine and sugar on the heart. It also illustrates the strong tendency towards denial of the possibility that favorite foods and drinks may cause problems. People tend to think that unless a food causes a readily identifiable symptom every time it is eaten in any quantity, it is not a likely cause of the symptom. This is not accurate. Though foods may act upon us in such an easily identified manner, the process is often more subtle. Our reactions depend upon the amount of the food ingested, when it was eaten last and in what quantity, what is was eaten with, and the overall status of the body at that time. An equal amount of a food causing no reaction once may cause a marked reaction the next time it is eaten.

In rotation diets, foods known to cause allergic reactions are eaten once every three, four, or five days; a food which when eaten daily caused reactions may perhaps then cause none. Allergy symptoms are caused by malfunctioning of the immune system, which produces antibodies in response to the allergenic food. The allergic reaction may then be strong if the food is soon eaten again, causing marked symptoms. When the food is not eaten again for several days, antibodies causing the allergic reaction dissipate, and any reaction occurring tends to be milder.

The heart symptoms above were a response to both caffeine and allergens (elements provoking antibody formation and an allergic reaction) in foods. Changes in blood sugar levels caused by sugar (caffeine too affects this) may interplay with these reactions. The acute heart symptoms, like acute symptoms that may occur in any system of the body, were directly caused by the foods.

Exercise.   Regular and controlled exercise is of particular benefit for problems with the heart and circulatory system; for full recovery it is essential. While parameters vary for each person, the heart should be taxed slightly beyond its customary workload for (at first) a short time, and daily. Very short walks are a good beginning for most people, at a speed not so fast as to cause any shortness of breath. If unaccustomed to walking, only a distance causing no strain or fatigue should be covered. The keys are commitment and regularity. As one grows stronger, length and intensity may be gradually increased.

Malignancies

People with cancer and seeking help usually feel a great deal of tension. Often pressure from different family members and physicians has been placed on the individual concerning the variety of possible treatments available. This dilemma can lead to confusion for the patient.

Controversy surrounding treatment of cancer with nutrition adds to his difficulty. The medical establishment condemns nutritional treatments of cancer. Surgery, chemotherapy, and radiation, the accepted treatments, usually alleviate symptoms of cancer for a time by destroying or removing cancer cells. But the underlying conditions that led to cancer are left unchanged, and cancer cells remaining continue to multiply.

Statistics concerning cancer survival are discouraging, but the actual situation is worse. Few individuals are encountered who are free of cancer several years after the initial diagnosis. Since an individual surviving five years after the initial diagnosis is counted as a cure, the official statistics are almost meaningless. Many people in the later stages of cancer today were originally diagnosed and treated more than five years ago. They count as cures in the statistics.

These people often seek alternative therapy through nutrition. Having exhausted conventional treatments, they hope that an alternative may help. Other people seek to use nutrition in support of their conventional treatments. This has become more popular as conventional medicine has recognized that optimal nutrition strengthens the individual and allows him to withstand chemotherapy with fewer side effects. And a few people decide from the start their best chance for survival is to avoid conventional treatment and search for a natural approach that will work for them.

For those having had (or in the process of having) conventional treatment, anything done to improve nutrition is in support of that treatment; nutrition should not be considered the primary means of treatment. For the individual who has had chemotherapy or extensive radiation, nutrition may be of only limited benefit. This was Dr. Gerson's experience, as it has been the author's. The basis of natural therapy is the strengthening of the immune system to enable it to reject the cancer. The capacity of the immune system to be so strengthened is apparently compromised by the poisonous chemicals used in chemotherapy.

Traditional foods diets reduce side effects of chemotherapy or radiation. Often individuals subsequently felt well for several months while continuing excellent nutritional programs. Unfortunately, in the several cases followed, tumors eventually reappeared.

This is why for the person receiving conventional therapy, nutrition should be considered only an adjunct to that therapy. The choice between conventional and nutritional therapy must be made at the outset. To expect nutrition to succeed after chemotherapy has failed is not realistic. Perhaps nutrition in conjunction with some other therapies may offer hope after conventional methods have failed.

The recent direction has been for more people to use nutrition as an adjunct to chemotherapy. While this diminishes side effects and helps make the person in the later stages of cancer more comfortable, it is unlikely to alter chances of survival significantly. And although such cases are not a fair test of the value of nutrition as therapy for cancer, the failure of such programs to increase survival may increase established resistance against nutritional therapy for cancer.

An extensive review of the problems inherent to conventional cancer treatment may be found in Ralph Moss's *The Cancer Syndrome*. While working as Assistant Director of Public Affairs at Memorial Sloan-Kettering Cancer Center in New York, Moss helped write a booklet on Laetrile which expressed opinions contrary to those of his superiors at Sloan-Kettering. He was fired the day after its publication, and he subsequently wrote the *The Cancer Syndrome*. The book is a revealing inside view of the cancer establishment, very helpful for one who may be questioning conventional therapy. Propaganda and misinformation about cancer and its treatment abound. Information about the realities of conventional treatment enables one to choose intelligently.

As with all diseases, no one treatment for cancer is best for everyone. For many people, conventional treatment is perhaps best, simply because they would never be able to go against conventional medical advice. Nutritional therapy for cancer requires personal commitment, discipline, and hard work; well meaning family members who believe it offers the best chances of recovery may not realize this. Unless the patient comes to understand and embrace a natural approach to disease and to cancer, nutritional therapy cannot succeed.

For the individual rejecting surgery, chemotherapy, and radiation, and willing to follow a rigorous nutritional course, nutrition offers the best chance of survival, in the experience of the author. Some such people have died, some survive for years with cancer, but with no sign of it worsening, and others recover completely.

Physicians writing earlier in this century reported that people with cancer typically survived many years unless operated upon, in which case death often shortly followed. A tumor is the body's way of segregating a diseased area, and when cut, cancer cells may spread much more rapidly than when the tumor is left alone. Cancer may be legally diagnosed only by a biopsy, presenting a dilemma.

Most people need to know what a biopsy will show before choosing a course of therapy, despite the risk involved. Others, particularly those sure they would choose natural therapy whatever a biopsy showed, may choose to avoid it. A number of people the author has worked with have made this choice, including women with breast lumps and men with lesions of the prostate gland, testicles, or breast, in every case with good results. An individual choosing this course should be highly motivated to follow a careful and thorough program. Even if he is not, however, we should recognize a person's right to choose to live out his life without being subjected to surgical dismemberment and an array of poisonous drugs.

The course of cancer, when treated through the kind of nutrition discussed, varies according to several influences. Among them are the stage of the cancer, the condition of the individual when starting nutritional therapy, the type of cancer, and the thoroughness with which the individual applies the recommended therapy.

Malignant Melanoma. One case is that of a man we'll call Konrad first seen a week after a diagnosis of malignant melanoma. A small mole on his arm had been removed and the biopsy showed stage IV melanoma (deep penetration of a highly malignant tumor below the surface of the skin into the underlying dermal layer). This type of melanoma has a poor prognosis. The treatment his surgeon had recommended was excision of the tissue around the area of the melanoma and removal of all lymph nodes in the arm and armpit, followed by extensive chemotherapy. Five year survival is less than 50 percent.

Konrad decided to have the surgical excision of the tissue around the area where the mole had been removed; a patch of skin about two inches square and one-half inch thick was removed. He declined lymph node removal and chemotherapy, and began a program of carefully planned nutritional therapy. His surgeon continued to see him monthly and, displeased with Konrad's decision to forego more extensive surgery and chemotherapy, offered the opinion that he had little chance of survival.

Konrad's therapy included many elements of the Gerson therapy. Fresh raw vegetable juices were made twice daily, yielding at least two quarts a day. Fresh organic vegetables and some whole grains were used. Liver juice was made daily, and coffee enemas were taken twice daily. Most vegetables were eaten raw. Fish was regularly eaten. Since dairy products of sufficient quality were not available, he used none.

Konrad did well, to the surprise of his surgeon (who eventually grew curious about his diet), and the melanoma has not reappeared; as of this writing, five years have passed. Konrad continues eating natural, organic foods, including a considerable amount of liver and fish, and he regularly makes raw vegetable juice. Over the past three years, the liver juice, coffee enemas, and many of the supplements used in the earlier stages of therapy have been reduced or stopped.

He considers himself recovered, but that he never will be "cured;" in other words, he must remain vigilant to avoid a recurrence. Gerson found some patients let the diet slide once cancer was no longer evident; almost invariably the disease subsequently returned. In individuals fighting cancer, tumors often diminish and increase in size according to how thoroughly programs are followed.

The author has met several people who recovered on the Gerson therapy in the 1950's, and has worked with several others who recovered in a similar manner, including a woman who recovered from breast cancer under the care of Max Warmbrand, a naturopathic physician and osteopath who practiced for many years in Connecticut and New York City until his death several years ago.

But by and large, cancer is difficult, and many people lose the battle. For the person who believes in it, natural therapy without the damaging effects of conventional treatments offers the best hope for recovery. Results seen are encouraging, but in the later stages of cancer, the most rigorous therapy may fail to halt the disease.

In-patient facilities for natural therapy enhance the chances of recovery, especially in more advanced cases. Gerson maintained such a facility, where his patients received help with the therapy and supported one another. A goal of the author is the establishment of such a facility in Connecticut.

Several clinics have been established for alternative therapies for cancer, mostly in Mexico and Europe. A number of promising therapies have been developed. The integration of the methods discussed here would almost certainly enhance the results.

Optimal diet for cancer seems to vary for each person. Some people have recovered on mostly raw food diets; others have used the mostly cooked foods macrobiotic program.

While many nutritional regimes stress a low intake of animal protein, the author has found animal source foods of the proper quality of benefit. For most people, as much raw food as possible is absolutely essential. The most important foods to choose from include sunflower and buckwheat sprouts and other raw greens, raw green juices, raw liver juice, salmon and other fish, and raw milk from grass-fed cows or goats if available.

One reason little is known with certainty about the best ways of approaching cancer is that few individuals with cancer find reasonable alternatives to conventional treatment. Until more people with cancer seek these alternatives, the problem will remain. The difficulty is increased by restrictions placed on medical doctors by the medical establishment about the ways they may treat cancer, making it difficult or impossible for them to use alternative therapies.

The person with cancer must look deep inside himself and choose how he wishes to live the rest of his life, whether that be for one week or fifty years. The therapy or combination of therapies best for him is that which is most attuned to judgments and emotions including (but perhaps going beyond) reason, common sense, and the conventional wisdom he may have accepted all of his life. The philosophy and ideas expressed in this book are intended to help clarify an understanding of why perhaps most of all when death is threatening, a return to a more natural way of living and eating may provide a better chance of survival than modern technology.

Prevention.   Prevention is the best way to deal with cancer. In many primitive societies, cancer was rare or perhaps even unknown; evidence indicates food was the primary protector. Current research has focused on individual nutrients such as vitamins A, C, and E, beta-carotene, and selenium, as cancer inhibiting factors. Extensive research has been done on the nature of carcinogenic substances.

For many people, two themes emerge. One is the idea that "everything is bad for you," and the other is the notion that large doses of nutrients thought protective against cancer are helpful. We all know people who attempt to avoid everything potentially carcinogenic or who dose up on the "anti-cancer" nutrients, or both. Others rationalize that since everything is bad for you and one can't avoid everything, why try—just eat whatever you want!

Avoiding carcinogens to the extent reasonable *is* reasonable, and traditional foods are rich in nutrients protective against cancer. Carcinogens are not the crucial issue, for if the immune system is sufficiently strong, one is protected. Traditional foods provide that strength.

Even a person who has for years eaten refined foods may avoid cancer. Of patients seen by the author over the years, several hundred have been followed for at least six months; these were people who embraced in whole or in part diets of traditional foods. Among them, not one has developed cancer during the time followed.

This is not coincidence. Cancer is apparently rare among people eating traditional diets, even in twentieth century America.

Rheumatoid Arthritis

Rheumatoid arthritis differs from osteoarthritis in that the immune system malfunctions and produces antibodies which attack tissues of the body, particularly in the joints. Similar autoimmune problems occur in other tissues in lupus.

These problems respond to careful and thorough nutrition. Rheumatoid arthritis is less common than osteoarthritis and often more difficult to treat. Patients are usually younger than those with osteoarthritis; the disease typically occurs in middle-aged and younger adults, and occasionally in children.

Extreme sensitivity to certain foods is usual, and for most people sugar is a problem. Fruits, milk, and cheese usually cause marked reactions. Some individuals using raw milk from grass-fed cows or goats, however, have not had adverse reactions.

One of the latter was a three-year-old girl first seen in 1981 one week after a diagnosis of rheumatoid arthritis. The joints of her wrists, fingers, and ankles were swollen, red, and painful, despite the use of aspirin. Her blood test was positive for rheumatoid arthritis. Offered steroid drugs, her parents elected to try nutritional therapy.

The swelling, pain, and redness in her joints were gone within a week of beginning the careful diet we worked out, and she no longer needed aspirin. She has been free of symptoms since, except for one period of several days in 1984 when she had some joint pain. Her mother explained the family had been careless with her diet for a few days prior. When she was returned to her usual diet, her symptoms again disappeared.

Unfortunately, rheumatoid arthritis is usually more difficult to treat. For some reason, most adults with this problem have found it difficult to follow a diet to the extent necessary for dramatic relief, more so than people with most other diseases. They have often expressed a feeling of being deprived when giving up rich, refined foods, and some would seemingly rather suffer the symptoms of the disease.

Even with careful compliance, progress may be slow. Much depends on the degree of destruction in the joints; the longer the disease has been established, the more difficult is treatment. Extensive use of steroids such as cortisone, common in those long with the disease, makes recovery more difficult. Nevertheless, many middle-aged and older rheumatoid patients find they may largely control their symptoms with attention to diet. Mild improvement in symptoms or even simply preventing the problem from becoming worse may be all some people desire; many choose to eat with some care in exchange for partial relief.

Those rheumatoid individuals making concerted and extended efforts to follow traditional foods programs that include elements of Dr. Gerson's therapy have made good to excellent progress. An unexpected problem has been adverse reactions to alfalfa sprouts, no longer recommended. Milk and cheese, coffee, fruit, fruit juices, refined flour products, and all sweeteners should be strictly avoided.

Results with the other autoimmune diseases have been similar; individuals who carefully follow the details of dietary recommendations have had marked improvements.

Herpes

An estimated 40 percent of the population now carry the herpes genitalis virus, and some 10 percent or more are thought to show at least occasional symptoms. The strength of the immune system influences the extent to which an individual carrying the virus shows symptoms, and strengthening the immune system through diet minimizes the chances of symptoms occurring.

A strictly followed traditional foods diet eliminates the symptoms of herpes. However, small amounts of certain foods may still precipitate attacks. Nuts are most likely to cause problems; even two or three walnuts or pecans, a few peanuts, or a little peanut butter may bring on symptoms a few hours later. Sugar too is suspect, though small amounts may be tolerated.

Nuts are rich in the amino acid arginine, thought to be responsible for precipitating the attacks. Why such small amounts of this natural food constituent should do so is a mystery. Nuts cause exacerbation of the symptoms of many different conditions, however, and are in general best avoided or used in only the smallest amounts.

Skin Problems

Eczema, psoriasis, and acne respond well to proper diet. Eczema often is an allergic skin reaction to certain foods, particularly dairy products and sweets. Improvements usually begin within days of eliminating these foods. Lasting improvement comes when following a traditional diet.

Psoriasis is chronic and recurrent; often arthritic symptoms accompany the silvery, scaly skin lesions. More intensive therapy is needed than in eczema. Elements of the Gerson therapy—raw vegetable juices, enemas, and raw liver juice—are helpful, for the juices and enemas cleanse the body of toxins that cause eruptions.

Acne too may be chronic and may take several months to clear. New eruptions become less marked than formerly, eventually no longer occurring. Cysts still present slowly dissipate. Hormones influence acne and symptoms often become worse at puberty and during menstruation. Several months may be required before the problem completely disappears, though complete care with the diet shortens the time. Fruits and sweets are best avoided, as are vegetable oils and commercial milk and cheese. Animal fats of proper quality are beneficial in cases of acne; fatty fish, certified raw dairy foods from grass-fed animals, and natural meat contain such fats. When natural meat or fish are not available, lamb may be used—commercial lamb is mostly range-fed and relatively free of chemicals and hormones.

Lesser skin eruptions many teenagers and young adults experience are mostly due to sweets, excessive fruits, processed fats and milk products, and a lack of fat-soluble protective nutrients. Vegetable oils, especially when used for commercial frying, affect the body's ability to metabolize fats normally. Citrus fruits and juices commonly cause the skin to erupt. Tomatoes too often cause this, and may affect mucous membranes; sores inside the cheeks and on the tongue are common during the late-summer tomato season.

We take these common foods for granted; it may be hard to believe they cause these symptoms, but they most certainly do, and many more. If the explanation for our ills were not so simple, perhaps modern medicine would find it easier to accept.

Gastrointestinal Diseases

Colitis.   An acute flare-up of colitis nearly always calls for a fast. If rectal bleeding occurs, a physician should be consulted to determine the cause. In ulcerative colitis, fasting until the bleeding stops allows the lesions to begin healing. This may take several days, but usually a day or two suffices. Warm water enemas are helpful; herbs may be used in the enemas to promote healing. Care must be taken not to insert the tip of the rectal tube beyond the anal canal (a maximum of two inches beyond the anal opening).

When one stops eating, peristalsis (the involuntary wavelike motion of the intestines which propels feces toward the anus) is greatly reduced, and feces stagnate in the large bowel. As water is reabsorbed across the bowel wall, they become hard and impacted. Enemas remove them, and the bowel is left clean; healing of lesions may then occur much more easily.

Once rectal bleeding has stopped, a diet of well cooked vegetables and broth, brown rice or other grains, and fish may be started. No other foods and especially no raw vegetables or fruits should be eaten. Chew foods well, and eat little at first; if no further rectal bleeding occurs, more food may be eaten. After a few days, eggs and meat may be tried if desired. Very small amounts of raw vegetables should be gradually introduced only if no symptoms occur; the amounts may then be slowly increased.

Individuals with colitis often have avoided milk and cheese because these foods aggravate symptoms. Consequently, deficiencies in calcium often occur; particular attention should be paid to this aspect of the nutrition.

Local fruits in season should be tolerated once recovery is complete, but care should be taken since overuse may precipitate a return of the condition. Citrus and other highly acid fruits such as pineapple especially aggravate symptoms, as do tomatoes. Milk and cheeses too must always be suspect.

Gastritis (inflammation of the stomach) and ulcers are treated in much the same manner as colitis. Again, if bleeding is present or suspected (dark stools are a cardinal sign), see a physician for a definitive diagnosis.

Coffee and alcohol increase the secretions of gastric acid, aggravating all gastrointestinal problems.

Hemmorhoids.   Hemmorhoids are a common problem requiring a somewhat different approach. They may be either internal (inside the anal opening) or external, and occur as early as the teen years.

The main cause is chronic constipation. Weakness of the blood vessels contributes; a hemorrhoid is actually a dilated rectal vein, and if the blood within it clots, the hemorrhoid is said to be thrombosed. These are the large, dilated, painful, inflamed, sometimes incapacitating hemorrhoids often given surgical attention.

In office surgery, the thrombosed hemorrhoid is incised and an attempt is made to remove the clot, an extremely painful procedure usually giving little relief, temporary at best. A hemorrhoidectomy is the more extensive hospital procedure in which hemorrhoids are surgically removed.

While an acutely inflamed hemorrhoid might ideally be treated by fasting, enemas are simply too painful. And without enemas, pressure exerted by stagnant and hardening feces within the bowel makes hemorrhoids worse. Although bowel movements are somewhat painful during the three to five days required for a thrombosed hemorrhoid to resolve, the best course is to begin eating an extremely high fiber diet immediately. Soft and voluminous stools result, keeping pressure exerted on the hemorrhoid by the large bowel to a minimum, since such stools may be easily passed without straining.

Even the worst cases of thrombosed hemorrhoids have been successfully treated in this way. The diet is mostly cooked and raw vegetables and whole grains. Cod liver oil is given to promote effortless bowel movements.

In one extreme case, a thrombosed hemorrhoid with a diameter the size of a quarter took five days to resolve. The patient was uncomfortable being on his feet for more than a few minutes at a time, and spent most of the five days on his back or in the tub taking sitz baths. After five days he began moving around a bit more, but two weeks passed before he could function normally.

Conventional medicine gives little recognition to the role foods play in gastrointestinal diseases. The digestive tract directly interfaces with foods, and in many people is the part of the body first and most easily influenced by foods. Belching, intestinal gas, indigestion, and often diarrhea speak of the eating of poor foods. Symptoms of more advanced gastrointestinal problems rarely come before these early warning signals have been ignored. The gastrointestinal tract indicates if foods eaten are well received, and a poor reception may indicate developing problems.

Hypoglycemia, Diabetes, and Weight Problems

These interrelated and often associated conditions are at least partly problems with carbohydrate metabolism. Avoidance of all refined carbohydrates, fruits, fruit juices, and sweeteners lies at the heart of the dietary treatment of diabetes and hypoglycemia. Weight problems usually revolve around the use of refined carbohydrates and unnaturally fatty foods.

Diets of mostly whole grains and vegetables control symptoms of hypoglycemia, but are improved by addition of substantial amounts of high quality animal source foods. Such a diet is most likely to reduce the craving for sweets.

The same is true in diabetes. The diabetic condition is chronic; improvement comes more slowly. Hypoglycemia may be an early stage of diabetes; both involve abnormalities in blood sugar. Eating traditional foods nearly always results in a reduction of the need for insulin in diabetics. Many individuals beginning a careful diet soon after a diagnosis of adult-onset diabetes have soon eliminated the need for insulin.

The main causes of overweight are refined carbohydrates, poor quality and unnatural fats, and lack of exercise, all of which depress thyroid gland function; this in turn makes the weight problem worse. Not only do refined foods provide poor nutrition and excessive calories; they also displace foods needed for a fully active thyroid gland and a fully active metabolism.

Fats of proper quality need not be avoided by a person with an overweight problem. Many people fail to lose weight eating unbalanced low fat diets which often lead to binge eating. A more reasonable approach uses foods needed for good health and a well balanced metabolism and allows weight to be lost naturally.

Headaches

Many people suffer regularly from at least occasional headaches. These headaches in nearly all cases disappear within the first few weeks of carefully following a traditional diet.

The reason is simple: almost all headaches, including migraine, are food related. Many are direct expressions of allergies. Like other organs, the brain may react to constituents in certain foods by retaining fluid and swelling, causing a headache. Similar reactions in the nasal sinuses may also cause headaches; milk and cheese are most often the offending foods. Eyestrain and fatigue can also play a role.

A persistent headache failing to end with careful dieting, or a headache following an injury, should be investigated by a physician, for headaches may be a sign of serious injury or disease. Much time and expense could be saved, however, by instituting a simple traditional foods diet for a few days before an extensive work-up is done in an attempt to determine the cause of headaches.

Cheese is the most suspect food in precipitating migraines. One middle-aged woman, however, suffered from severe migraines once or twice a month for over thirty years before finding they ceased when she stopped drinking alcohol. She was not a heavy drinker, taking a drink or two a few times a week. The drinks did not always precipitate a migraine. But they sometimes did, for when she stopped drinking entirely, the migraines stopped. In the years since, she has had headaches only on some days after the rare occasions when she has had a drink or two the night before.

Anxiety, Emotional Disturbances, and Mental Illness

Thinking is as biological as digestion. Disturbances of the mind must ultimately have a biochemical explanation, though we may be unable to provide it. Nutrients profoundly affect some mentally disturbed states, and reactions to foods may cause such states. Suger induced hypoglycemia, for example, is often accompanied by depression, anxiety, or both.

Weston Price found no mental illness in primitive cultures where the people ate only their traditional foods. In studies of inmates in American jails, reformatories, and mental institutions, he discovered that large majorities, often approaching 100 percent, had deformities of the dental arch and other marked abnormalities in the shape of the skull. His work paralleled that of other investigators; he was not the first to discover these correlations between changes in the shape of the skull and criminal behavior, mental backwardness, and abnormal mental states.

Price's work suggests dietary changes have led to anatomical changes that have resulted in increased incidence of these problems. Given that anatomical changes have occurred in large segments of the population, we are left with the issue of how the foods eaten influence the mental state of an individual, whatever anatomical equipment the individual might have (this taken in terms of potential as dictated by the physical capacity of the brain).

In the experience of clinicians working with natural foods, the mental state of an individual may sometimes be profoundly influenced by dietary changes. Feelings of greater stability, calmness, and confidence are common in patients embracing a whole foods diet. Among patients specifically seeking help for mental disturbances, results are mixed. Many are unable to follow the details of a thorough program. Among those who have, particularly those suffering from anxiety and depression, many have experienced relief and others have had no improvement. It is impossible to know who will or will not respond.

Many factors besides foods affect the state of mind of individuals with marked mental and emotional problems, but food can be a profound and even a dominating influence. Some of the early proponents of megavitamin therapy were physicians using vitamins for people suffering from schizophrenia and other mental illnesses. The use of traditional foods in a carefully controlled diet would significantly enhance the responses of individuals institutionalized for these problems.

What of how foods affect future generations? The mental well-being of western society requires us to abandon refined foods that have led to degenerative changes in the shape of the human skull which often (perhaps usually) accompany mental disease. Though this may be difficult to believe, the evidence about us is difficult to ignore.

Candidiasis

Candida albicans is a yeast microorganism found in the normal human organism; it is concentrated on the skin and mucous membranes. Antibiotics, sweet foods, and oral contraceptives are among the influences affecting the amount of *Candida* occurring in an individual; overgrowth of *Candida* is called candidiasis. The orthodox viewpoint holds that candidiasis occurs only as either a localized yeast infection (as in the vagina) or as a systemic illness that may occur when the immune system breaks down in debilitating chronic illness. However, a growing number of physicians believe that overgrowth of *Candida* may lead or contribute to a wide variety of symptoms and conditions, including most of those previously discussed in this chapter.

Chronic yeast infections are thought to be capable of affecting any system of the body. Because the drug nystatin has activity against *Candida* and seems to have little other effect, it is often prescribed for individuals thought to be suffering from candidiasis. Often a yeast-free and sugar-free diet is prescribed in conjunction.

In the author's experience, symptoms of candidiasis disappear when the dietary principles explained in this book are carefully followed, without the use of nystatin. This usually occurs in spite of the use of small amounts of yeast-containing foods such as apple cider vinegar, beer and wine, and certain breads. In extreme cases, all yeast-containing foods are eliminated for a few weeks, and nystatin may give more rapid relief. Certainly nystatin has proved useful for many patients unwilling to follow a sufficiently careful natural foods diet, though relief it gives often disappears when the drug is stopped.

Other Conditions

People sometimes ask about the nutritional treatment of uncommon and seldom seen conditions. They tend to think their problem will not respond to nutrition, despite evidence of successful cases. This thinking results in part from the feeling people often have that their own diet is quite good and thus can have little to do with their problem.

Even for these individuals, a committed effort to follow the program outlined has usually led to significant improvements. This includes both people with well-known conditions such as multiple sclerosis, muscular dystrophy, epilepsy, macular edema, cataracts, and glaucoma, and those with other seldom seen chronic and debilitating diseases. Even those with some conditions usually thought of as entirely genetic, such as Down's syndrome, have shown some improvements in both overall health and mental function.

Price's evidence indicates the occurrence of such genetic conditions is profoundly influenced by the parents' nutrition and could be almost entirely prevented if their nutrition prior to pregnancy, and the woman's during pregnancy, was optimal. His observations are in conflict with the views of most geneticists, who have largely rejected the concept that nutrition affects the genes themselves. Recent research and discoveries, however, have provided theoretical models for how the genetic material outside the nucleus of the fertilized egg may be directly affected by the mother's nutrition. This non-nuclear genetic material is now known to reside in the mitochondria, the energy-making part of the cell.

This research provides an explanation for Dr. Price's observations, and indicates the conventional thinking about nutrition in genetics has been erroneous. As with controversy in medical circles over the role of nutrition in health and disease, we may hope that what common sense, empirical observation, and traditional wisdom tells us is right will eventually be proven to the satisfaction of those who control policies affecting millions of lives.

* * *

The development of chronic disease is influenced by a person's genes, but the fundamental and underlying cause is the slow breakdown of the body as it is poisoned by foods for which it is not adapted. A host of other influences affect this process, particularly physical activity and the mental and emotional state.

Treatment of all disease is thus accomplished in a similar manner. Recovery involves understanding natural laws governing human nutrition, and the physical and psychological needs of each individual. To help oneself, these things must be well understood; to help others, they must be well communicated. For the physician, the foundation of such communication is best built in his own good health. This is the meaning of the ancient words, "Physician, heal thyself." With those words, we turn to the concluding chapter of part I for an examination of the relationships between individuals, physicians, and goals in health.

11

Relationships

Individuals
Physicians and
Health Goals

*T*hough food is the dominant subject, this book is about health, and this chapter is about relationships involved in a search for health. Challenging but realistic goals may be established once one understands what may realistically be expected; thus the placement of this subject at the end rather than the beginning of part I. An understanding of one's health goals and a sound relationship with a physician who is sympathetic toward those goals may form a basis for utilizing the information about food to be presented in part II.

To progress toward better health, one must make decisions. Reasonable decisions are based on information, and the most basic information required for decisions about health is a solid answer to the question: Where do I stand now?

An individual with a problem who has not been examined should see a physician. A detailed knowledge of one's current condition provides both a baseline for measuring improvements and a means of deciding how seriously the business of improving health should be taken. Even when under a physician's care, one may ask oneself questions the physician may not ask. Done thoroughly, a self-assessment complements a professional medical assessment. At times the latter may not define or diagnose the problem; an individual may nevertheless realize something is wrong and seek other opinions or take appropriate nutritional measures independently.

Self-assessment questions may relate to growing older without fear. One might ask, "Is my body feeling as if it will carry me through for the duration without becoming diseased?" We all grow old; with time we see not as far, run not as fast. When the biological clock inside has run its course, we die.

This does not frighten us. But disease does, and rightly so. Old age and death are as natural as life. Disease is not.

A gentle suggestion: in taking stock, ask questions that help us learn to live in health. Success may bring genuine happiness and peace of mind.

Working With A Physician

A physician may help in a search for health. Although most doctors think more in terms of disease than in terms of health, a working relationship with a caring and competent doctor who is respectful of individual needs and goals enables one to understand medical conditions and make reasonable decisions about courses of treatment.

A physician's first duty is to use his medical expertise to gather information for assessing his patient's status. This is the purpose of a thorough medical history and physical examination, and of laboratory tests and any special diagnostic procedures.

Doctor is the Latin word for teacher; the physician's next duty is to explain his findings clearly and simply. If he understands the broad spectrum between robust good health and overt disease, and recognizes the numerous sub-clinical problems people eating modern diets develop, there will be much to talk about. A doctor with this knowledge may help one prevent early symptoms from developing into major problems.

Most physicians find conditions satisfactory if no problems treatable with drugs or surgery are present. But when such conditions are discovered, the individual style, personality, and character of the physician greatly influence subsequent events.

Almost every doctor realizes that whatever the condition, choices about methods of treatment exist. But because most also believe strongly in some particular method, each tends to recommend his particular method to patients. While this is understandable (often the physician has little knowledge of alternate ways of dealing with the problem) the most competent physicians are aware and knowledgeable about methods outside of their own area of expertise. When telling a patient of a medical problem, such a physician is willing and able to explain the existing options. If his particular approach is the one most suited for the individual and his problem, this will become apparent. The patient is free to make an informed choice.

This issue is complex even before bringing in the matter of treating disease through nutrition. Surgery and drug therapy are commonly a matter of one physician's opinion over another's; hospital studies have shown that patients receiving certain drugs or surgical procedures statistically fared no better—or fared worse—than those with similar conditions receiving no treatment. Often there is considerable debate between physicians over whether a given condition in general, or a given patient in particular, should be treated surgically, pharmaceutically, or not at all (nutrition, alas, is seldom considered).

Most conditions commonly treated with drugs or surgery are indeed treatable through nutrition, and this complicates matters further. Many physicians do not accept this, or accept it only on the most limited basis.

Without the knowledge and experience to treat medical problems in this manner, most physicians cannot offer the alternative of treatment through proper nutrition to their patients.

The realization that one may know more about these matters than one's physician can be a matter of life and death. To his evaluation of the situation, one must add one's own. For some people, the recommended course of drug or surgical treatment is the most appropriate course to follow. For others with the discipline, knowledge, tenacity, and courage to steer their own course, there are times when it is not.

This is not a recommendation that anyone embark on a course of self-treatment for a serious medical problem; the help of a competent and understanding physician may be immeasurable. But there are times when a recommended drug or surgical treatment is not in the best interest of an individual patient. The discerning patient must be prepared to recognize when this is the case.

Seek out a physician understanding of this. Usually a doctor who takes the time to know his patients as individuals is responsive to these issues. Long ago and far away, most of us had a family doctor, a general practitioner with whom we grew up. He knew us well, our families, histories, and idiosyncrasies. In this age of the specialist, too often a medical problem is seen as an isolated issue in a single part of the body, rather than as a signal that the body will break down further if one does not change one's ways. In years past we were more willing to listen, and general practitioners and naturopathic physicians were willing to give us these frank appraisals we needed to hear. Perhaps their time has come again.

The Significance of the Medical History and the Physical Exam

The body is an integrated whole and the symptoms we suffer relate to one another and to how we live. For the physician, the medical history begins a process similar to putting together a jig-saw puzzle, whether the patient has come for preventive care, has been previously diagnosed elsewhere, or is ill with undiagnosed symptoms and signs (symptoms are subjective feelings, while signs are objective and physically detectable or measurable). All of these cases may be equally challenging, because the proper questions elicit responses revealing patterns in the puzzle that soon give shape to a picture remarkably unique for each individual.

And yet, patterns of problems are seen in much the same form in many people. Which pattern dominates at a given time in life is determined by an interplay of genetic background, ways of reacting to stresses, and individual dietary and exercise habits. We call these patterns diseases, symptom complexes, diagnoses, illnesses. These labels are useful when used to organize information; they help relate problems to one another and ultimately to causes and solutions. But a physician should not forget that the names are but labels, and whatever the label, each individual's set of medical problems is unique.

Information gained in the history helps shape the physical exam. While circumstances necessarily dictate the thoroughness of the initial exam, a physician must know an individual's physical condition well if a solid and cooperative relationship is to be established. A competent physician observes, measures, and intuitively senses hundreds of bits of information in a fifteen minute examination. The meaning of symptoms discovered in the history may be explored, clarified, and amplified. The possible need for special laboratory tests or further diagnostic procedures may be investigated and determined. Out of this process comes a sense of the individual's overall condition.

The medical history and physical exam thus generate a record of where an individual stands medically; laboratory tests and special diagnostic procedures clarify and enlarge upon that record. A description of symptoms with their history, physical findings, emotional state, pertinent family history, dietary history, exercise habits, and current medications—this information is all relevant. The physician working with an individual in this manner requires at least forty-five minutes for the first visit. The information generated may be used to begin creating an appropriate plan reflective of the individual's needs and goals.

Health Goals

Set goals. Achievements come with goals and a realistic means to reach them. Determine the specifics and plan timetables; one must then take these goals seriously.

Be realistic, but take on challenges. Health goals may involve foods, feelings, plans for self or family, or the elimination of troubling conditions—but whatever the goals are, know they are possible. Unlike any other aspect of life, one has complete freedom about what one eats from this moment until death. Health is one result of wisely exercising that freedom; others include greater self-control and freedom in other areas of life.

Welcome change—including the changing of goals. Defeat leads to destruction only when nothing is learned. Learn, and change. Learning to eat as one knows is best takes time, and the modern world does not make this easy. Achieving health is a genuine challenge.

The enemy is apathy. We sometimes ask, what is it all for? We love family, friends; yet in some moments we wonder, why bother? What is it for, then: the food, the exercise, the caring?

For self. When it's not for anyone else, each person does it for himself. To run fast and free on a mountain ridge, or walk peacefully on a quiet beach; to be free forever from the surgeon's knife; to feel strong and confident of one's body; indeed, to understand that "the most supreme instrument in life is a perfect body." Goals may intertwine health and independence; a feeling of physical and psychological strength may become a sustaining force.

That which is for oneself and that which is for the people we love are sometimes inseparable. When one acts in harmony with his own deepest spirit, he acts for all, including himself. Eating traditional foods attempts to harmonize with the human spirit; by selecting living foods we can establish this bond. The times we succeed, feelings of apathy are replaced with feelings of strength and love—feelings we may even in apathetic moments choose to make a part of our goals.

* * *

With these thoughts on the relationships involved in setting and achieving health goals, we conclude part I of *Traditional Foods Are Your Best Medicine*. We have reviewed historical, anthropological, and evolutionary aspects of traditional foods; current and historical research into the health effects of these foods; and clinical experience relating to the use of these foods in treatment of acute and chronic disease.

One goes through three overlapping processes in learning to use traditional foods as medicine. In the first, knowledge and understanding are acquired through study. Then one finds the desire and the will to put the information into practice. Finally, one must find sources and secure the foods one has decided are necessary. In part II of this book, we integrate these processes in examining traditionally raised foods, and the production methods which make modern foods inferior. Understanding the differences between traditional and modern foods helps provide the motivation to set and achieve health goals, and serves as a guide to eating naturally.

II

TRADITIONAL VERSUS MODERN FOODS

A Guide to Natural Eating

12

Fish and Shellfish

As wild creatures, fish and shellfish live in their native environment, eat their natural diets, and are among the foods we are best adapted to eat. But because environmental pollutants may contaminate them, they should be selected with care. This chapter provides an overview of the pollution problem and of influences affecting the quality and flavor of seafood in general, while Appendix 1 provides details about individual fish and shellfish.

Many highly toxic pollutants contaminate coastal waters and even the deep oceans. These chemical compounds and heavy metals accumulate in the fats of fish. Many shellfish particularly concentrate pollutants because they constantly filter water. Thus fatty fish and shellfish are often avoided by many people; in recent years, a general fear of cholesterol and all animal source fats has added to concerns. In the case of fish, shellfish, and naturally raised animals, this fear is unfounded. But the problem of pollutants in fish and shellfish remains.

Water Pollution

People have always used waterways for waste disposal. In earlier times, fewer people used less chemicals and created less sewage; many chemicals now widely used did not even exist. Today sewage, industrial wastes, detergents, and other pollutants (many highly toxic) are discharged into rivers, lakes, and oceans.

Treatment of sewage fails to remove adequately nitrates and inorganic phosphates. These major pollutants lead to eutrophication, an excessive growth of algae which decays in slow moving estuaries, rivers, and bays. The resultant foul smelling substances are toxic to fish, shellfish, and other wildlife which live in these coastal areas or must pass through en route to breeding grounds.

Agricultural fertilizers and spray residues include chlorinated hydrocarbons such as DDT and organophosphates such as parathion and malathion. Organophosphates are related to nerve gases developed in Nazi Germany during World War II. These substances all reach water via seepage and runoff. Wind carries mercury and other poisons in dust which is blown from chemical factories near waterways. Discharge of wash water and industrial wastes, dumping of trash and highly toxic chemicals, and oil spills are the other principal modes of contamination of coastal areas.

The principal industries contributing to this are the paper industry in the Pacific Northwest, Alabama, and Mississippi; chemical plants in the Gulf and middle Atlantic states; and the oil industries in New Jersey, Louisiana, Texas, and California. All are concentrated at seashores or on large rivers, and only about one-fourth of all wastes discharged receive any type of treatment. Mercury, nickel, fluoride, oil, cement, white lime, caustic soda, hydrocyanic acid, and lactonitrile are among the many items discharged in large quantities. In a 1965 report of the Environmental Pollution Panel of the President's Science Advisory Committee, the latter two chemicals were reported to have killed Gulf Coast fish within twenty-four hours at levels below .3 parts per million (ppm). Many similar cases could be cited.

Drums containing highly toxic materials, especially chlorinated hydrocarbons, have been dumped a few miles offshore from major coastal cities. They eventually leak.

Millions of tons of oil have been spilled into the world's oceans in the past twenty years, mostly in coastal areas. Oil-laden sediments resulting move considerable distances with bottom currents. As long as seven years after a spill, oil has been shown to be incorporated into the body tissues of crabs in sufficient quantities to drastically affect their behavior, reproductive capacity, and ability to survive.

Mercury and PCB's (polychlorinated biphenyls) are two industrial pollutants of particular concern because of their ubiquitous presence in the environment. In 1968, Swedish health officials warned people not to eat fish from fresh and coastal waters more than once a week because of the presence of mercury in the tissues. In 1970, Canadian and American officials ordered a stop to fishing in Lake St. Clair and Lake Erie for the same reason. Chlorine plants, pulp and paper factories, and the electrical industry are the chief contaminators.

Mercury is also used in agriculture; at least one million of the six million pounds marketed yearly in the United States wind up in croplands. Although the Food and Drug Administration prohibits the sale of foods containing mercury, tests show grains, apples, eggs, milk, and other products contain levels in the range of .01 to .1 ppm. The World Health Organization suggests a maximum of .05 ppm.

Once in waterways and the sea, mercury is absorbed into plankton and moves up the food chain. Highly carnivorous species which live for several years and grow large acquire the most dense concentrations. Although living in open ocean, tuna and swordfish are especially susceptible; the metal concentrates in the fats of these large, fatty, carnivorous fish.

PCB's are used in transformers and capacitors, as hydraulic and heat-transfer fluids, as plasticizers and solvents in adhesives, and as sealants. In the 1970's, four thousand tons entered waterways yearly, largely through sewage, leaching of industrial fluids, and from landfills and dumps. An outbreak of illness in 1968 in Japan was called Yusho, or rice oil disease, because the patients had eaten rice oil contaminated with tetrachlorobiphenyl (a PCB) which had leaked from the pipe of a heat exchanger during manufacture of the oil.

The patients numbered about one thousand. They developed darkened skin, a cheeselike discharge from the eyes, severe acne, numbness, nerve pains, swollen joints, edema, and jaundice. Among eleven live and two stillborn babies born of these patients, all but one showed at least some of these symptoms. The disease lasted in many cases for more than three years. Shortly before these people began to become ill, seven hundred thousand chickens had been contaminated and died of the disease.

The patients had each consumed from .5 to 2.0 grams of the PCB; fat tissue from the skin contained from 13.1 to 75.5 ppm of the substance. One-tenth of a teaspoon equals .5 grams.

Thus great harm may be done by small amounts of PCB's. Concentrations may vary widely within the same area. While samples of Hudson River water contained from .3 to 3.0 parts per billion (ppb), sediments in the river bottom showed values up to 13,000 ppb (equal to 13 ppm). Most species of North Atlantic fish show a range from .01 to 1.0 ppm in their tissues, but this is much higher in seafood taken from waters near industrialized areas. While apparently some PCB's and mercury are found in seafood from even the most remote waters, a dramatic difference in the concentration of poisons is based on the life history of the seafood consumed.

Species spending most of their lives in deep waters far out at sea are most likely to be least contaminated; coastal species living in polluted waters are most contaminated. Shellfish and fatty fish especially should be from relatively unpolluted waters.

Pollutants become more concentrated in fish which are higher up the food chain, making smaller species more desirable. Smaller, deep water fish include herring, sardines, and anchovies; the smaller salmon such as pink, coho, sockeye, and Atlantic; some members of the cod family, including scrod, hake, haddocck, and pollock; and mackerel, pompano, red and yellowtail snapper, striped bass, butterfish, squid, octupus, and tilefish, among others. Tuna, bluefish, swordfish, and king salmon are best eaten when taken from waters off coastlines in unindustrialized areas. A wide variety of anadromous fish (oceangoing species returning to rivers to breed) are best eaten when taken in the unpolluted bays and rivers of unindustrialized and lightly populated areas, as are freshwater fish from similarly located lakes and streams.

The habitat of most commonly eaten shellfish is coastal waters. Since all are bottom dwellers, and since bivalves such as oysters and clams constantly pass water through their systems to filter nutrients, shellfish in contaminated waters concentrate undesirable substances. A knowledge of the waters shellfish are taken from is thus imperative in judging their desirability. Good fish merchants know where their stock is from.

Quality and Flavor

A small fish market is located on the docks of the fishing village of Menemsha on Martha's Vineyard Island off the coast of Massachusetts. The cement floors are always wet from a recent rinsing, a sea breeze blows through open windows, and out the back door one sees fishing boats tied up at docks. Fish eyes shine and scales glisten; dead fish on ice in glass cases are so fresh they look almost alive, and all one smells is the ocean and the faint sweet fragrance of prime seafoods.

That is quality.

When examining a whole fish, first look at the eyes, which should be clear and full. If milky and sunken, look no further; this fish is not fresh. The flesh when pressed should be firm, rather than soft; one's fingers should leave no indentation. A clean fragrance, unblemished skin color, and bright red gills confirm the diagnosis of fresh fish. Fillets or steaks should appear clean, crisp, moist, and firm; yellowing, a dried out appearance, or any strong odor indicate lack of freshness.

Less oily species generally keep well longer than those with a high oil content. Few species have more than about 15 percent fat content; those that do include herring, mackerel, and some varieties of salmon at certain times. The fat content varies greatly with both the diet of the fish and the season, most species being prime in fat and flavor in autumn. The seasonal variation is greatest among larger fish.

Any species may be excellent in one area and poor in another. The presence of pollutants in the water, various types of algae, the foods available to the fish in the locale, seasonal variations in fat content, freshness, seasoning, and method and amount of cooking all combine to determine whether a given fish lives up to the potential for the species.

The author considers seafoods to be one of our most important traditional foods and at the core of a traditional diet. Appendix 1 details the characteristics and habitat of most of the important seafoods and is designed to aid in selecting fish and shellfish for optimal health and eating pleasure. A warning about preservatives sometimes used on fresh sea-foods is included.

The catch of fishing boats once filled the world's dining tables. We turn now to the foods which for modern people have largely replaced fish and shellfish as dietary staples, as we examine the production of modern meat, fowl, and eggs.

13

The Production of Modern Meat, Fowl, and Eggs

*K*nowledge of foods used by our ancient ancestors, primitive cultures surviving into the twentieth century, and contemporary hunter-gatherers known free of chronic disease shows that meat, fowl, eggs, milk, and milk products may form a substantial part of an optimal diet, if of the proper quality. Evidence was detailed in previous chapters.

Differences between traditional and modern versions of these foods warrant close examination. In this chapter, the methods of the modern meat industry will be examined: the living conditions of animals; antibiotics, hormones, and feeds routinely used throughout the industry; and the inspection and regulatory systems for meat. The products themselves will also be examined, as we learn how meat has changed in the last thirty to forty years.

Naturally raised animals warrant an equally thorough examination. A few livestock producers raise animals without using drugs, chemicals, pesticides, or hormones. In the next chapter, we'll see how the quality and quantity of the fat in these animals differs from that of conventionally raised animals.

Controversy about the meat industry centers on the use of antibiotics and carcinogenic hormones, but perhaps even more significant is the effect of an animal's diet and of its exercise upon the composition of the meat produced. Fats in wild grazing animals have been shown by laboratory analysis to be significantly different from those in conventionally raised domestic cattle. Analysis has also shown similarities between fats in naturally raised cattle and those in wild grazing animals.

The quality of eggs, milk, and milk products is based in these same influences—animals must be well exercised, and range and barnyard fed, if they are to produce top quality food. Pasteurization and homogenization also have profound effects on milk and milk products. Here again, comparing and contrasting information about conventional products and naturally produced counterparts provides a basis for making informed choices.

144

In recent years, many people have decided to eat less meat. Reports commonly appear in the media about antibiotics, chemical residues and female hormones in animals, dangers of cholesterol and fats, shoddy inspection procedures, and a host of other confirmed or possible problems with meat. Truly, meat consumption is down. But many eating less meat would leap at the chance to have venison or other wild game, without thinking twice about the cholesterol content (which happens to be the same in wild meat as in domestic). And though many others may not have a taste for it, most people intuitively know wild game is healthy food.

Several influences affect an animal's life and the composition and quality of its meat, among them its food, the use of drugs and toxic chemicals in its care and feeding, and its access to fresh air and exercise. An awareness of the connection between food and health takes us the next step to the realization that the composition of the meat we eat profoundly affects us.

The Production of Meat

Calves nurse from cows that have been fed hay grown with chemical fertilizers derived from petrochemicals and heavily sprayed with pesticides. Cows are usually fed a synthetic protein supplement. Pastures utilized in feeding cows are generally heavily sprayed and chemically fertilized.

When two months old, males are castrated and all calves are implanted with a growth stimulating hormone (typically a female hormone). Because diarrhea is common at this age, many ranchers mass treat calves with antibiotics; when calves are weaned at seven months of age, more are used to control possible respiratory ailments. At that time, animals are again implanted with a hormonal growth promotant, wormed, and dipped in a toxic insecticide bath to kill scabies-producing lice. Farmers, by law, must dispose of residual liquids at licensed toxic waste disposal sites.

From this point on, low levels of antibiotics are constantly added to feed rations. For some undiscovered reason, this stimulates growth, as do hormonal implants.

Beef cattle typically weigh about six hundred pounds when fifteen months old, when another hormonal implant is made. Fly control procedures are employed in grazing areas; insecticides are spread by tractor-driven sprayers, or by aerial spraying of animals with crop dusting aircraft. Eartags impregnated with insecticide are often used. The ears are the place of choice for hormone and insecticide implants because humans do not customarily eat an animal's ears.

Animals go to feedlots for ninety days of fattening when about eighteen months old; again they are wormed, dipped, and implanted with a hormone. Fly control insecticide procedures are intensified because of crowded quarters, and a larger dose of antibiotics is used in feed because of the great danger of infectious disease. Respiratory disease is especially difficult to control; dust kicked up by thousands of cattle is hard on the animals' lungs.

Because pregnancy in heifers in feedlots is highly undesirable, recent development of a drug causing pregnant heifers to miscarry has been welcomed by feedlot operators; many routinely inject all incoming heifers. The drug, called Lutalyse, is a synthetic analogue of a naturally occurring prostaglandin which helps regulate the reproductive cycle. Specifically, Lutalyse brings on ovulation, which in a pregnant heifer induces miscarriage.

The active ingredient has the same effect on the human female reproductive tract. The label states: "Women of childbearing age...should exercise extreme caution when handling this product." A veterinarian wrote in a column in *Beef Magazine:* "...pregnant women should not even handle the bottles as they could cause abortion and changes in the menstrual cycle...just from absorption through the skin." The manufacturer states no residues of Lutalyse are ever found in beef. Can we be sure?

Antibiotics

Many millions of years ago certain microorganisms developed the ability to elaborate compounds which can inhibit the growth of, or kill, competing organisms; we call these compounds antibiotics. Other organisms in response developed the capacity to resist the effects of the antibiotics; many resistance strategies were developed over the course of evolution.

With the development and increased use of antibiotics in the 1940's, resistant strains of microorganisms greatly increased, and doctors began finding that bacteria resistant to one or more antibiotics were causing disease in susceptible individuals. By the late 1960's epidemics of such diseases, including typhoid and dysentery, had occurred in several places around the world.

This has been attributed in part to overuse of antibiotics in humans. However, a large and growing number of scientists believe the use of very large quantities of antibiotics in domestic animal production is a major cause of this worldwide increase in the number of disease causing pathogens resistant to antibiotics. These scientists believe antibiotics added to animal feed are creating drug resistance in livestock bacteria that is transferable to human bacteria. The Japanese microbiologist who discovered the mechanisms by which these "resistance factors" operate (and his work has been confirmed by a host of other researchers) wrote nearly twenty years ago in *Scientific American* that the overuse of antibiotics might well make them useless. By all accounts, the problem has since become much worse.

In the late 1940's, researchers at Lederle Laboratories accidentally discovered that animals grew more rapidly when their feed contained low levels of antibiotics. Publication of experimental results and marketing efforts followed shortly, and by 1954 nearly five hundred thousand pounds of antibiotics were added to livestock feed yearly; about nine million pounds a year are added now. In 1980, American Cyanamid alone (the parent company of Lederle) sold $120 million worth of drugs for animal use in this country, and $265 million worth abroad. About half were tetracycline based feed additives. Many other companies are involved; in 1980, American farmers spent $242 million on antibiotic feed additives. Virtually all of America's conventionally raised poultry, 90 percent of hogs, and 70 percent of beef cattle are raised on feed dosed with antibiotics.

Money makes powerful lobbies; the drug and cattle industries have successfully blocked efforts of hundreds of scientists and physicians to prevail upon the government to stem the use of penicillin and tetracycline as feed additives. These efforts have been backed by an array of published documentation about the seriousness of the problem. Among countries banning use of antibiotics in livestock feed and regulating all use of antibiotics on animals are Great Britain, Norway, Sweden, Denmark, West Germany, the Netherlands, and Czechoslovakia. The United States does not regulate the use of antibiotics on animals or in their feed.

The issue of residues of antibiotics and other drugs in meat is more difficult to track and measure than the resistance problem; residues may only be discovered when tests are run, and by then the carcass has usually gone to market. Violative levels of antibiotics and sulfur drugs are often found in inspected animals. Continuous use of small amounts of antibiotics in feed, and periodic use of large doses to control disease, assures that even if levels in excess of allowable amounts are not present, trace amounts of the drugs, their conjugates, and their metabolites will be present in the meat (these conjugates and metabolites are compounds the drugs are converted to within the animal; they are little understood and are not measured).

Hormones

A number of natural and synthetic sex hormones cause livestock and poultry to gain weight more rapidly and with greater feed efficiency.

Used in increasing amounts since the early 1950's, these hormones have drastically changed the way animals are raised.

The endrocrine system consists of tiny hormone-producing glands which, with the nervous system, regulate metabolism. Active in minute amounts, hormones change delicate balances within the endocrine system by exciting cells in tissues sensitive to them. This excitation can be a trigger inducing the growth of cancer. Though we have evidence the effects can be devastating, some of these substances have not been in use long enough to demonstrate the long-term effects of increased body loads.

Diethylstilbestrol (DES) was for many years the most widely used of these hormones in both livestock and humans. An inexpensive synthetic estrogen, it was extremely popular in the cattle industry; in tests with steers, DES increased weight gain 15 to 19 percent and feed efficiency 7 to 10 percent.

But in the late 1960's, physicians for the first time found clear-cell adenocarcinoma (cancer) of the vagina in girls and women under the age of twenty-five. Ensuing studies revealed that in the majority of cases, their mothers had been prescribed DES during pregnancy for the purpose of preventing miscarriage, a common treatment given an estimated three to six million women from 1941 to 1971.

Incredibly, DES therapy for pregnant women continued even after DES had been shown to cause cancer in tests with laboratory animals, at levels close to those periodically detected in the inspection of meat from animals raised on DES. Detection methods do not reveal levels of various conjugates and metabolites of DES, which may be the substances doing the actual damage. This is a severe limitation of testing for residues of toxic substances used in raising animals; the problem of residues is likely much more severe than tests indicate.

Despite limitations, by the early 1960's testing procedures established that DES was present in meat, and it was to be banned under the Delaney Clause. This legislation, a 1958 amendment to the Federal Food, Drug and Cosmetic Act of 1938, states "...no food additive shall be deemed safe if it is found to induce cancer when ingested by man or animal..." However, in 1962 Congress passed another amendment specifically allowing continued use of DES in livestock. And it continued to be used to treat threatened abortion in women. Only upon publication of reports of cancer in young women as described above did pressure leading to the eventual banning of DES begin to mount.

Other incidents had occurred. For a time in the 1950's, DES implants were used in caponizing male chickens. Dogs eating waste from the processing of these chickens, and some men and boys eating chicken necks, began showing signs of feminization (the implants were in the chickens' necks). The FDA banned use of implants for caponization, and the USDA bought some ten million dollars worth of contaminated chicken and destroyed it. Other reports in medical journals describe young children developing breast enlargement after exposure to DES in products accidentally contaminated with the substance.

In Puerto Rico, where DES continues to be used, a virtual epidemic of premature sexual development, with grossly enlarged breasts in young children of both sexes, and ovarian cysts and precocious puberty in girls, occurred in the early 1980's. Hundreds of children were treated by physicians who eventually linked the problem to overuse of DES in locally produced chicken. In Puerto Rico, drugs such as DES are sold over the counter for animal use with no veterinary prescription needed.

The chicken producers were selling over five hundred thousand pounds of chicken each year to the school lunch program. Then while the plight of hundreds of sick children was being publicized, the weight of the chickens suddenly and mysteriously dropped from about four pounds each down to two to three pounds. Other evidence implicated meat and milk producers. The FDA and other regulatory agencies were uncooperative with attempts by physicians to convince the agency to investigate the suspect producers; nothing was ever proven.

A happy ending: in the vast majority of children, symptoms largely disappeared once the ingestion of suspected products ceased. Orville Schell's fine investigative account of this story, related in his book *Modern Meat* (much of the information in this section on the meat industry comes from Schell's research), paints a poignant picture of the pathos of the children and the callous unconcern of the industries and regulatory agencies involved. Whichever food producer was most to blame, the overuse of DES was almost certainly the cause of the problems.

Returning to America: the FDA finally banned DES feed additives in 1972 and implants in 1973. As a result of the livestock industry's legal maneuvering and appeals, the ban did not go into effect until July 13, 1979, when further sale and shipment of DES became illegal. Stocks on hand were to be usable until November 1, after which further use was illegal.

In March of 1980, the FDA discovered over fifty thousand head of cattle in Texas had been illegally implanted with DES after the ban. Throughout the spring, the count rose; the final tally showed 427,275 head of cattle in 318 feedlots in twenty states had been illegally implanted after the November 1 deadline. Illegal sales of DES had been made by forty-nine drug distributing companies after the sale deadline date. How many cattle were illegally implanted and not discovered is unknown. Another series of violations was discovered in 1983.

The FDA never prosecuted anyone for any of these violations of the law. Concepts of law and order are rather selectively applied in our country today.

Since DES was banned, cattlemen have chosen from a variety of somewhat more expensive similar drugs, including chemicals similar in structure to estrogens, and combinations of estradiol and progesterone (two hormones normally produced in minute amounts in the mammalian female body). The market is lucrative; over 99 percent of conventional feedlot cattle are implanted. Because the substances now used are naturally occurring hormones, attempts to regulate and monitor use have become less restrictive; the drug and cattle industries are being left to monitor themselves.

The danger of these hormones is somewhat subtle. Only tiny amounts of residual substances in meat are ingested, amounts that may only be a small percentage of the same substance normally found in the female body itself. This may seem harmless enough, but the endocrine system is very delicate; small amounts of hormones may have profound and long-lasting effects. We are dealing with the unknown; the effect of small doses of hormones over extended periods of time has simply not been investigated. Given the track record of the drug and cattle industries and the federal regulatory agencies involved, the possibility these substances will be irresponsibly overused cannot be ignored.

We could reasonably conclude the possibility is a probability. Particularly in the cattle industry, a callous disregard for the dangers of drugs, pesticides, and hormones used in modern meat production has been noted by investigators; it seems part of the macho image of cowboys. A callous disregard for the law—seen in many quarters as an intrusion of the federal bureaucracy—has apparently prevailed.

The Feeding of Modern Animals

Antibiotic additives in livestock and poultry feed, and the spraying of feedlots with insecticides to control flies, is not the end of the chemical infestation of meat production. Recently, new products called oral larvacides have been used to control flies. These organophosphate insecticides are added to feed and pass through the gastrointestinal tract, making the animal's manure toxic to fly larvae. The manufacturers admit "small amounts" are absorbed, but claim they are metabolized and leave no residues exceeding the allowable levels in meat. Organophosphates are related to nerve gases; while some are thought to be relatively innocuous to mammals, others are deadly.

A partial list of substances that are fed to animals raised for food includes waste scraps and dust from plants manufacturing cardboard containers; waste matter from Frito-Lay plants; shredded cardboard, including the petroleum-based wax coating; waste paper, including additives such as ink, glue, clay, and plastic used in its manufacture (the ink contains carbon black, mineral oil, and hydrocarbon resins, many of them carcinogens); orange peel pulp (rich in insecticide residues); and cooked garbage (fed to pigs in many hog-producing states, and containing nearly anything one can imagine—many pigs in northern New Jersey receive New York City's garbage every morning). A subindustry revolves around recycling these cellulose-containing materials for animal feed; the digestive system of ruminants converts cellulose into energy. An array of synthetic flavoring and aroma agents are used to make many of these "foods" palatable to animals.

Among substances recently tested by government, industrial, and university agricultural researchers for use as animal feed additives are: cement dust (the beef was reported by researchers to be tastier than that from cattle fed conventional foods); manure (during fattening, steers were fed diets of up to 60 percent manure, with no reported adverse affects on the flavor or composition of the meat); dried sludge from sewage plants (this may never be used because of the so far insurmountable problem of buildup of extremely toxic substances in the sludge); and plastic hay which expands in the digestive tract to provide roughage. When fed diets of mostly grains, cows require a small amount of hay to prevent problems from developing in the rumen, the first of their four stomachs. Plastic hay is designed to fulfill this requirement and eliminate the need for fresh hay. These products and a variety of mold inhibitors, flavoring agents, and bactericidal agents may soon be added to the list of non-foods already used to grow and fatten animals for human consumption.

Veal Calves

The feeding of veal calves is particularly illustrative of practices which are designed to produce a desired commercial product. This intent shows no regard for either the effects on consumers or the life of the animal. Newborn calves are taken from their mothers and chained in crates twenty-two inches wide by fifty-four inches long. Here their entire lives are spent; they may not stretch, turn around, or even lie down in a natural position.

Animals are never let out of these crates, and are kept in the dark to reduce movement. Total lack of exercise prevents development of muscles and speeds weight gain. Many are injured and sick; no straw covers wood slatted floors, resulting in leg injuries. Respiratory and intestinal diseases are common.

Chloramphenicol, a drug illegal in veal production but extremely difficult to detect, is reported by the USDA to be used often. This contributes to anemia that is deliberately induced by using feed rations deficient in iron. The light-colored meat resulting is sold as premium or milk-fed veal. Animals are given no solid food and are deprived of drinking water, inducing them to drink more of their milky liquid feed and gain weight faster.

Pig Factories

About 80 percent of the over ninety-five million hogs born in America each year are raised in large, indoor confinement, factory-farm facilities. After weaning at three weeks of age, animals are put in wire mesh cages or small cement pens, where they remain until reaching a weight of about fifty pounds. They are then moved to "finishing pens," where each animal has about six square feet of space. As with veal, slatted floors devoid of straw or bedding material result in injuries. Hogs grow to over two hundred pounds in these facilities.

In many facilities, confinement areas are located directly over manure collection pits; resultant fumes are described as overpowering. Research done within the industry found that over half of the people working in these facilities develop chronic bronchitis. At least fourteen workers are reported to have died suddenly from "acute respiratory distress and systemic toxicosis." Disease induced in animals makes constant administration of antibiotics necessary; other research within the industry found that some 70 percent of the hogs show symptoms of pneumonia.

The Egg Industry

Over 95 percent of eggs are now produced in factory-farms where laying hens live four or five to the cage. The quarters are so cramped—the cages commonly have a floor space of about twelve by eighteen inches—that animals cannot make the motions of their fundamental behavioral needs, much less walk about or build nests. Competition for space is fierce, injuries common, and cannibalism widespread. Feeding and watering is completely automated. Density is such that up to two hundred and fifty thousand birds may be confined in one building. Veterinary care is non-existent; high disease and mortality rates are considered acceptable because hens are cheap to replace.

Inspection

Orville Schell interviewed many of the nation's fifty-five hundred meat inspectors, several USDA officials, and many individuals who have investigated the meat industry. He quotes a veterinarian who is a federal meat inspector: "Sometimes we'll find cancer....sometimes we'll get batches of bad animals....Some of the slaughterhouses out there are just killing sh--. They don't care. They buy junk cows at ten cents a pound and sell them at ten times that amount. What the hell! They can afford to have a few carcasses condemned."

Violative residues of antibiotics and sulfur drugs are common. Prostaglandins and natural estrogens are not checked. No inspections are done on farms or at feedlots, so it is impossible to know if an animal was heavily dosed with any toxic substances shortly before being shipped; detection depends on random samples and luck. Withdrawal periods from many drugs are required by law before animals may be legally shipped for slaughter. Violations often occur, but only a small percentage are detected; even then the animal has usually gone to market by the time test results are known.

Much of this abuse occurs because the effectiveness of inspection suffers from lack of funds and a deliberate policy by top officials to downgrade the inspection system. In a 1983 report entitled "Return to the Jungle" (Upton Sinclair's *The Jungle* triggered the first meat inspection law to be passed in 1906), Kathleen Hughes from the Center for Responsive Law points out that many newly appointed officials in the USDA came to government directly from the meat industry. This situation has its analogue in the FDA, where the ranks of top officialdom have long been filled by appointees who were previously drug company executives. Subsequent changes in regulations made it more difficult than ever for meat inspectors to do their jobs properly. The government failed to fill 10 percent of the inspectors' jobs authorized by Congress, resulting in increased work loads in slaughterhouses. Demands were made to speed up inspections, and regulations were instituted making it more difficult to reject carcasses.

In a 1982 letter to *The Federal Veterinarian*, the Arkansas chapter of the National Association of Federal Veterinarians stated that the job of field vets in the Meat and Poultry Inspection Program had been undermined and circumvented by the program's management. It is stated thusly: "...they apparently respond to pressure exerted by Washington politicians on behalf of the meat and poultry industry." Other indications of serious problems include the statement of a retired federal meat inspector to the House Agriculture Committee: "Lax enforcement allows contaminated products bearing the mark of inspection to be sold all over the world and at home." A 1981 report of the Government Accounting Office stated that in visiting sixty-two meat-packing plants, GAO inspectors found a "high incidence of unacceptable ratings" and a "large number of deficiencies."

As assistant secretary of agriculture during the Carter administration, Carol Tucker Foreman was in charge of meat inspection. In 1983, she stated before a congressional committee: "There is a good chance the American public consumes meat with violative residues of carcinogenic and teratogenic chemical residues with some regularity." (Teratogenic means causing abnormal fetal development.)

A few other reports from Mr. Schell:

—In 1981, the USDA's Program Review Branch of the Food Safety and Inspection Service found adulterated or misbranded meat in 20 percent of meat-packing plants inspected.

—In 1983, a former supervisor for the USDA's meat grading program charged in a formal complaint that illegal abuses dangerous to the public existed in the inspection program. Among practices he observed to be prevalent were the use of spoiled meats in production of frankfurters and baloney, and grossly diseased livestock to make products for human consumption.

—A television report in 1983 alerted the USDA that a Colorado meat packer with a twenty million dollar contract to supply beef to school cafeterias had been slaughtering diseased and dead cattle, some reportedly contaminated with pathogenic bacteria.

—The president of a New York packing company was in 1983 convicted of slaughtering dying and diseased cattle. He did not go to jail for this felony, receiving instead a suspended sentence, probation, and a fine.

—Two companies in Pennsylvania were indicted in 1984 for allegedly buying sick and dying animals as pet food, and then reselling them as food for hospital patients, school children, and air force personnel.

These rather terrifying reports demonstrate the desirability of knowing the sources of one's foods well. Substitution of chicken for beef is no improvement; chicken are heavily treated with hormones and drugs. Allowed no exercise, they live their lives in small cages and never see sunlight. Cancer is found in many when they are slaughtered.

Appearance in the media of stories such as those above, and the red herring of the extended, extensive, and misleading cholesterol scare, have been major causes of a decline in meat consumption; the wonder is that consumption has remained as high as it has. While America may continue eating large amounts of meat because of a callous national indifference to our collective health, a greater influence may be simply that eating meat is very natural for most people. We by and large enjoy it; meat tastes good and feels satisfying. Humans have always been what some anthropologists call "opportunistic carnivores"—when meat is available, it is eaten. Modern day hunter-gatherers go to great lengths to insure a steady supply of meat, even when unlimited amounts of more easily obtained plant foods are available; the capture, sharing, and eating of meat is accorded almost mystical qualities.

Many people today may desire meat because they lack the nutrients provided by natural meat—not necessarily protein, but other, fat-soluble nutrients, as discussed in previous chapters. Although modern commercial meat does not supply those nutrients, the desire for meat remains. When told meat is bad for health, we perhaps instinctively reason, "If meat is so bad, how did we make it this far as a species?"

The answer lies in the meat's quality, which in turn is a direct reflection upon the quality of the lives of the animals. Modern mass-produced animals do not produce meat of traditional quality. No private individual, stable, zoo, kennel, or even research facility may legally treat animals as they are commonly treated on factory-farms. Pressure from the agribusiness and pharmaceutical lobbies has explicitly excluded farm animals from protection under the federal Animal Welfare Act. Thus individuals producing the nation's meat have complete control over the treatment and feeding of animals. No laws require any consideration for the welfare of animals. Laws relating to the quality of meat as it affects the health of consumers are concerned only with preventing tainted meat from reaching consumers; they do not reflect any understanding of what constitutes natural meat with its attendant health benefits. Ironically, the interests of animals and consumers are coincident, for healthy, naturally fed, and humanely raised animals provide healthy food.

Since early in the evolution of animal life, animals have utilized other animals in the struggle to survive. The earliest humans ate animals; as we evolved, the capture and consumption of animal life became increasingly important in the unfolding story of the most magnificently developed animal yet to inhabit the earth. Ancient cave drawings and paintings, traditions surviving into the cultures of modern day hunter-gatherers, and the rich folklore of a myriad of ethnic cultures all indicate that the killing of animals has always been done with the utmost respect and even love for the animal to be eaten, be it wild or domestic.

Most modern production of meat, fowl, and dairy products is a travesty on this rich and uniquely human heritage. By what right do modern people do this to animals—we who call simpler cultures savage, barbaric, primitive? By eating these animals we unthinkingly participate, perhaps because we think we have no choice.

But an alternative does exist. Humanely raised and healthy meat is available, for a growing number of people are raising food animals naturally. Healthy meat is good food, well worth the extra effort needed to secure it. Naturally raised meat, fowl, and eggs are the subjects of the next chapter.

14

Naturally Raised
Meat, Fowl, and Eggs

Growing numbers of farmers and ranchers throughout America are carrying on a traditional American industry—the raising of animals without the use of chemicals, hormones, or drugs. Others attempt this to the extent feasible; finding feed grown without pesticides or chemical fertilizers when adequate range is not available (winter in the north, summer in dry areas) can be difficult. Nevertheless, an increasing amount of meat, fowl, and eggs produced mostly or completely without chemicals, hormones, or drugs is becoming available.

Defining Organic

Naturally distrustful of commercial claims about products, people often ask how one may know if foods are produced as claimed. Most states have not yet passed laws regulating foods claiming to be "organic" or "natural," and often one must rely on knowledge of the label or on the integrity of the merchant selling the food. A merchant thorough in investigating his products knows their strengths and limitations.

California and Oregon, however, have passed laws regulating the labeling of these foods. Producers in other states may choose to adhere to these standards. By so doing, their products may be sold in California and Oregon as certified organic foods; in other states the producer may use this certification to demonstrate the validity of his claims. For a full explanation of the California organic foods law, see Appendix 4.

Every producer of natural meat and fowl has different policies. Some go beyond the California law in terms of care taken in raising animals and in purity of products. For example, one ranch in Colorado has raised beef cattle for nearly one hundred years and has never used chemicals, hormones, or drugs on their animals or crops (the occasional animal requiring antibiotic therapy for a health problem is not sold as naturally raised and organic). This ranch provides retailers with letters and testimonials from veterinarians, feed suppliers, and other people they do business with demonstrating the purity of their beef.

This particular ranch is the first to be authorized by the Food Safety and Inspection Service of the United States Department of Agriculture to label their beef as follows: "Feed used is always hormone and stimulant free, no artificial ingredients, only minimally processed. The USDA does not permit preservatives in this product." The Service made this authorization after checking documentation from inspectors, feed dealers, and an animal nutrition consultant. As of this writing, this is the only natural label in the United States that has this USDA approval, and as such sets a standard.

Other similar products are available, and others will appear, as more people become aware of the health benefits of naturally raised meat and fowl. Demand is rising; the beef described is now sold fresh in some natural foods stores and even in some supermarkets.

Natural Diet For Animals

Hormones and antibiotics aside, what distinguishes one animal from the next is exercise and what it eats. Meat, fowl, eggs, and dairy products are of most benefit when from animals which have lived outdoors eating their natural diets. This means beef and lamb raised on grass, barnyard chickens and their eggs, and milk products from pasture-fed cows and goats. These foods and fish are rich in fat-soluble protective nutrients; their fat composition is similar to that of wild game.

Fowl and Eggs

While chickens sold as "organic" or "naturally raised" may indeed be free of chemicals and drugs, most are raised in henhouses. Conditions are roomier than for conventionally raised chickens, and the diet may be organic grains, but the animals still have little or no exercise and are not eating their natural diet. Free-run chickens eat greens, insects, and worms. Grains are used as supplemental feed, particularly in cold months, but do not predominate. As with beef, a diet of mostly or all grains changes fat composition. Free-run chickens are leaner, their fats more polyunsaturated, and their skins a golden yellow color due to the rich supply of carotenes in fresh greens.

Most fertile and organic eggs are from confined chickens. While superior to conventional supermarket eggs, they do not compare with eggs from free-run chickens. The latter have a bright yellow-orange yolk, a noticeably thicker and stronger shell, and a distinctly enhanced flavor.

Eggs may be blended raw with milk or yogurt, flavored lecithin, and vanilla extract into a tasty eggnog drink.

Egg shells are an obvious and excellent source of calcium. Simply pulverize them to a fine sand-like powder in a blender with water and pour the powder off with the water into a cup. The powder settles and may be taken with a spoon and washed down with water. Bones are equally rich in calcium. Though now unconventional, these foods have traditionally been used to build healthy bodies. Like an animal, an egg is a whole and balanced food, meant to be utilized in full. Using these foods eliminates the need for calcium supplements.

Beef

Tests performed by Oregon State University scientists compared beef from growers raising animals on mostly mother's milk and grass, with little or no grain, with USDA choice beef. Eight different cuts of each were analyzed for total fat content and for calories per pound. Naturally raised beef averaged 7.3 percent fat and 1050 calories per pound; USDA choice beef averaged 30.0 percent fat and 1674 calories per pound. For fattier cuts (flank and brisket) the difference was only a factor of two. For leaner cuts (shank, round, rib, chuck, plate, and loin), USDA choice beef was from five to nine times fattier than naturally raised beef.

The grass-fed animals were particularly lean because they were not grain fattened and because they were slaughtered at ten months of age, rather than the usual eighteen. Fat content of naturally raised beef varies considerably; most producers feed animals grains for three months to fatten them for slaughter. Animals fed only grass have yellower fat, due to carotenes; grains make the fat whiter. The fat content of the grass-fed animals above is nearly as low as that of African grazing animals.

Most consumers of natural beef do not necessarily want such lean meat. The leaner meat is, the more it tends to be tough and chewy, especially cooked rare; most people prefer meat more tender. By feeding cattle grains for varying periods before slaughter, producers control the grade of the beef. USDA grades, from fattiest to leanest, are prime, choice, good, standard, commercial, and utility. Generally, the fattier the beef, the more tender, tasty, and expensive it is and the more grains the animal has been fed.

Organ Meats

Organs, particularly liver, have rich concentrations of many nutrients. But because the liver purifies the blood, it concentrates substances not naturally present in an animal. While the liver is one of the best parts of a naturally raised animal, these substances are a problem in conventionally raised animals.

Brain is seldom eaten in America today; in other cultures, and here in earlier times, it was a delicacy. Some physicians have made use of brain in therapeutic diets. It is now known to be a rich source of DHA (docosahexaenoic acid, very similar to EPA and likely involved in many of the same key metabolic pathways). Francis Pottenger recommended brain in an eggnog recipe so it could be eaten raw; liver too was used raw blended with juice. These foods may be used with excellent results, sometimes in these raw recipes but also lightly broiled.

Heart is extremely lean and muscular, but very tender when lightly cooked. The flavor is similar to that of steak. These and other organs are often available in stores carrying naturally raised meat and fowl, sometimes fresh but often frozen. Organs may be priced rather reasonably because of little demand; the author has seen them advertised as pet food and sold for a dollar a pound, ironic because in times past, Indians of the far north ate the organs and left the muscle meat for their dogs.

Lamb

Lamb is of special interest because conventionally raised lambs are relatively clean while at pasture; they are not usually implanted with growth promoting hormones, nor are they routinely fed antibiotics. In feedlots antibiotics are administered in the feed. Naturally raised lamb are often shipped to slaughter straight from the range, without being feedlot fattened on grains.

The way lamb is raised may be why Pottenger found lamb of particular value. Among his many publications was an article appearing in the *Journal of Applied Nutrition* in 1957 entitled "Therapeutic Effect of Lamb Fat in the Dietary." He notes lamb fat, particularly lightly cooked or raw, is extremely beneficial for individuals suffering from dry skin or dry hair. Pottenger attributed the benefits to polyunsaturated fats of animal origin, structurally different from those of vegetable origin. EPA had not yet been discovered; Pottenger empirically found that foods we now know are rich in EPA had great therapeutic benefit.

He wrote that the nutritional value of animal fats depended on various influences: the species of animal, whether or not it had been castrated, the age at slaughter, and the feeding methods used to rear the animal, including the use of chemicals in feed and of hormones. Precisely because lamb is quite fatty and was ideally raised on all counts, it was well suited for individuals with problems related to deficiencies of unsaturated fats of animal origin. Pottenger did not observe the same benefits when beef was substituted for lamb. Lamb was cooked rare, no more than two minutes on a side at 450 degrees F. for a one-inch chop.

He also wrote that in using substantial portions of lamb and of brain—both very fatty—even in people with initially high cholesterol and tri-glycerides, he never encountered increases. Instead, levels invariably went down. Parallels with recent discoveries by physicians working with fish oils are striking, and further demonstrate why animals raised on their natural diets provide food for building strength, resistance to disease, and longevity.

Vilhjalmur Stefansson's 1928 Experiment

The Arctic explorations of Vilhjamur Stefansson were described in previous chapters. We now return to the geographical and gastronomic adventures of this particularly carnivorous early twentieth century man to see what he can teach us about traditional meat.

In his Arctic explorations, Stefansson and his men succeeded in living for months at a time in good health, free of scurvy, on a diet of nothing but seal and occasionally polar bear. During many extended visits to the Arctic between 1906 and 1918, Stefansson lived on nothing but meat, fish, and water for an aggregate of over five years.

The prevailing view then as now among dietitians and medical people was that a mixed diet of animal and vegetable foods was necessary for health. Stefansson's revolutionary views and the narrative of his experience were viewed with skepticism. As he put it, many people expressed opinions amounting to "you are likelier to meet a thousand liars than one miracle."

Stefansson was quite well known for his Arctic exploits, and when a group of doctors asked to examine him extensively for evidence of ill effects from his years of living on an all meat and fish diet, he agreed. A committee failed to find any of the supposed harmful effects, and published their findings in the *Journal of the American Medical Association* (July 3, 1926) under the title "The Effects of an Exclusive Long-Continued Meat Diet."

An experiment was subsequently organized whereby Stefannson and a colleague from his Arctic days were to live exclusively on meat and fish for one year in New York City. The organization administering the experiment was the Russell Sage Institute of Pathology. The committee in charge included physicians, professors, and administrators from Harvard, Cornell, and Johns Hopkins Universities; from The American Museum of Natural History; and from several other institutions. The research work, including several weeks of full-time monitoring of the men in Bellevue Hospital (at the beginning and end of the year), was done by a team of physicians headed by the Medical Director of the Russell Sage Institute of Pathology. During the intervening months, Stefansson and his colleague came daily to the hospital for analysis of blood and excretions, insuring that if the men cheated on the diet the physicians likely would detect it.

The experiment was concluded in January, 1929. Both men came through the year in excellent health. All tests for any detrimental changes detectable by physical or laboratory examination were negative. The only problem Stefansson had was during early days of the experiment when physicians asked him to eat only completely lean meat (chopped fatless muscle). Within two days, he became ill with diarrhea and "a general feeling of baffling discomfort." This had also occurred in the Arctic once when for three weeks he ate only caribou so thin there was no appreciable fat behind the eyes or in the marrow (caribou are normally about 5 percent fat). Still, he did consume some fat then by eating tendons and the soft ends of bones, and he assumed that was why symptoms did not occur until the end of that three-week period. They appeared much sooner in New York because there was almost no measurable fat in the chopped fatless muscle.

The symptoms disappeared within three days of introducing fats—the sirloin steaks, brains and other organs, fish, and other meats constituting the diet for the year. Fish bones and rib ends were eaten for calcium. The diet was not really high in protein, for analysis showed 75 percent of calories to come from fats.

Stefansson did not get scurvy, either in the Arctic or in New York. Confirmation of his explanation for this appeared in a 1977 article in *American Anthropologist* entitled "The Aboriginal Eskimo Diet in Modern Perspective." The authors state Stefansson's appraisal forty years earlier of the vitamin C nutriture of those Eskimos living in the far north was accurate: "...if you have some fresh meat in your diet every day, and don't overcook it, there will be enough C from that source alone to prevent scurvy." These Eskimos had no plant foods available most of the year.

Stefansson wrote those words in describing the New York experiment and some of his Arctic experience in a three part article called "Adventures in Diet" that appeared in *Harper's Monthly Magazine* in November and December of 1935, and January of 1936. This fascinating account provides a lucid example of the need to avoid preconceived notions about diet, and does much to dispel the idea that meat and animal fats are necessarily unhealthy.

The 1977 article mentioned above reported that after careful analysis, the aboriginal diet of Arctic Eskimos (consisting mainly of land and sea mammals and fish, and virtually lacking plant foods) was found "capable of furnishing all the essential nutritional elements when prepared and consumed according to traditional customs....There is no history among Eskimos of the epidemic vitamin deficiency diseases which afflicted some cereal-based food cultures."

These accounts of the adequacy of an all meat and fish diet for Stefansson, and for primitive Eskimo groups, are not meant to suggest an all meat and fish diet would be appropriate for the reader. Genetics undoubtedly play an important role in these accounts; some individuals are likely much more suited than others to metabolize large quantities of animal source food. The point rather is that for some individuals, large quantities of meat and fish are compatible with excellent health. Evidence presented throughout this book indicates that substantial amounts of animal source food are required to build strength, optimal resistance to disease, and longevity. The quality of such foods is a prime consideration.

Meat Stefansson ate in New York City in the 1920's was in many respects more similar to the wild game he ate in the Arctic than to meat generally available today. Beef cattle were to a much greater extent grass fed, hormones and pesticides were not used in animal production, and antibiotics were yet to be discovered. The innovations of modern meat production described earlier have since taken place. Although many cuts of meat Stefansson ate during the experiment were fatty, the fats were of a different composition and quality than those in today's meats, almost certainly containing significant amounts of eicosapentaenoic acid (EPA) and other beneficial fatty acids not found in modern conventionally produced meats.

Conventionally produced dairy products are similarly lacking in these beneficial fatty acids; modern mass production methods unfortunately have taken much that was good out of once good foods. As with meat, however, a growing number of producers are making high quality dairy foods available. In the next two chapters, we will examine conventionally and alternatively produced milk and milk products.

15

Conventional Milk
and
Milk Products

*I*deally, change may proceed rather slowly in early stages of dietary adjustments. Food preferences result from a lifetime of likes and dislikes, habits, and culturally ingrained responses to foods available in different situations; though much needed, change may come with difficulty. Drug or alcohol problems must obviously take priority over changes in diet. Sugar too can be druglike and addictive; it must be largely eliminated if substantial progress toward better health through natural foods is to be made.

For many people the elimination of conventionally produced milk products is as important as the elimination of sugar is for others. These foods too are addictive in that most people use them habitually and find them difficult to give up. These are considered healthy foods, and the assumption is well founded; for past generations, natural milk, cheeses, and butter were available and were indeed excellent foods.

Today's conventional products, however, do much harm. Often symptoms of fatigue, nasal congestion, colds, and allergy are directly caused by milk or cheese and disappear rapidly when both are eliminated from the diet. Other symptoms are subtly and indirectly related to these foods, and a host of other chronic problems developing over the years are greatly influenced by milk products.

Several technical and well documented arguments can be made against the milk, cheese, yogurt, and butter seen on supermarket shelves. These arguments involve pasteurization, toxic residues, fat composition, homogenization, and synthetic vitamin D.

Pasteurization

Though necessary for public health reasons (because the health of cows producing milk is so poor and because milk is kept so long before consumption), pasteurization denatures all enzymes and heat-labile nutrients, changing the chemical structures of proteins and fats in the milk.

163

Heat-processed milk, cheese, and yogurt create allergies in consumers, though the symptoms may not be recognized as allergies. Reactions to pollens, molds, dust, and other environmental substances are usually linked to these and other dietary influences.

Commercial interests dictating food production have made certified raw milk impossible to obtain in many parts of the country. Scare tactics have been used to convince the public that all raw milk is dangerous. Pasteurization enables quantities of milk to be collected, shipped long distances, and stored. This is impossible with raw milk, which if not used fresh has traditionally been made into soured milk products. As a result, raw milk has always been locally produced.

Concern for consumers' health appears in milk advertisements, but this does not reflect reality. The production of food is a business, be the food milk, meat, cereals, vegetables, fruits, or candy bars. Profits are placed before concerns about consumers' health. As a result, modern milk is poor food.

Toxic Residues and Fat Composition

Modern cows are routinely fed antibiotics and feed grown with pesticides. They are subjected to insecticides, drugs, and other chemicals. These substances appear in their milk.

The fat composition of milk and milk products reflects the fat composition of the animal giving the milk. The same problems occurring in beef—excessive total fats and saturated fats, and inadequate polyunsaturated fats, particularly EPA—occur in conventionally produced milk. Such milk is an entirely different food than milk from grass-fed, chemical-free animals.

Homogenization

Homogenization breaks down fat globules in milk, causing them to remain dispersed. Evidence indicates this practice produces substances in homogenized milk which damage arterial walls. Kurt Oster, M.D., chief of cardiology at Park City Hospital in Bridgeport, Connecticut, has written extensively about this. His thesis is that the enzyme xanthine oxidase (XO), found in milk fat, is normally not absorbed into the bloodstream from the intestines when unhomogenized milk is drunk. The homogenization process emulsifies fats in milk, releasing the XO and making it available for absorption. Individuals using homogenized milk have high levels of XO in the blood, while those using only unhomogenized milk, skim milk, or no milk have very low levels. XO is thought to act chemically to scar arterial walls, with subsequent deposition of fatty material on the scars contributing to the development of atherosclerosis.

Oster and many other physicians, including Dr. Kurt Esselbacher, chairman of the Department of Medicine of the Harvard Medical School, who has publicly expressed his full support of Oster's overall concept, believe homogenized milk is a major cause of heart disease in this country. Finland, which also uses the homogenization process on nearly all of its milk, has a heart disease rate comparable to ours, lending further support to the xanthine oxidase concept. Countries where little homogenization occurs, such as France, have heart disease rates less than half that of ours and Finland's.

Synthetic Vitamin D

Vitamin D_2 (irradiated ergosterol) has for many years been added to most commercial dairy products; it is also commonly used in multi-vitamins. Years ago, when cows spent most of the year outdoors eating grass, natural Vitamin D and carotenes gave butter, particularly summer-made butter, a naturally bright yellow color. Such butter, however, did not store and ship as well as a lower vitamin, less yellow butter; over the years the quality and vitamin content of butter has dropped as the color faded—as cows came to spend less time outdoors eating grass and more indoors eating grains. Eventually, yellow dye was added to most butters.

Vitamin D is a complex of several vitamins existing in certain animal fats. One of the complex, vitamin D_3, is produced by the action of sunlight on skin. Vitamin D_2 is a synthesized approximation of vitamin D_3, with a slightly different biochemical structure than its natural counterpart. Studies have suggested vitamin D_2 is more active than vitamin D_3 in stimulating calcium metabolism. Clinical experience with arthritis patients and others with problems involving calcium utilization has demonstrated that synthesized vitamin D, whether in milk, other foods, or vitamins, contributes to health problems. Failure to include adequate sources in the diet of the full complex of natural vitamin D and fat-soluble nutrients associated with it in nature further contributes to problems.

In the 1930's, several studies linked irradiated ergosterol with calcification of the placenta and other problems in pregnancy. Results published in medical journals caused some concern at the time, but these warnings and those of Weston Price and others about dangers of synthetic vitamin D have gone largely unheeded.

Several years ago, grossly abnormal calcium metabolism led to the death of at least one infant in England when for a short time the amount of irradiated ergosterol added to milk was increased from four hundred international units (IU) to one thousand IU per quart. The infant dying from this highly unusual abnormality was the first reported death due to "idiopathic hypercalcemia of infancy" (high levels of serum calcium due to an unknown reason). The addition of irradiated ergosterol to milk in England was subsequently stopped.

In the past several years, a synthetic form of vitamin D_3 (made from the fat in sheep's wool by a complex process) has in many places been added to milk instead of vitamin D_2. Little is known about differences between this form of vitamin D and that which occurs in nature.

* * *

The adulteration of milk has made a liability out of a delicious traditional human food. Professionals in the fields of medicine and nutrition are evenly split between the pros and cons of drinking conventional milk; resulting confusion makes it difficult for the lay person to choose foods wisely and is cause for concern in light of the problems to which adulterated milk contributes. Sadly, the public cannot win; avoiding conventional milk and milk products may lead to calcium deficiency, while using them contributes to the problems detailed in this chapter. The use of other calcium-rich foods and food supplements, or both, by those avoiding milk and milk products is one viable alternative. Another is the use of certified raw milk and butter and raw milk cheeses, discussed in the next chapter.

16

Certified Raw Milk Butter and Raw Milk Cheeses

*N*ot everyone agrees milk or milk products should be part of the human diet after infancy. Human milk is designed by nature as the perfect food for human babies, but the argument has been made that just as all other species drink no milk after weaning, neither should we. Many adults have difficulty digesting milk, particularly pasteurized milk, and most milk products. Many others develop chronic allergies from using these foods. While this lends credence to arguments against milk, such reactions are usually due to the poor quality of conventionally produced milk and milk products. While for some individuals genetic influences play a role, for most the body's reaction to milk depends largely upon the quality and state of the particular milk used.

Milk in History and Evolution

Domesticated animals were first used for milk eight to ten thousand years ago; until then, the only milk humans used was from the breast. This proved adequate through millions of years of evolution, and we no doubt could live in health without milk today.

The Swiss of the Loetschental Valley were among the few traditional groups Weston Price studied who used milk products (the others were certain African tribes, including the Masai). The Valley people used raw, whole milk (both fresh and cultured), cheese, and butter, all in substantial quantities. Milk was from healthy, grass-fed animals, and was used unpasteurized and unhomogenized. Such foods clearly can play a major role in a health-building program for the individual genetically enabled to utilize these foods well.

Yet we could attain optimal health without dairy foods. Price discovered groups with complete resistance to dental decay and chronic disease using no dairy foods; their diets invariably included other rich sources of calcium and other minerals. The soft ends of long bones were commonly chewed, and the shafts and other bones used in soups.

Modern medicine is discovering the importance of a substantial intake of calcium. For example, several recent studies have linked high blood pressure and other problems with chronic subclinical calcium deficiency. Paradoxically, other problems are associated with high consumption of conventionally produced dairy foods; this has not gone unnoticed by researchers, nutritionists, and physicians. The importance of the quality and freshness of milk products lies behind the paradox. This concept has not been considered in attempts by the medical community to explain the health effects of dairy foods.

Milk from domesticated animals became important as a human food several thousand years ago. With domestication and settlement, fewer animals were available; as man roamed less, he hunted less, eating more grains and vegetables. Milk replaced animal bones as the chief source of calcium and some other minerals.

In indigenous cultures where adults use milk, often it is used as cultured or clabbered milk. This is similar to homemade raw yogurt, and is partially predigested—much of the lactose (milk sugar) has been broken down by bacterial action. This process must be accomplished over a period of several hours in the stomach when fresh milk is drunk; yogurt or clabbered milk is much more easily and quickly digested than fresh milk.

Many people with a history of allergic reactions to milk, even raw milk, can use and enjoy clabbered raw milk. Similarly, though pasteurized cheeses cause problems, small amounts of raw milk cheeses often do not. Considerable individual differences exist; some people are much more adapted for these foods than others. Milk products from pasture-fed animals almost never cause allergic reactions and are superior to those from animals fed mostly grains. Unfortunately, such food is difficult to find.

Adaptations in evolution are always the effects of particular causes. Humans developing the ability to digest milk into adulthood possessed a survival advantage; such change is the basis of evolution. Those who can digest milk may best use this advantage, and avail themselves of high quality certified raw milk and cheeses. These foods provide variety and are enjoyed by most people; they are a reasonable dietary option. Other sources of calcium and fat-soluble vitamins are available and are usually needed; in most areas, the lack of superior dairy products from grass-fed animals makes it wise to use even raw milk products no more than moderately.

Utilizing Raw Dairy Foods

The following guidelines for the use of dairy products are suggested for those wanting to utilize these foods:

—If using commercial dairy foods, eat none for a week before introducing certified raw milk. This gives the body an opportunity to clear itself of antibodies causing allergic reactions to milk products, allowing the best chance to react well to high quality raw milk foods.

—Then try some raw milk, clabbered raw milk, or homemade raw yogurt. In many adults, any milk causes allergic reactions—nasal congestion, postnasal drip, or diarrhea or loose stools several hours later. Certified raw milk available in many places is produced neither organically nor from grass-fed animals. Individuals reacting poorly to such raw milk may well not react to milk from grass-fed animals. Equally, the test of taste shows there is no comparing milk from grass-fed animals with that from animals fed mostly grains and hay. In many cases, one is best off using no milk or very little if milk from grass-fed animals is unavailable.

—Clabbered raw milk or homemade raw yogurt may be made from any certified raw milk; allergy reactions to these foods are much less marked than to the milk itself. Clabbered milk is made by allowing raw milk to stand in a warm room for forty-eight to seventy-two hours. Fermentation increases with time, and more curds separate as the taste becomes stronger. Initial addition of a yogurt culture viable enough to grow in unheated raw milk results in a more yogurt-like consistency and flavor.

—Butter does not cause allergic reactions. As a concentrated food, butter should be used only moderately. The best butter, made from grass-fed animals, is a darker yellow.

—Raw milk cheeses too are highly concentrated foods and are best used moderately. Some find even raw milk cheeses to constipate or cause allergies; as with milk, the feeding of the animal is paramount. When cheeses are from milk from grass-fed animals, problems have not been observed to occur.

Because milk contains sodium, so too do cheeses. Low-sodium cheese has no added sodium.

Raw goat's milk cheeses are usually the healthiest. Compared to cow's milk, goat's milk is more similar biochemically to human's milk. Goat's milk cheeses are sometimes produced organically, and because goats feed on grasses, weeds, and shrubs, they are likely to graze a lot and eat less grain than cows.

Raw milk cheese should not have been heated to over one hundred degrees to coagulate the curd. Natural cheeses are not ground, melted, or mixed with anti-mold chemicals, preservatives, and a variety of food additives, as are most conventionally produced cheeses. An organic cheese is made from milk from organically fed animals and should be free of pesticide residues; some producers order laboratory tests periodically to insure this is the case. Raw milk cheeses are required by law to be aged for at least sixty days. Since this insures that no viable harmful microorganisms remain in the cheese, aged raw milk cheeses may be sold even in states where raw milk may not be legally sold for human consumption.

Availability, Certification, and Safety

The availability of these foods varies from region to region because of restrictive laws; many states prevent the sale of raw milk for human use, and of raw butter. Laws prohibiting the certification and sale of these foods hide in the cloak of public safety but are the result of lobbying by the dairy industry to protect commercial interests. Raw milk of a quality suitable for market cannot be mass-produced on huge farms by cows that are little more than antibiotic filled milk machines, living far from the land nature intended grazing animals to feed upon. Raw milk cannot be shipped in tanker trucks, processed in plants, and distributed in super-markets far from where it is produced, as can commercial milk. Nor will raw milk keep for weeks on a shelf.

Raw milk from healthy animals is outstanding food for many people, particularly growing children. In states where raw milk is certified by government agencies, certification assures healthy animals and milk produced under sanitary conditions. Government regulations and enforcement are stringent about the production of raw milk, which is allowed bacteria counts only a fraction of those allowed in milk to be pasteurized. Such certified raw milk is safer than conventionally produced milk, for any problem in the pasteurization process—they occasionally occur—leads to contaminated milk. This is why outbreaks of salmonella and other problems have been traced to pasteurized milk and cheese several times in recent years, and never to certified raw milk, raw butter, or raw milk cheeses.

The Superiority of Raw Milk

Studies by eminent physicians and scientists, including Francis Potten-ger, have clearly demonstrated the superiority of raw milk as compared with pasteurized. Raw milk contains vital heat-labile nutrients not found in pasteurized milk. The medical establishment and public health authorities have failed to recognize that a deficiency of these nutrients has substantially contributed to the development of the epidemic of diseases plaguing modern civilization.

Production of raw milk should be carefully inspected and certified by public health agencies; poorly produced and controlled raw milk can lead to serious diseases, particularly in susceptible individuals. But many state health agencies, under political pressure from the dairy industry, have simply prohibited the sale of all raw milk and raw butter, claiming all such products are dangerous to the public. This is not true; the history of certified raw milk in this country shows raw milk and raw milk products are not dangerous or harmful when an adequate certification procedure is enforced. The public has been robbed of the right to good food, and the industry and government agencies responsible have convinced us they are the protectors of public health. The dairy industry meanwhile counts profits (much of which comes from government subsidies, i.e., our taxes) as national health deteriorates.

Food is big business. Interest groups profiting have deliberately made it difficult to eat simply and naturally; traditionally produced milk, cheese, and butter are difficult to find. Only if we support the few dairy farmers producing natural products of the highest quality will this begin to change. Like organic vegetable farmers discussed in the next chapter, organic dairy farmers remain a minority. But good quality raw milk cheeses (though not necessarily raised organically) are available in many natural foods stores, and many states have certification programs for raw milk and raw butter. By educating legislators and demanding the highest quality foods for ourselves and our children, more and more states will follow the lead of those with laws regulating the production of certified raw milk and raw milk products; demand in California is such that these foods are available in many supermarkets.

California is also one of the few states with a law regulating the labeling of organic foods. In the next chapter, the basic differences between the way foods have traditionally been produced, and the way most foods are currently produced, are presented as we compare and contrast organic farming with modern chemical agriculture.

17

Chemical Versus Organic Farming

*P*eople often ask if there is really much difference between produce available in supermarkets and organically grown produce sold in some natural foods stores. Simply—yes. But only when some details are understood does the answer have much meaning. An examination of how food is conventionally produced today and how food has traditionally been grown makes the difference clear.

Chemical Agriculture

Imagine driving across America's heartland, seeing thousands of square miles of midwestern farmland. Travel in the mind's eye through citrus country of Florida, apple and cherry groves of upstate New York and New England, fields of vegetables in valleys of Oregon and Washington, and everywhere in between along back country roads where farmers grow our food. A picture of great beauty emerges; rural America remains very lovely.

But the loveliness is tinged with a lingering sadness, for hundreds of millions of pounds of poisonous pesticides are sprayed on the land every year. And though this land is vast, one realizes it is nonetheless finite and perishable.

Many of these poisons work systemically and become part both of the soil and of plant tissues. Farmers consider this advantageous; they need not reapply them after a heavy rain. The more familiar ones legally found in foods coming to market include aldrin, captan, chlordane, DDT, dieldrin, lead arsenate, lindane, malathion, methyl bromide, and parathion. Allowable amounts vary; chlordane, for example, is allowable in concentrations up to only .3 parts per million. The maximum allowance of such a minute amount provides testimony of the toxicity of this substance. No one will argue these agents are not incredibly toxic in tiny amounts. Given the documented performance of the FDA in enforcement (consider the DES affair) and the agency's admitted lack of manpower to test adequately both the pesticides and the foods themselves for residues, the established limits on concentrations are not particularly reassuring.

Production of food was once the province of small farms owned by a large percentage of our people. Now, it is big business. In a land once producing food with considerable love, care, and attention to concerns of consumers, little thought is now given beyond the expedient and the maximally profitable. One need not elaborate on the obvious.

Consider, however, the results. The land lies essentially raped. Insects have grown increasingly resistant to pesticides; larger amounts of toxic chemicals are used, killing insect predators and thus destroying natural checks. Meanwhile, more and more petrochemically derived fertilizers are used in attempts to maintain high yields. Humus reserves have been depleted; the living organisms of the soil have been killed. This circle has made most farms as dependent on chemical fertilizers and pesticides as an addict is on drugs.

Herbicides are used on weeds; fungicides are used in fields to control fungus diseases and in storage and transport to control rot. Fumigants are sprayed on stored foods to kill insects. An estimated twenty-five hundred (no one is sure of the actual figure) additional chemicals are added to foods in processing.

Tests of these substances, when they are tested, are made individually. But interactions of two or more chemicals have unpredictable results, often resulting in greater toxicity than results from use of one alone. Effects of potential carcinogenic agents are equally unpredictable; the development of cancer often takes many years or even decades from the time of exposure to carcinogenic agents.

The latest threat to the integrity and safety of our foods is a coordinated effort by government officials and the nuclear industry to create a multi-billion dollar a year industry to irradiate nearly half the food Americans will eat by 1990. The details of this plan are presented in Appendix 3, "Food Irradiation—The Latest Threat to Our Foods."

Organic Farming and Living Soil

An organic agriculture is more than the absence of negative and harmful influences. In the early 1900's, a man whose work changed the shape and substance of many buildings Americans live and work in wrote of the need for an organic quality in architecture. He borrowed a word from the organic farming movement because he envisioned an architecture in touch and in scale with nature, as the living soil is with the plants it nurtures.

The man was Frank Lloyd Wright. He called his vision for buildings and the spaces they define "organic architecture," and to be in one of his buildings is to know why. His buildings nearly live and breathe; being in or around them constantly reminds one of the heights to which the human spirit may soar.

An organic agriculture truly does live and breathe. The soil teems with microorganisms that give vigor and resistance to plants, with worms to aerate the soil and insect predators to control pests. High in humus and nurtured with natural fertilizers, a living soil provides plants with strength to resist disease and insects, as well as superior taste and nutritional value.

More farmers are realizing their own interests are no more served by chemical agriculture than are the public's, and as they change to organic methods, more naturally grown foods will become available. Conversion of chemically overworked soils is not easy; such soils are often reduced to a state not conducive to organic growing. This is one reason organic foods initially may cost more to produce. Prices have come down in recent years, however, and are in many areas competitive with conventionally grown crops. A recent USDA report on organic farming (based on a study of sixty-nine organic farms ranging in size from a few to fourteen hundred acres) concluded that organic farming is competitive economically with chemical farming.

Certainly problems exist in the organic movement. Laws and regulations are needed in many states to insure that the consumer is getting what he believes he is getting. Demand in some areas is so light that little organic produce is available, and what is available, particularly in the winter months, may not be fresh. Cooperative efforts, education, and increased desire for good foods will solve these problems. Only by understanding the issues involved and voting for organic foods with our food dollars can we build an agriculture providing high quality foods while sustaining resources for the future.

Healthy traditional and so-called primitive cultures discussed in previous chapters ate plant foods that were nourished by virgin soils or a carefully and naturally maintained traditional agricultural system; this was an integral part of their success. Naturally grown foods are one of the primitive influences needed to solve modern problems.

Organically grown vegetables are sometimes available in natural foods stores, or seasonally directly from growers; they may complement the conventionally grown vegetables many of us often must settle for because of the difficulty and expense of obtaining organically grown vegetables. The place and importance in the diet of vegetables in general, and of specific vegetables in particular, are considered in the next chapter.

18

Vegetables

*T*raditional diets place considerable emphasis on animal source foods. These foods have always provided certain essential nutrients unavailable in foods in the vegetable kingdom. Traditional cultures and contemporary hunter-gatherer societies invariably have customs and rituals surrounding the use of certain animal source foods.

This is not to deny, however, the importance of plant foods in traditional diets. In all regions (except the northernmost Arctic), plant foods, either cultivated or gathered, play a vital role. Generally, the closer to the equator, the larger a role for plants in terms of calories. For most people in the temperate zones of North America, a diet in which a majority of the calories are provided by plant foods is appropriate. The precise proportion varies with individual tastes and needs, and indeed tends to vary within the individual seasonally and throughout life.

Though this chapter is quite short, do not be misled; vegetables are essential. A healthy diet may be built around raw vegetables.

Green Vegetables

One large raw vegetable salad, or two of moderate size, ideally appears on each day's menu. This translates into a large consumption of fresh greens, which are with high quality animal source foods the most important items in the diet. If one suffers from gastrointestinal disease, one should use raw greens with extreme caution if at all in the early stages of dietary treatment (see chapter 10 for details). Others may begin eating salads slightly larger than those currently eaten, and slowly increase the size. Body and mind may then gradually adapt to larger amounts of raw vegetables. Use desired varieties of lettuce and sprouts, celery, parsley, and other palatable greens and raw vegetables.

A small amount of dressing helps make a salad enjoyable; virgin olive oil and unpasteurized apple cider vinegar or lemon juice are preferred ingredients. For many people, a salad of moderate size at both lunch and dinner may be preferable to a large salad at one meal or the other. Canned sardines packed in water or sild sardine oil are for many a healthy and enjoyable addition to salads.

Cooked greens also provide many nutrients. Broccoli, kale, and sometimes dandelion and other greens are readily available. Regular use of quantities of vegetables containing oxalic acid is discouraged; these include spinach, beets and beet greens, swiss chard, and rhubarb. Oxalic acid is found in most kidney stones. Although it is a normal metabolite, its presence in stones indicates a disorder in its metabolism and excretion; eating quantities of these foods may contribute to the development of this problem. While there is no proof this is so, a prudent course calls for selecting other vegetables containing no oxalic acid. A policy of using indigenous foods also limits use of the oxalic acid-containing vegetables.

Using Indigenous Foods

Foods most suited for an individual are those indigenous to the type of climate in which his ancestors evolved and lived. We of European ancestry are not biologically equipped to utilize foods indigenous to the tropics and the subtropics in any substantial quantity. Vegetables rich in oxalic acid are of tropical origin and have been used in northern climates only in recent centuries. This may seem a long time, but ancestors of humans (except those of African descent) migrated out of Africa into more northern climates over one million years ago. People of European descent evolved and developed under the influence of foods native to northern and temperate parts of the world.

Adverse effects from foods of tropical origin are commonly seen clinically. Many very popular foods are not indigenous to northern and temperate climates. These include citrus and other tropical fruits and their juices; the nightshade (*Solanaceae*) family of vegetables, including tomatoes, potatoes, eggplants, and green peppers; many nuts, including cashews; and the oxalic acid vegetables listed above. For many people, these foods constitute a major portion of the diet, and a variety of symptoms and clinical problems often result. Improvement invariably results when use of the offending food or foods is reduced sufficiently or discontinued.

Sprouts

Sprouts are rapidly growing fresh young greens, the equivalent of fresh cut greens from the garden. Ideally sprouts make up a major part of one's salads, especially sunflower seed, buckwheat, and clover sprouts. The latter are available in most health food stores and many supermarkets. While most sprouts are grown without soil, sunflower seed and buck-

wheat sprouts require at least an inch of soil for growth. Both are sometimes seen in natural foods stores growing in flats, and both provide a
rich supply of nutrients, including chlorophyl, alpha-linolenic acid, and
raw food enzymes. Both may be easily grown at home, either in the
garden or in flats indoors under plant lights.

Other grains, legumes, and seeds may be sprouted; many are seen in
both supermarkets and health food stores. Sprouted legumes such as
peas and chick peas are for many people difficult to digest and cause gas.

People with autoimmune disease, particularly rheumatoid arthritis and
lupus, have noted aggravations of symptoms when eating alfalfa sprouts.
Some clinicians suspect aggravations may be caused by other sprouts as
well, particularly other sprouted grains (alfalfa is a grain). Clover, sunflower, and buckwheat are grasses rather than grains. No problems have
been noted using their sprouts.

Clover sprouts have a milder, sweeter taste than alfalfa sprouts and
are available in many natural foods stores and supermarkets. They may
be easily sprouted at home. Soak seeds in water in a glass jar for twelve
to twenty-four hours, then cover the opening with cheese cloth and a
rubber band and rinse and drain several times. Stand the jar at a sixty
degree angle with the open end down in a dish or pan. Left this way,
excess water drains out. Rinse every eight to twelve hours. Edible sprouts
grow within two days; within four to five they are mature and ready to
refrigerate. To turn them green and greatly increase vitamin content,
leave sprouts moist in the sun for a few hours before refrigerating.
Sprouts are at times the closest that one may come to having a garden.
Most people who try them grow to like them.

Sea Vegetables

Edible seaweeds stand near the top of tables listing foods according to
nutrient density. Rich in many vitamins and minerals, they especially
concentrate iodine, critical in thyroid gland function and lacking in the
diet of many Americans. An excellent source of trace minerals, sea vegetables have always been widely utilized by traditional coastal cultures
and even inland people who bartered for it.

Dulse and nori are the most easily used edible seaweeds now sold
commercially; both are customarily eaten raw, either alone or in salads.
Nori is also used in traditional Japanese sashimi, rolled with rice, vegetables, and often raw fish.

Dulse sold in natural foods stores is harvested off the coast of Canada
from the cold waters of the northern Atlantic, dried, and packed into
plastic bags. It is very thin, and a little goes a long way; a fraction of a
bag may be cut up or pulled apart and sprinkled throughout a salad.

Like dulse, nori is not processed with heat. Japanese have farmed the ocean for nori for centuries by seeding rope nets which are stretched between buoys just below the ocean's surface. In a few months, the ropes are pulled aboard ships and the nori is sucked into machines. The mash is slowly dried on shore at low temperatures in flat, square forms. The paper-thin sheets which result are sold in various places throughout the world.

Nori is grown in coastal Japanese waters, while the dulse available comes from northern Canadian waters far from major population and industrial centers; the latter seems preferable. The flavor of seaweeds may seem a little strange at first, but dulse quickly becomes a welcome addition to raw vegetable salads. Nori is best used in sashimi and other traditional Japanese dishes.

Other sea vegetables available are usually cooked; they include wakame, kombu, and hijiki. Usually they are used in vegetable and grain dishes and soups.

Kelp is available as both tablets and powder. If other sea vegetables are not eaten regularly, kelp may be taken as a supplemental source of iodine and trace minerals.

Other Vegetables

Carrots, green beans, peas, corn, cauliflower, squashes, onions, and garlic are among other vegetables available. Most are good lightly steamed or raw in salads; they may also be used well cooked in wintertime soups and stews. These vegetables should usually be cooked as lightly as is palatable; many find fresh corn delightful raw.

The Nightshades

Foods from the nightshade family may be occasionally enjoyed, but problems occur with regular use of these foods. Garden-ripe tomatoes in late summer taste good, but when eaten in quantity they cause many people to develop small sores in the mouth and on the tongue, and often skin problems. Like all minor symptoms, these should not be ignored; they yield clues about how foods affect the body.

Tomatoes, like citrus fruit, tend also to aggravate gastrointestinal problems. Potatoes cause marked intestinal gas in many individuals, and some people note indigestion whenever eating green peppers. Eggplants too may cause a variety of seemingly unrelated symptoms.

Perhaps it may seem an overreaction to largely avoid these foods because such symptoms occur in some people, but there are other reasons. The green parts of the nightshade plants are poisonous—everyone knows not to eat tomato vines, for example. Centuries ago, the fruits of the plants as well were considered poisonous; only in the past few hundred years have they been used as foods. Plants from the *Solanaceae* family contain a glycosidic compound similar to a metabolite of vitamin D_3 (a compound made in the body from vitamin D_3). When grazing on these plants, animals develop stiff legs and a number of symptoms indicative of calcium problems; the compound obviously detrimentally affects their calcium metabolism. Literature about animal husbandry from all over the world reveals that each culture has a name for these symptoms in animals, and in each case, their cause is the same—grazing on plants from the nightshade family.

Avoiding the nightshades is not the sole solution for arthritis or any other serious problem. But evidence indicates these foods play a role in arthritic and other diseases. The nightshades are indigenous to tropical and subtropical climates; our ancient ancestors did not have these foods. A prudent diet emphasizes other foods and limits tomatoes, eggplants, green peppers, and potatoes to at most occasional use in small quantities.

Raw Vegetable Juices

Fresh raw vegetable juices are best prepared from greens and carrots. A piece of apple may be juiced to sweeten the mixture a bit. Raw juice is excellent therapy for most chronic problems; the concentration of nutrients in juice without the bulk of the vegetables allows ingestion of a much larger amount of enzymes and other raw food nutrients than if the vegetables themselves were eaten. Juices are best freshly prepared and drunk at least thirty minutes before meals to avoid interference with the digestion of solid foods. Fresh raw juices are often available in natural foods stores and at juice bars; they make excellent snacks.

* * *

Whole grains will be discussed in the next chapter. Essential in the diets of many contemporary traditional agricultural cultures, whole grains were at the heart of the natural foods movement that spread throughout America in the 1960's. For many people interested in natural foods, vegetables and whole grains form a substantial part of the diet; this has been necessitated by the move away from conventionally produced meat and dairy foods. We have seen that foods other than whole grains, paradoxically including meat of the proper quality, are even more natural candidates to be dietary staples than are grains. We will now attempt to integrate these divergent streams of influence in considering the place of whole grains and foods made from whole grains in a contemporary traditional diet.

19

Whole Grain Foods

Whole Grains

Among people Weston Price studied in the 1930's and found immune to dental decay, only those in the Loetschental Valley of Switzerland and on the islands of the Outer Hebrides off the coast of Scotland used whole grains (rye in the Loetschental, oats in the Outer Hebrides) as an essential part of the diet. The people of Georgian Russia, Vilcabamba, and Hunza also use large quantities of whole grains. Evidence presented in chapter 5, however, indicates grains may play too large a role in the diet of many people in Vilcabamba and Hunza.

The place of whole grains in the diet, even those carefully grown without pesticides and chemical fertilizers, has been debated for many years by people interested in anthropology and nutrition. Grains became a staple in the diet of some humans beginning only about fifteen thousand years ago, when settlements first appeared around the edges of wild grain fields and people first learned to domesticate these plants. Many of us are descendants of ancestors who first used grains fewer than two thousand years ago. Anthropologists tell us we are biologically the same as we were at least forty thousand years ago. We thus evolved to our present biological state on a diet that did not include grains.

Most of the cultures Weston Price found to have immunity to dental and chronic disease used no grains. Grains have become a staple over the past fifteen thousand years in agrarian societies the world over—yet Price's work also showed that hunter-fisher-gatherer societies enjoyed greater strength and immunity than their grain-eating agricultural contemporaries. What role should grains play in our diets today?

The author recommends whole grains as an option for part of the diet. Grains are convenient—they store and travel easily, and they are relatively inexpensive. They are high in fiber and easily prepared. Their inclusion in the daily diet works well for most people. Grains are not essential for a healthy diet, and their excessive use at the expense of high quality animal source foods and raw vegetables is detrimental, but when properly grown and simply prepared, they are reasonably included.

The grain most easily prepared with the least cooking is toasted buckwheat, or kasha. The inedible outer hull of the buckwheat groat has been mechanically removed and the raw groat lightly toasted. Indigenous to northern Russia, kasha is a hearty food, rich in a more complete protein than any other grain, and considered the most strengthening of the grains. The buckwheat plant is actually classified botanically as a grass rather than a grain.

Because the toasting process has partially cooked kasha, it may be prepared in a few minutes—simply mix one part kasha to one part hot or boiling water and let stand a few minutes. Kasha is convenient when traveling; it is not perishable and can be prepared by simply adding hot tap water.

Brown rice is the most commonly recommended and used whole grain. Available in both short grain and long grain varieties, short grain is traditionally considered more strengthening. Mixing in a little wild rice (gathered largely in northern Minnesota and Canada where it grows in shallow lake bottoms) adds a distinctive flavor. Brown rice is subject to oxidation at high temperatures and is best kept airtight and refrigerated or in a cool place.

Millet is a grain of Middle Eastern origin, highly nutritious and with a distinct flavor of its own. Millet, whole oats, hulled barley, and whole wheat all may be cooked much as brown rice is; simply boil water (two parts water to one part grain), add grain, return water to a boil, then simmer until done, about thirty to forty-five minutes. Oats are also available as steel-cut oats—chips of whole oats which cook in about twenty minutes. Cracked wheat is the equivalent in wheat. The available whole and cracked wheat are winter wheat. While wheat is the most traditionally American grain and is rich in protein, most people prefer the flavor of brown rice, toasted buckwheat, and millet for cooked whole grains, favoring wheat in breads.

Oat meal (rolled oats) has been flattened and partially cooked; it may be quickly prepared, but it is nutritionally inferior to steel-cut or whole oats. Bulgur wheat, another popular item in natural foods cookery, is like millet of Middle Eastern origin. Unlike millet, it is not a whole food, for before being cracked, it has been boiled, with considerable loss of nutrients. It too is quickly prepared, as is pearled barley. In the abrasive process used to make pearled barley, the fiber content and over half the protein, fat, and minerals of the whole barley kernel are lost. Similar losses occur in the production of cous-cous (semolina) from wheat. With the exception of oat meal, these are refined foods rather than whole grains.

Foods Made From Whole Grains

In addition to whole grains, which remain fresh and in their natural state until cooked and eaten, a host of foods made from whole grains are available. These include breads, flours, pastas, and pastries.

When grain is made into flour, its nutrients are exposed to oxygen. Certain nutrients, particularly vitamin E, are very much susceptible to destruction through oxidation. Other, little understood effects result in loss of vital nutrients. Many animal experiments have demonstrated a great difference between the effects of fresh whole grains or freshly ground flour and those of flour not completely fresh.

Visitors to Hunza have observed that when traveling about the country, natives carry small hand mills for grinding wheat to make fresh chapattis, small loaves of bread which are a dietary staple. They do this rather than grinding flour at home and making chapattis before leaving, or even carrying flour with them. Food is scarce, and the Hunzas recognize the need to utilize their grains in the most efficient possible manner—completely fresh.

Breads made from sprouts without the use of flour are available in natural foods stores. Sprouted grains are less subject to oxidation than flour and are rich in nutrients. Various grains are sprouted and made into loaves, either plain or with small amounts of sea salt, lecithin, yeast, and other natural ingredients. The finest are slowly baked at low temperatures to insure minimal destruction of heat-labile nutrients.

Scores of sizes and shapes of whole grain pastas are available, most made from whole wheat flour and, in some products, spinach or artichoke flour. Like whole grain breads and sprouted whole grain breads, these foods are useful, especially for individuals and families making a transition from refined foods and becoming accustomed to the taste of natural foods. Simply cooked whole grains day after day may prove unpalatable; whole grain products provide an important alternative for those who enjoy them.

Another important alternative is provided by fresh fruit, discussed in the next chapter. Fruit, like grains, is thought of as a dietary necessity, but is best considered an option appropriate in some circumstances and not in others. An explanation of this blasphemous proposal follows.

20

Fruits, Nuts, and Seeds

Fruits

America loves fruit—orange juice for breakfast, fruit at lunch to help keep weight down, fruit for snacks, fruit for dessert. Especially for many health conscious people, fresh fruits and fruit juices are considered important foods and are eaten daily all year.

Fresh fruit supplies raw enzymes, vitamin C, and potassium. Vitamin C is partially destroyed by cooking, and fresh fruit is an important source for many people, though it may be equally well supplied by other raw foods, especially vegetables. Potassium too is abundant in vegetables. Because many people eat few vegetables and little raw food, fruit has become a major source of vitamin C, potassium, and vital heat-labile nutrients. As a result, many people feel better eating fruit and eat substantial amounts.

The question, however, is whether raw food nutrients might be best supplied by other foods, and if so, what then should be the place of fruit in the diet? Could excessive fruit, while supplying much needed enzymes, be simultaneously contributing to the development of problems? And what of fruit juices?

Consider the place of fruit in the diet of our ancestors. *Homo erectus*, the ancestral human species preceding and leading to the development of *Homo sapiens*, is thought to have developed in Africa and then migrated throughout Europe and Asia around one million years ago. By the time this migration took place, men were hunting cooperatively and meat played an important if not dominant role in the diet. Food gathering was also important in the mixed economy of early man, and in Africa fruit undoubtedly was an important food. But as migrations spread north, fruit must have played a diminishing role. For hunter-gatherers of Europe and northern and central Asia, fruit came to be a small and insignificant part of the diet. Even among modern-day African hunter-gatherer and herdsmen tribes, fruit plays a role secondary to that of animals and wild vegetables.

For our European forefathers, berries were available in summer, and other temperate zone fruits, in fall. Seasonal patterns are much the same in most of America. But now we use tropical and subtropical fruits all year long. Heat-processed juices, devoid of the enzymes found in fresh fruit, are consumed in large quantities.

Such consumption patterns are not part of the diet we are genetically programmed to eat. Our physiological responses to food are simply not adapted to handling large quantities of fruit, especially tropical fruits and juices, and these foods in particular contribute to the development of serious problems.

Gastrointestinal diseases, including ulcers and colitis (particularly the acute phases), are aggravated by citrus fruits and juices, as are skin diseases. Also, many arthritic patients are aware their symptoms are worsened by these foods.

Symptoms due to hypoglycemia—low blood sugar—are aggravated by fruit juice, dried fruit, and sometimes fresh fruit. An eight-ounce glass of fruit juice has the fruit sugar of several pieces of fruit, and is rapidly absorbed; the body must immediately metabolize this sugar. Dried fruits have much the same effect. Extracted fruit juice does not appear in nature, and the body has no effective way of handling any substantial amount.

In whole fruits, the fruit sugar is much more dilute and more slowly absorbed. Fruit is digested over some time, usually thirty to sixty minutes, and the body has time for a much more measured and controlled response. When ripe and fresh fruits are eaten in moderation, the metabolic response is good. Even quite a large amount of some fruits may be eaten occasionally without problems by people in good health. Melons in particular seem to be well handled in quantity when eaten alone.

Fruit eaten in quantity with other foods causes gas or indigestion or both. Grapes, apples, pears, bananas, and dried fruits may cause gas even eaten alone in quantity. Excessive gas is a clear sign the body is reacting poorly to foods.

Generally, those recovering from health problems are wisest to avoid fruit entirely for a time. Later, small amounts may be gradually introduced when temperate zone fruits are in season. People of European ancestry living in southern parts of America are no more prepared genetically to consume tropical and subtropical fruits or fruit juices than are people living in the north; a few years, or even generations, does not change one's genetic equipment and physiology.

Once accustomed to a traditional diet, one has little desire for fruit from the end of the fresh apple season in the fall until berries appear in late spring. When an abundance of raw food nutrients are supplied by proteins and vegetables, there is no need for fruit. Cravings for fruit seem to disappear when eating quantities of high quality animal source foods. Fruit that is eaten seasonally is immensely enjoyed. An occasional glass of unpasteurized apple juice (available frozen from some natural foods stores, or juiced fresh at home) makes a pleasant and healthy treat.

In traditional Chinese medicine, all fruits are yin; tropical fruits and all fruit juices are extremely yin. Excess yin may result in discharges— diarrhea or inflammation of the bowels, acne and other eruptive skin diseases and rashes, colds, and many other problems. Yin foods of good quality are most appropriate at the most yang time of the year—summer—for yang is hot, and yin foods help balance the heat. In considering the place of fruits in the diet, this rather inexact concept of yin and yang is a useful tool; the author's clinical and personal experience confirms traditional wisdom. This concept of balance is helpful in choosing fruits. Let fruit consumption ebb and flow with the seasons. Foods which are sometimes beneficial may at other times be harmful.

Nuts and Seeds

Though often thought of as protein foods, most nuts and seeds supply far more calories from fats than from proteins. Their high oil content makes them highly subject to oxidation and rancidity, especially when shells or husks have been removed. Eaten in substantial amounts, nuts and seeds invariably create quantities of intestinal gas. Many unsuspecting people suffering with this embarassing problem, and fond of snacking on nuts and seeds, have discovered that it was not due to "nerves" or some other undefinable cause; it disappeared when nuts and seeds were eliminated from the diet. Flatus is especially marked when nuts and seeds are ingested together with dried fruit, as in popular granola mixes.

A more serious problem occurs in people with herpes. Symptoms of genital herpes may be completely controlled by avoiding refined foods and following a traditional diet. Very minor symptoms—a few tiny spots with some itching, lasting only a day or two—occur if there are occasional and minor dietary transgressions. Major outbreaks may be triggered, however, by eating even a few nuts. The amino acid arginine, prevalent in all nuts, has been implicated; but the fattier varieties such as cashews, pecans, walnuts, and peanuts for some reason particularly seem to aggravate the problem. Seeds may have a similar effect. An occasional almond or two seems to be tolerated.

Nuts have been a limited part of the food supply for many traditional cultures. Perhaps when carefully stored they are a reasonable food taken in small quantities, but by and large they seem to cause nothing but trouble.

Sesame and sunflower seeds have been advocated because they supply the same polyunsaturated fatty acids found in vegetable oils. Seeds, however, cause the same problems nuts cause, though on a somewhat smaller scale because usually fewer are eaten.

Vegetable oils are ubiquitous in many prepared foods. A discussion of vegetable oils (and several other food and non-food items), many of which contribute to the development of heart disease and other chronic illnesses, is the subject of the next chapter.

21

Other Foods
Seasonings
and Beverages

*T*he extent one uses the items discussed in this chapter depends on how long one has eaten mostly unrefined foods, how simple one wishes to keep the diet, and how serious one's health problems may be. These items are not nutritionally necessary but are useful in adding variety and additional taste to basic foods. Individuals with chronic health problems are advised to use them minimally at most, while those in good health usually can use small amounts of some and moderate amounts of others without problems. For everyone concerned, caffeine, refined flour, and sugar should be consumed no more than occasionally.

Vegetable Oils

Manufacturing Methods. Commonly used salad and cooking oils include safflower, peanut, soy, corn, sesame, sunflower, and olive oils. Two general methods of oil extraction are used: the vegetable, nut, or seed may be pressed mechanically, and it may be treated with a chemical solvent.

In the latter method, the solvent is subsequently separated from the extracted oil. The solvent commonly used is hexane, a petrochemical. The oil is then bleached and saponified (treated with an alkaline agent to produce soap). The soap is then taken off, and the residue processed further. Resulting oil has been subjected to high temperatures many times during these processes. The last series of steps involves up to forty to fifty filtrations to deodorize the oil and remove impurities.

Resulting oil is devoid of many natural substances found in more simply made oils, including chlorophyll, lecithin, carotenoids (substances occurring in most plants that may be converted into vitamin A in the body), vitamins, and minerals. Vitamin E is found in plants from which oils are extracted; it protects the oils from oxidation. Removal during refinement results in oils highly subject to rancidity, which is why petrochemically derived preservatives such as BHT (butylhydroxytoluene) are added. While some claim BHT helps preserve *us* and delays the aging process, safer methods are available. Animal studies show BHT has a wide range of toxic effects, and it is a suspected human carcinogen.

Oils initially extracted by pressing may subsequently be solvent extracted and go through these bleaching, saponification, and filtration processes; they may still be labeled cold pressed, a term with no legal definition and without clarification meaningless. A label stating an absence of preservatives shows some Vitamin E is present, indicating a simpler refinement process than that used for most supermarket oils.

The pressing method may be used to produce an unrefined and truly cold pressed oil. Heat produced is minimal when pressing is done slowly and carefully. An unrefined oil is clear and shows sediment in the bottom of the container. Such oils contain the full complement of substances natural to them, and the label may state the vitamin E content.

Conventionally produced oils are heavily used in most prepared and restaurant foods, and in condiments such as salad dressings. Biochemically, they are strikingly different from carefully made, unrefined oils, and they do the body harm.

Olive Oil.   The vegetable oil most suited for regular use is olive oil. For many years, olive oil was maligned because it is the most saturated of vegetable oils, but evidence indicates unsaturated vegetable oils are the more damaging fats. The oil of the olive, used for thousands of years, has returned to its place as the traditional salad and cooking oil.

Oil should not be overheated. Even the finest oil should be used moderately, for oil is a highly concentrated food. A maximum of a tablespoon or two a day is a sound guideline.

The first pressing of olives is done with gentle pressure, and temperatures produced are not much above room temperature. Oil thus extracted is sold as "extra virgin;" that from the next pressing is sold as "virgin." Oil from subsequent pressings of pulp and pits is processed with high heat and chemical solvents, and is sold as "pure" olive oil.

Vinegar and Lemon Juice

Because vinegar is so acidic, it does not spoil rapidly and requires no preservatives. Organic varieties of both brown rice vinegar and apple cider vinegar are available. Vinegar with olive oil is excellent on salads. In cooking soup bones, vinegar lends acidity to help leach calcium into the soup.

The lemon represents a compromise in a position against use of tropical and semitropical foods. A squeeze of lemon does much for fish, salad, or mineral water. The small amounts used have never been noted to cause the problems associated with using quantities of citrus fruit and juices.

Honey and Other Sweeteners

Because honey is a naturally occurring sweetener, many people think eating substantial quantities is beneficial, or at least harmless. Maple syrup is often thought of similarly, though what one buys has been concentrated by boiling the sap that flowed from the maple tree. Sweeteners such as molasses, brown sugar, corn syrup, dextrose, turbinado sugar, fructose (also called levulose, or fruit sugar), and others are often represented as being less harmful than sugar itself.

Of all these, only raw, unrefined honey is unconcentrated. Honeycomb, bee pollen, and royal jelly all have been shown to contain many vitamins, minerals, and other natural substances that may have medicinal qualities. Much has been written about the supposed and nearly magical qualities of honey and these other products of bees. Thus folklore and the inherent appeal of its sweet taste combine to make honey a most attractive food.

Honey contains the simple sugars fructose and glucose, and a sizable amount of sucrose. White sugar is nearly pure sucrose. Sucrose is rapidly broken down in the body to glucose and fructose. Glucose is the form of sugar circulating in the blood and used by cells of the body to produce energy; glucose and sucrose in foods both cause a rapid rise in blood sugar. Fructose is utilized in a slightly different manner and is thought to cause a somewhat less rapid rise in blood sugar (fructose, however, causes a more rapid increase in serum triglycerides and perhaps in uric acid).

In many people, particularly those using sweeteners habitually, a pronounced rise in blood sugar leads to a subsequent drop to below the normal fasting level. This is hypoglycemia, or low blood sugar. Weakness, fatigue, and a variety of other physical and mental symptoms may result.

All sweeteners, honey included, are more or less equally capable of causing low blood sugar. Furthermore, all usually exacerbate symptoms of whatever conditions may be present. Put simply, whatever is wrong, sweets of any kind make it worse. This includes not only the sweeteners listed, but also fruit juices and dried fruits.

The author has not seen an exception—substantial amounts of these concentrated sweets worsen one's condition. In relatively healthy individuals, a teaspoonful of honey—or sugar—or a baked sweet good ("natural" or otherwise) is harmless on occasion. In individuals with chronic conditions, even seemingly small amounts often cause a flare-up of symptoms. This may well be related to overgrowth of *Candida* (the yeast microorganism discussed in chapter 10) in many individuals with chronic diseases. Small amounts of sweets usually lead to larger, further insuring the provocation of symptoms. But the work of Dr. Melvin Page showed that even small amounts of sweeteners have dramatic effects on the blood.

Dr. Page, a dentist very knowledgeable in the field of nutrition, kept careful records of thousands of patients for many years. He studied relationships between dental decay, the ratio of calcium to phosphorous in the blood, and the ingestion of sweets. He found even a one-ounce dose of honey, fructose, or sucrose to have a pronounced effect on the ratio of calcium to phosphorus in the blood; sucrose had the most pronounced effect (fructose—fruit sugar—had the least). He found this ratio was invariably elevated in individuals developing dental decay.

This is interesting in light of Weston Price's discovery that the saliva in the mouths of decay-free native people had certain consistent characteristics in the ability to dissolve calcium and phosphorous—characteristics not found in the mouths of individuals eating refined foods. The calcium and phosphorous content of the saliva, of course, is directly influenced by the content of these two elements in the blood. Page's work thus directly complemented Price's—both men showed that disturbances of calcium and phosphorous metabolism occur in tooth decay. We may infer that these same disturbances effect the condition of the entire body.

Thus reasonable work has given indications why the human body reacts so poorly to sweets. Francis Pottenger's work demonstrated that gross skeletal changes occurred in cats fed sweetened foods—again we see disturbances of calcium and phosphorous metabolism.

What of the argument that honey is a natural food enjoyed by humans since the dawn of mankind? Likely true, but wild honey was generally a rare treat available in limited quantities, especially in more northern climates. The taste for sweets largely disappears in individuals not consuming them. Early humans probably had neither the desire nor the opportunity to use much honey. They likely learned this was a food to consume sparingly.

Herbs and Seasonings

Many organically grown fresh and dried herbs, seasonings, and spices are available; no problems have been observed with their use. Dried herbs are best purchased whole and then ground at home. Conventionally grown and produced ground herbs, seasonings, and spices contain some or all of the following: fillers, anticaking agents, artificial coloring, preservatives, monosodium glutamate (MSG), and pesticide residues. Reactions to these various extraneous substances may occur.

Culinary herbs go well with natural foods. Many commonly used herbs also have medicinal properties useful in helping alleviate symptoms of acute or chronic disease.

Black pepper is one seasoning best avoided; it irritates the intestinal tract. Cayenne red pepper, used in moderation, does not have this effect.

Salt.   The most commonly used and widely misunderstood seasoning is salt. Salt restriction is often advised for those with high blood pressure; this benefits some and not others. High blood pressure has many causes, and excessive salt is simply one contributory factor in some individuals. The foods eaten play an important role in the sodium content of the diet, for different natural foods vary widely in sodium content. Yet salt added to food in cooking and at the table weighs heavily in the total amount of salt consumed.

Foods of animal origin have much more sodium than vegetables, grains, and fruits. Humans require a minimum amount of sodium, thought to be from two to five grams per day (five grams is about a teaspoonful). If too little is supplied in food, some must be added; this biological necessity did much to determine where early agriculturists settled. A diet with any substantial amount of animal source foods includes adequate sodium, while a vegetarian or largely vegetarian diet must be supplemented with small amounts.

Few inland areas have readily accessible salt; the earliest farming villages tended to grow up around places that did. Cultures that did not often went to great lengths to get salt. Some Chinese drilled deep into mountains and with bamboo pipes brought up brine from salt deposits. Inland farmers in many places relied on river boats and caravans to bring salt. Salt in ancient times was the most valuable single commodity in commerce. At least one writer has pointed out that where salt was plentiful, democratic and independent societies tended to develop, and where it was scarce, those who controlled the salt controlled the people.

So salt has a history as old as mankind, and it is not necessarily an evil substance. The problem now is its high usage in processed foods. Canned vegetables, for example, have hundreds of times more sodium than fresh unsalted vegetables. Salt is added to nearly all processed foods; the taste buds grow used to it, and the unsalted comes to taste plain.

The typical American diet contains six times the salt of a typical hunter-gatherer diet, which is about one-third meat and two-thirds vegetable matter, usually with no added salt. In many hunter-gatherer and fishing cultures, however, some salt was used in drying and smoking game animals and fish, with no associated problems.

Individuals eating moderate to substantial amounts of animal source foods should not add salt to foods and should minimize use of heavily salted items such as pickles, olives, and canned fish. This is particularly important for those with chronic problems. The less animal source foods are eaten, the more appropriate the use of tamari or previously salted foods. Salt content in smoked fish and other salted foods varies greatly from product to product. In smoked fish, the subtler, more time-consuming smoking methods use considerably less salt.

Traditionally, soy sauce (also called tamari or shoyu) is made by allowing soybeans, and often wheat, to ferment in water and salt (in wooden barrels, often cedar). Organic brands are free of the additives, pesticide residues, and sugar found in conventionally produced soy sauce. A small amount—a teaspoonful or so—in vegetable soups, or on rice and vegetables, adds flavor and is especially appropriate on days when not much animal source food is eaten. Those choosing to eat little in the way of animal source foods may use up to a teaspoonful or two daily, depending on the condition and specific diet of the individual.

Alcoholic Beverages

A Few Words About Alcoholism.   In considering health effects of liquor, wine, and beer, one should remember these are not only drinks but also drugs. For many individuals, some combination of genetic and environmental influences makes alcohol in any form dangerous. The physical ravages of alcohol abuse are well known. More insidious are the mental processes involved, the ways in which addiction plays on the mind.

Alcoholism begins in the mind, though physiological idiosyncrasies may predispose some individuals. Ultimately alcohol takes over not only the mind but the body as well. The inclination for this particular form of self-abuse is stronger in some than others, but anyone drinking enough can become addicted to alcohol.

Recovery involves a commitment not only to stop drinking, but also to attempt to change certain aspects of personality that led to drinking. If such commitments are not made, the individual sooner or later drinks again. Actively seeking help through Alcoholics Anonymous provides the best chance of rehabilitation for the alcoholic ready to work at recovering. Though there is some debate, the vast majority of recovered alcoholics and counselors working with alcoholics believe that once an individual has been physically addicted to alcohol, he can never drink again without eventually drinking heavily. Acceptance of this is the first step in recovering from an acutely addicted state.

Most alcoholics deny to themselves and others any problem with alcohol. And if it's not a problem, why seek help? An anecdote popular amoung heavy drinkers sums up the attitude: "Who says I have a problem with alcohol? I get drunk, I fall down, I get up. No problem."

Nothing in this section on alcoholic beverages should be taken to mean those recovering from alcohol abuse should consider using small amounts of alcohol. The author wishes also to warn of the fine line that for many separates the regular use of small amounts of alcohol as a tasty beverage, relaxant, and mild mood enhancer, from the beginnings of dependence and eventual abuse.

If alcohol in any way prevents the achievement of goals and one's full potential to live happily, the line has been crossed. Addiction per se may not be present, but allowing a damaging drug to replace positive things in life reveals a weakness. It is a very human weakness—the simple desire to slip into a drug-induced state of relaxation, rather than using one's time to pursue active goals and find more positive ways to relax.

If alcohol plays a significant role in one's life, an honest examination of attitudes may be helpful. An experiment many people find enlightening involves abstinence from alcohol for a month. It is normal for even a light and occasional drinker to miss alcohol the first week or two. But the individual missing it more and more into the third and fourth weeks, and anxious for the month to pass, discovers alcohol apparently is quite important. Those without dependence generally do not miss alcohol by the end of the month and subsequently experience no particular desire to drink on other than special occasions.

Health Considerations. Some medical studies suggest people having a drink or two a day enjoy better health and live longer than those abstaining. Some enjoy citing this information while drinking two double scotches a night, with three or four ounces of whiskey in each. The studies, however, refer to standard one-ounce drinks, or the equivalent in beer or wine (a small glass of wine or a bottle of beer each contain less than an ounce of alcohol). Other more recent studies, however, indicate that no measurable health benefits are derived from alcohol.

Centenarians in Georgian Russian enjoy homemade vodka and wine. Both are made from unheated grapes and are rich in enzymes and minerals, while low in alcohol content. This is a most beneficial way to enjoy alcoholic beverages. Moderate use of alcohol is apparently not incompatible with a healthy and long life.

Though not recommended, even a somewhat immoderate use of alcohol may exist without extreme consequences. A case in point involves the lifelong history of a gentleman always fond of strong drink. About twelve years ago, he suffered considerably with repeated attacks of angina pectoris, chest pains thought to relate to spasms of the coronary arteries and relieved by nitroglycerine. He has since then followed many suggestions found in this book, eating fish several times a week, taking cod liver oil and vitamin E daily, and walking several miles most days (he gradually built up the walking). By no means a model patient, he eats a fair amount of refined foods, and daily, during the twelve years since the angina began, and for at least twenty-five before, he has had at least two or three and an average of five to six ounces of liquor—and sometimes more.

He has had no angina pain in over ten years, and he now is seventy-one years old. Medical textbooks state that on the average, a heart attack, often fatal, occurs within five years of the first symptoms of angina.

Liquor does the gentleman no good, and alas, he may drop dead tomorrow or show symptoms of chronic liver disease. But despite the limitations of his diet and the stress of excess alcohol, protective nutrients and regular exercise have enabled him not only to escape a heart attack but also to lead a fairly vigorous and active life. He is no genetic miracle, for his father died of a heart attack in his early sixties, and he himself while in his thirties suffered a mild and nearly symptomless stroke, from which he fully recovered. The point is that however one chooses to live, learning and applying a few age-old nutritional principles may enhance health and lengthen life.

Regular use of hard liquor is not a wise practice; the weight of physiological evidence indicates that, in all but the smallest amounts, alcohol acts as a poison. An individual not regularly drinking liquor notices a marked effect upon ingesting even an ounce or two, and continues to feel sluggish the next morning. Because alcoholic beverages are not regulated by the FDA, a wide variety of toxic ingredients found in liquor and in most wines and beers are not listed on the labels. These substances include ammonia, asbestos residues, coloring and flavoring agents, glycerin, hydrogen peroxide, lead residues, mineral oil, methylene chloride, plastic, pesticide residues, and sulfur compounds.

Many people enjoy an occasional beer, especially in hot weather. German law allows only the use of hops, malt, and water in the brewing process; imported German beers are thus quite pure. Some other imported beers (and several American beers also) are made from only natural ingredients without the use of chemicals or preservatives, as are a few American and imported wines.

Ingredients and equipment for making wine and beer at home are available. Unlike commercial beer, home brew need not be pasteurized before bottling; thus enzymes natural to the fermented raw product are left undisturbed. Advances in the equipment, techniques, and raw materials available have made it possible to home-brew beer healthier than any available commercially for a fraction of the cost. Carefully made, such beer may equal the taste of the finest imported beers.

Caffeine-Containing Drinks

Caffeine is found in coffee, cola drinks, and a number of nonprescription drugs. Closely related compounds include theobromine, found in chocolate and cocoa, and theophylline, found in tea. A twelve-ounce Coca Cola contains about the same amount of caffeine as a cup of instant coffee (about sixty-five milligrams), and a chocolate bar contains nearly half that amount of theobromine.

Intake of caffeine and related compounds above one's individual limit causes caffeinism. Extreme nervousness, poor sleep, abnormalities of the functioning of the heart, intestinal and stomach upset, and irritability are among possible symptoms, which are indistinguishable from those of anxiety neurosis. These symptoms may be evoked in adults by doses of caffeine and related compounds beginning at about two hundred milligrams a day—the amount found in three cups of instant coffee, or two cups of percolated coffee.

A seventy-pound child drinking one coke and eating one candy bar ingests nearly one hundred milligrams of caffeine and theobromine. By weight, his dose is equal to or greater than that of the adult consuming two hundred milligrams. Many children suffer from caffeinism, which may manifest as hyperactivity or other behavioral problems. Effects of caffeine and related compounds depend on the dose and on the weight and tolerance of the individual user.

Withdrawal symptoms occurring when frequent users stop ingesting caffeine include headaches and drowsiness. Nearly everyone stopping caffeine experiences these symptoms, often for as long as a week. Headaches usually begin within twenty-four hours of the last dose. Caffeine is a potent and highly addictive drug.

Caffeine aggravates ulcers (and other stomach and intestinal conditions) by increasing stomach acid secretions. Marked effects on the heart and circulatory system are likely why studies have shown coffee drinkers are at increased risk for heart attacks. Other studies have shown increased risks of pancreatic cancer and cancer of the bladder. Pregnant women are urged to curb caffeine consumption because caffeine enters the placenta and effects the growth and development of the fetus; several studies have linked birth defects with caffeine consumption.

Methylene chloride, commonly used to remove caffeine to make decaffeinated coffee, was found by government researchers to cause liver cancer in mice when given in high doses. An alternative method (the water-drip Swiss process) decaffeinates without use of methylene chloride or other carcinogenic chemicals.

Coffee is stimulating and imparts an alert and pleasant feeling. Driving on a long trip may be an occasion to use coffee to keep alert and avoid drowsiness; if driving all day, one might have three or four cups. Coffee in this situation has survival value—it makes one a better driver when attention to the road is required for several hours. One using coffee only on such occasions may find that the next day, the "high" feeling imparted by caffeine is missed, and one longs for a cup of coffee. The feeling passes within a day or so, but the experience helps one understand how people become addicted to caffeine.

By and large, coffee and caffeine are best avoided. Caffeine aggravates a wide variety of medical problems and is likely involved in the development of these problems as well.

Refined Flour and Sugar

How white flour and sugar adversely affect the human body has been detailed in many excellent books. The issue of why we go on using them long after we're fully aware of the effects is more difficult to understand.

The need to conform is real; we tend to comply with friends and social norms. We rationalize by calling foods we know weaken us a treat, then saying a little bit won't hurt. We realize regular use of all but the smallest amounts of liquor and foods containing refined flour and sugar is harmful; still we want them. Perhaps too many lives lack meaningful and exciting activities human beings have traditionally enjoyed, and as a substitute, food and drink become irrational entertainment. Though this is natural enough on occasion, there is little doubt we overdo it.

Life is change. Eating traditional foods consistently causes changes, among them a marked decrease in the desire for strong drink and foods with white flour and sugar. The reasons are physiological—the well-balanced body and mind have less desire for poor foods, and a rich supply of high quality animal source foods reduces the taste for sweets.

Most people find it easier to eat no sweets at all. When constantly trying to eat small amounts, one is always attempting to decide how much is too much. Memory of the sweet taste constantly lingers. A decision simply to be done with it ends daily decisions and mind games. Within a month or two one stops thinking about sweets as memory of the taste fades a bit. At this early stage, even a taste usually augments one's desire. Success comes only with continued abstinence; with time the taste for sweets is lost. Some even eventually find it possible to eat sweets occasionally with no thought of them the next day—if one still wants them at all. But for most, sweets are like Pandora's box—best not opened by mere mortals unless prepared for difficulty.

Meaningful and enjoyable activities—family life, time spent with friends, sports, hobbies, challenging work, gardening, hunting, fishing, a thousand other things—may replace the entertainment value often demanded of foods. Food is both a fuel and a pleasure, and the highest octane is necessary for maximum pleasure, not only in eating, but in all elements of life. One may love the foods one uses, and yet not hesitate to modify the diet as new things are learned.

Tastes grow accustomed to simple foods over time; the natural flavors of traditional food become more satisfactory than the salty and sweet tastes of refined food. The eating is enjoyable, but a greater pleasure lies in the performance of the body. Securing the best foods for self and family is the most basic and primitive element of life, the one from which all other functions were derived. Were this a priority for our culture, it would be a different world indeed.

One eating well need not be preoccupied with food; securing the finest foods becomes a reflex and a necessity. A number of things may be enjoyed as much as eating, and a few considerably more.

Everyone trying to eat a more natural diet goes through a process of learning not to want refined foods. Commitment and time are needed— and the realization that the products of factories and a poisoned agriculture are halfway foods, macabre and twisted perversions of the living foods nature designed the human body to thrive on.

Because we all have eaten so many of these halfway foods for much of our lives, the subject of the next chapter—vitamins, minerals, and food supplements—is of importance to many of us. Recognizing modern foods are lacking, we take supplements. Many of the most helpful supplements are concentrates of superior foods. Supplemental vitamins and minerals may often be of additional benefit, particularly when prescribed in conjunction with dietary changes. We will see, however, the problems inherent in relying upon pills to provide good nutrition.

22

Vitamins
Minerals
and Food Supplements

Vitamins in Foods Versus Laboratory Vitamins—
How Natural Are "Natural" Vitamins?

*V*itamins may be extracted from foods or synthesized in biochemical or biological processes. Some synthesized vitamins used in pills and added to many foods are not biochemically identical to their counterparts in nature.

An example is vitamin D$_2$, or irradiated ergosterol. Irradiation of primary grown yeast with ultraviolet light produces this compound. Since this is a "natural" process, irradiated ergosterol is often called a natural vitamin. It is added to milk, many other food products, and vitamin supplements, particularly those formulated without the use of animal products.

Irradiated ergosterol is not the same as vitamin D$_3$ produced in the body when ultraviolet light strikes the skin, and richly supplied in fish oils, milk fats from animals feeding on fresh greens, and liver. Nor does vitamin D$_2$ supply the complex of D vitamins found in these foods; indeed, it does not occur in nature. A synthesized biochemical approximation of D$_3$, vitamin D$_2$ has similar biological effects, but with subtle, little understood, yet highly significant biological differences (which were discussed in chapter 15).

The literature and labeling tactics of vitamin companies lead one to believe vitamins labeled "natural," "organic," or "from natural sources" are isolated from foods. This is the case for certain forms of vitamins A, D, and E, but except for the products of one or two companies, it is not so for the other vitamins. The exceptions are high priced and of low potency; they are actually food supplements which are rich in vitamins.

All other vitamins are manufactured—synthesized—by a few large companies (Hoffman La Roche and Eastman Kodak are two of the giants) in much the same manner. The companies then sell vitamins to other companies which formulate them into pills.

Deceptive labeling tactics are often used to trick consumers into thinking vitamins were derived from foods. Vitamin C, for example, might be labeled "ascorbic acid from sago palm." Dextrose, a form of sugar which contains no vitamin C at all, is extracted from sago palm and used as the base molecular material for a complex laboratory process that synthesizes vitamin C. Or the label might say "vitamin C derived from the finest natural sources." True, but the vitamin C was synthesized. It might also say "with rose hips and acerola," which are then used as the base material for the tablet or capsule. But a swallowable tablet of rose hips or acerola can contain a maximum of about 40 milligrams of truly natural vitamin C; the rest is synthesized.

Labels usually proclaim "natural" B vitamins to be derived from yeast. But companies manufacturing yeast add synthetic B vitamins to food fed to the yeast during its growth, and then fortify the yeast further with additional synthetic B vitamins when it has grown. This allows a yeast of any B vitamin potency desired to be produced and used to formulate vitamin pills with "B vitamins derived from yeast."

Nutritional yeast sold as a food supplement has nearly always been produced this way. Ammonia too is generally added to the growth medium of the yeast, just as it is used in chemical farming—as a nitrogen fertilizer to increase protein content in the finished product.

The different B vitamins used in these processes are all laboratory synthesized, with the occasional exception of vitamin B_{12}, which may be chemically refined from a bacteria. The only truly natural B vitamin supplements are dessicated liver and yeast grown without addition of B vitamins.

Vitamins A, D_3, and E are the only vitamins extracted from foods. Molecular distillation is used to extract A and D_3 from fish liver oils, and E from vegetable oils or by-products of their refinement. Synthesized vitamin E is different biochemically from natural vitamin E; the former is incompletely utilized by the body and may even disrupt the metabolism of natural vitamin E.

Antioxidants—Vitamin E, Vitamin C, and Selenium

Vitamin E.   Vitamin E is among the most important of nature's antioxidants; it protects cell membranes from a host of damaging events. The absence of whole grains and liver, traditional foods rich in vitamin E, from the modern diet has resulted in widespread deficiencies. Much evidence demonstrates this has significantly contributed to the modern epidemic of heart disease and other problems.

Vitamin E is the one vitamin or mineral the author regularly recommends in amounts well beyond those found in foods. Two hundred IU or more of supplemental vitamin E per day is appropriate for nearly everyone. Individuals with a history of hypertension should take only one hundred IU daily during the first month and monitor the blood pressure; this vitamin sometimes raises it a bit initially. This is thought to be due to strengthening effects upon the heart.

Vitamin E also helps protect fats in cells throughout the body from oxidizing effects of free radicals, molecules thought to be involved in the development of chronic degenerative diseases (particularly heart disease and cancer), as well as in the aging process itself. Many modern foods, particularly vegetable oils high in unsaturated fats, increase free radical formation, as do food additives, pesticide residues, and air pollutants.

Eating refined foods during a considerable part of one's life creates a chronic deficiency of vitamin E. How much supplemental vitamin E is ideal is difficult to determine. The RDA of eleven to fifteen IU was arrived at by averaging the amount found in the diets of several thousand people surveyed; it reflects the modern norm rather than an optimal intake. Price's immune groups consumed at least ten times the amount of both fat-soluble and water-soluble vitamins modern diets provide—and their air was clean. Known functions of vitamin E, and the poor quality of modern air (particularly city air), imply that ten times the RDA should prudently be considered a minimal intake.

Several fractions of vitamin E occur in foods; the alpha is the most active, at least in protecting the heart and circulatory system. Other fractions, however, are thought by some biochemists to be equally important in protecting against oxidative processes involved in the aging of cells. Certainly the beta, gamma, and delta fractions would not complement the alpha in the body and in foods without a purpose. Vitamin E containing all of these fractions is called mixed tocopherols.

Expect to pay more for natural vitamin E, be it alpha tocopherol alone or mixed tocopherols, than for synthetic. Mixed tocopherols are always natural. Synthetic vitamin E is labeled "d,l-alpha tocopherol," and is a mixture of the "d" and "l" forms. Only the "d" form is found naturally in foods and the human body. Labels on both natural and synthetic forms must list the amount of alpha tocopherol present; with the synthetic, half of the listed amount is the "l" form. Vitamin E labeled "d-alpha tocopherol" is natural and contains only the alpha fraction.

Vitamin C.   Vitamin C is another antioxidant which may be judiciously supplemented at times. Hunter-gatherer diets provide an estimated four hundred milligrams daily, similar to that found in any traditional diet rich in greens, sprouts, and raw foods. Those in urban areas might best double that amount as protection against pollutants.

Selenium.   Selenium is a trace mineral with antioxidant properties; it too is poorly supplied in modern foods. Selenium functions together with vitamin E in many biochemical processes. The importance of selenium's role in protecting against cancer and other chronic diseases and the lack of selenium in modern foods has been well documented by Richard Passwater in his 1977 book, *Selenium as Food and Medicine*. Regular use of a modest amount as a supplement—one hundred to two hundred micrograms per day—is prudent as a means of bringing up the body's reserves. Seafood and organ meats are rich sources.

Food Supplements

Food supplements may be used in lieu of vitamin and mineral pills to provide nutrients for individuals with special needs, and more generally to provide enhanced nutrition by supplying nutrients lacking in modern foods.

Food supplements are concentrates designed for regular use as a supplement to the diet. Most are dried foods or extracts. Examples are cod liver oil, dried kelp (in the form of tablets or powder), dessicated liver tablets and other dried organ concentrates, bone meal, and lecithin granules. High quality food supplements are an excellent means of supplying specific nutrients.

Cod Liver Oil.   The most important of these special foods is cod liver oil. Lack of nutrients found in fish oils is a major reason most Americans suffer with symptoms caused by faulty mineral metabolism, for certain of these nutrients help control mineral metabolism. Eicosapentaenoic acid (EPA), deficient in modern foods, is also concentrated in fish oils. Details on the use of cod liver oil may be found in chapter 7.

Calcium.   Special foods rich in calcium and other minerals, for example organic bone meal and oyster shell calcium, may be used in conjunction with cod liver oil in helping to correct problems with mineral metabolism. Amounts recommended vary with the diet and needs of each individual. Generally, if one does not consume significant amounts of certified raw milk or raw milk cheeses, bones, or egg shells, up to one thousand milligrams of supplemental calcium should be taken daily.

A substantial amount of calcium is consumed in traditional diets. Our hunter-gatherer ancestors ate at least twice the calcium we do, and usually much more. Agricultural cultures were richly supplied with calcium in raw dairy products and green vegetables. Use of animal bones in making soups and stews is universally practiced by traditional cultures. Immune groups Weston Price studied ate from four to eight times the present Recommended Daily Allowance (RDA) of eight hundred milligrams. A recent USDA survey revealed a majority of Americans fall short of even the RDA.

Iodine.   Another nutrient in short supply in the diet of many Americans is iodine. Price found people in immune groups invariably consumed many times the trace amounts found in most American diets and recommended by the government.

Much of our food is iodine poor because it is produced far from the oceans. Historically, goiter belts throughout the world have occurred in inland areas—regions where a substantial part of the population suffered from the enlarged thyroid gland resulting when the gland grows in an attempt to utilize what little iodine is present in the diet.

Goiter is a symptom of hypothyroidism or myxedema—chronic, grossly low thyroid function. Iodized salt has helped alleviate the problem, but many Americans suffer from chronic subclinical low thyroid function, not necessarily so marked as to cause a goiter or be detected by blood tests, but nonetheless causing symptoms and contributing to the development of chronic diseases. Eating liberal amounts of foods rich in iodine—seafood and sea vegetables—guards against this. Supplemental kelp tablets or powder may also be used to supply iodine and trace minerals found in the sea.

Other Concentrates and Extracts.   Other special foods used at times include raw glandular products (liver, heart, brain, and others glands prepared from naturally raised animals by freeze-drying, thus preserving enzyme content), alfalfa tablets, lecithin granules, and marine lipid concentrate, rich in EPA and DHA.

Megavitamin Supplements Versus Traditional Foods

Vitamins are sometimes used in concentrations hundreds of times greater than found in foods. When taken in large doses, vitamins are being used for drug-like effects—effects beyond those caused by the normal amounts of vitamins supplied in foods. At what level of supplementation such effects may be said to begin is somewhat arbitrary, varies for different vitamins and individuals, and even varies in an individual as his needs change.

Generally, however, when vitamins or minerals are taken in amounts more than ten times the recommended daily allowance, the possibility they may have drug-like effects must be considered. Traditional diets contain at least this amount of vitamins and minerals, but in the balanced form natural to foods. A few individuals because of biochemical individuality require large amounts of certain vitamins, the lack of which in them may lead to disease; while large doses of required vitamins may be of benefit, the needs of such individuals usually are best met with an optimal traditional diet.

Even when megavitamin therapy (supplementation beyond ten times the RDA) does give relief to an overriding symptom, other problems correctable only by superior nutrition remain. Though borderline vitamin and mineral deficiencies are common and lead to many symptoms and diseases, attempts to balance the effects of eating fragmented foods with large doses of synthesized vitamins and extracted minerals provide at best limited relief. For recovery, the natural vitamins, minerals, enzymes, and associated nutrients found in high quality whole foods are necessary. While some synthesized vitamins, particularly the B vitamins and vitamin C, are biochemically equivalent to their natural counterparts in foods, biochemical differences exist for others, some of which were discussed above.

Beyond known biochemical differences, one may question the ability of laboratory chemists to manufacture nutrients with the same effects as those in foods. What of unknown synergistic effects of other nutrients associated with vitamins in foods? Clinical experience confirms that a large intake of vitamin pills is usually to no avail; when the pills stop and the proper foods begin, recovery begins.

Research into possible long-term effects of taking man-made or extracted vitamins in potencies far beyond those in foods is sparse. Vitamin companies certainly are not doing any. Though little is known, we do know dependencies develop in at least some circumstances. Pregnant women taking large doses of vitamin C may cause scurvy to develop in the child after birth by creating a dependence in the foetus. Vitamin B complex deficiencies may be similarly created. This causes one to pause before using or recommending large doses of vitamins, though at times large doses may be helpful. Certain problems in pregnancy, for example, respond well to megadoses of vitamin B₆—though the problems are better solved with proper diet. Megadoses of vitamin E may be of great benefit in heart disease. And the use of vitamins C and E and of several food supplements rich in vitamins, minerals, and other nutrients may be an integral part of a program aiming to neutralize the effects of environmental pollutants and optimize health.

Minerals are elements, and as such cannot be synthesized; whatever the source, calcium is calcium. The way in which minerals are biochemically arranged with other molecules is thought to be of importance in the way they are absorbed, transported, and utilized, and a wide range of prices exist for mineral supplements formulated in different ways.

Mineral supplements should not be taken in amounts beyond ten times the RDA, and even ten is rather high. Most supplements are designed to supply amounts roughly equivalent to the RDA's, though some contain more. Modern diets are often deficient in minerals, and while supplementation may be of benefit, it should be approached cautiously. Disproportionate supplements of one or several minerals may disrupt the body's mineral balance. Using special foods and food supplements rich in minerals and natural vitamins is the superior way to supply the body in need with these nutrients. Many nutrients impossible to identify, formulate, extract, and encapsulate are then consumed.

Traditional foods diets supply optimal amounts of all vitamins, minerals, and associated substances, known and unknown, in the exact balance and proportions nature has designed over the ages. Vitamin and mineral supplements used in conjunction with such diets may be of additional benefit, especially in an individual depleted of reserves by years of inadequate diet. Sometimes specific problems respond more quickly when vitamin and mineral supplements addressing specific needs are used.

Relief occurring through vitamin and mineral supplementation alone is incomplete, however. An individual may achieve marked relief from particular symptoms, but unless the diet is corrected, other imbalances soon occur, and with them, other problems. Supplements are best used only in conjunction with proper diet, even in treatment of problems which may be aided somewhat with supplements alone. A deeper and more lasting healing occurs when recovery is based on multiple factors present in proper foods rather than on a particular ingredient the body is most obviously and sorely lacking. Traditional foods are indeed your best medicine.

Epilogue

Toward a Philosophy of Natural Living

As a child, I loved animal stories, especially those by a turn of the century chronicler of the Indians and wildlife of North America, Ernest Thompson Seton. Years later, these words of Seton were rediscovered in a little book entitled *The Gospel of the Red Man:* "The culture of the Red man is fundamentally spiritual; his measure of success is, 'How much service have I rendered my people.'"

Such a philosophy may be the foundation of a natural way of life and the basis of happiness. Health and inner peace reflect and are reflected by a helpful and cooperative attitude. This is not to say we should not be well rewarded in our work for our helpfulness and our cooperation. If we are not, how may we well serve our families and friends?

But we serve ourselves and our people best when our considerations are not overly material. Good food is expensive; so is a pleasant home and land in a clean environment. These things we have a real need for, and it takes money to buy them. But chasing dollars to purchase many of the amenities of civilization is a questionable pursuit. Might we be happier in the garden, taking a walk, chopping wood, or playing with children, than watching television? Could the money used for an expensive car be better spent? Are our many possessions worth the time away from simpler pursuits—time which could be spent with family and friends, at hobbies, learning, playing sports?

People of earlier cultures developed highly accurate prescriptions for living happy and healthy lives, lives generally untroubled by the depression, loneliness, and personal turmoil marking many lives today. From these people, from men and women who studied and lived among them, and from healers who have understood, followed, and taught nature's laws, we have had passed on to us certain truths about food, attitudes, and ways of life that may enable us to live in relative health and happiness, despite the turmoil we see about us.

"Most men," Winston Churchill once wrote, "occasionally stumble over the Truth, but most pick themselves up and continue on as if nothing had happened."

Information is of little value until and unless it leads to action. Developing one's own philosophy of natural living can only come with attempts to live by principles judged reasonable. Choice must be followed by commitment. The reward may be one's own unique and satisfying way of coping happily with the modern world, one I personally would find overwhelming were it not for the semblance of understanding gained from studying our past.

Appendix 1

Seafood
Characteristics
and Habitat of
Popular Fish and Shellfish

This appendix presents information about seafoods useful in understanding and selecting fish and shellfish for both enjoyment and maximal health benefits. Particular attention is paid to the issue of how one may determine which species, and individuals within a species, are likely to have been least affected by water pollution. Consideration also is given to the relative amount of fats found in different species, to aid in judging which may be richest in EPA and other marine lipids. There are sections on saltwater fish, shellfish, and freshwater fish, with listings in each arranged alphabetically. Raw fish, smoked fish, roe, stocks, and preservatives sometimes used on fresh fish and shellfish are discussed in the final section of this appendix.

Much of the information in this section is distilled from A.J. McClane's *The Encyclopedia of Fish Cookery*, a beautifully photographed and written reference work by one of the world's true experts on seafood.

SALTWATER FISH

Anchovies

Anchovies are often seen along the seashore traveling with other small fish, including silversides and small herring. The canned product is heavily salted, packed in oil, and sometimes smoked. A rich and distinct flavor is characteristic.

Bluefish

Like tuna, swordfish, and striped bass, bluefish is a fatty Atlantic Ocean species known to concentrate pollutants in fatty tissues; polychlorinated biphenols (PCB's) have been found in blues in recent years. An oceangoing species, bluefish also spend considerable time close to shore. Accounts written one hundred years ago describe multitudes of bluefish in inlets and harbors of New York and New Jersey, and even today they arrive in coastal northeastern waters in legion numbers every fall. Their razor sharp teeth are designed for predation; because they live on other fish, they concentrate the small amounts of PCB's found in smaller fish.

But the life habits of bluefish are such that for several months of the year on the East coast, uncontaminated bluefish are available. Blues migrate from south to north in spring and summer and reverse direction in fall and winter, ranging from Florida to New England. Particularly in spring, baby bluefish are caught on the Carolina coasts and shipped north where they are filleted and sold. These fish often weigh less than a pound and have lived in clean waters. Blues found to be contaminated were larger and taken in more northern waters, particularly along the New Jersey coast.

Bluefish may be strongly flavored; small young fish are less so. Like all highly predacious fish, blues contain enzymes that spoil the meat rapidly if the fish is left ungutted without ice for a few hours. And the high oil content necessitates particular care when they are shipped. When well cared for, these fish cook to a soft texture, with a long flake, and an unmistakably distinct flavor. Broil bluefish enough to flake cleanly; broiling one side for a few minutes in a hot oven suffices for small ones, while larger fish require baking, or broiling both sides a few minutes each. Blues also sauté nicely; try this with butter, onions or garlic, white wine, tamari (soy) sauce, and seasonings.

Butterfish

So called because of the high fat content, butterfish is found in both of our oceans and the Gulf of Mexico. Butterfish is reasonably priced, and when taken in clean waters is an excellent find. The flesh is firm, large-flaked, and sweet. A mixture of oil and water rich in fatty acids comes off in cooking; it may be used on rice or vegetables, or in soup. The Pacific species is sometimes marketed as Pacific pompano. Butterfish are small, generally under twelve inches, and are sold as fillets.

The Cod Family

An extension of the Continental Shelf, the Grand Banks are a series of shoals running about four hundred miles from the southeast coast of Newfoundland to Georges Bank east of Massachusetts. Warm Gulf Stream waters meet the cold Labrador Current along the Banks; the resulting plankton growth forms the basis of the ocean ecology that has supplied countless fish to both sides of the North Atlantic for hundreds of years. Cod, haddock, pollock, and halibut form the bulk of the fish taken; all but halibut are members of the cod family.

A constant fog is created by the meeting of the warm and cold currents, and the shallowness of the banks (average depth two hundred feet) builds huge seas. Many men have died catching cod for the world's dinner tables. For centuries, cod was a staple throughout the northern rim of the Atlantic, cooked fresh every conceivable way, made into chowders, cakes, and puddings, or salt-preserved for months. The entire fish was used; the roe, cheeks, tongue, and air bladder were considered delicacies. The liver and its oil have for centuries been used medicinally.

Cod was so important economically that for centuries it was found on coins, corporate seals, letterheads, legal documents, stamps, and even wind vanes. And of course, we have Cape Cod.

Cod is a lean fish. The flesh is firm and white and will flake cleanly apart along lines of cleavage as soon as it has been cooked through. The head, liver, and roe all make excellent eating.

Cod is actually a family of fish; the major members are the Atlantic cod, haddock, hake, and pollock. The Atlantic cod is by far the most numerous, and the one most commonly referred to as cod. The largest recorded weighed over two hundred pounds, caught in 1895 off the Massachusetts coast.

Today, cod over ten pounds are graded large. Those weighing 1 1/2 to 2 1/2 pounds are called scrod; their mild flavor make scrod broiled with butter and lemon juice one of the easiest fish for an unenthusiastic fish-eater to enjoy. Broil fillets in a very hot oven for just a few minutes, until the flesh just flakes apart with the touch of a fork. Small fillets need not be turned over. The flesh is delicate and tender, the flavor, mild with a touch of sweetness. There is not a hint of the strong fishy taste oilier species may have when not completely fresh and properly prepared.

Haddock is similar in both appearance and taste to cod, but generally smaller, usually weighing from two to five pounds. Like cod, it is a deep water species. Hake is even smaller, generally less than two pounds; the flesh is coarser and somewhat stronger tasting. Pollock has a similar taste and generally weighs four to five pounds; it is sometimes called Boston bluefish.

Cod and these other members of the cod family fulfill the author's criteria for healthy eating—they are of moderate size and thus fairly low on the food chain, and they spend most or all of their lives far out at sea. Two members of the cod family not recommended are ling cod (burbot), a freshwater fish found mainly in deep lakes and in some rivers, and tomcod, a small shallow water coastal fish caught mainly in brackish estuaries and rivers.

Dolphin (Mahimahi)

Not to be confused with the fascinating and often entertaining mammalian dolphin (a member of the porpoise family), this fish has a magnificence of its own. The author remembers well watching them caught on a fishing boat off the coast of Florida when he was a boy. Leaping high above the ocean's surface when hooked, the dolphin, often three to four feet long, flashed brilliant greens, yellows, and shades of red as they fought for freedom. Occasionally one would escape, throwing the hook; for these beautiful fish, one could not help but feel glad. Most, though, were drawn inexorably to the side of the vessel where a waiting crewman would pierce the loin with a gaff and toss the fish unceremoniously on the deck. Writhing, thrashing, slowly losing the rainbow colors that come when dolphin are feeding or excited, the dolphin died on the deck. Catching dolphin is for many a bittersweet experience.

No mixed feelings are experienced, however, when it comes to the eating. Dolphin meat is wonderful—white, firm, moist, and sweet. A wide-ranging species found in tropical and subtropical seas the world over, dolphin was almost never seen in markets until recent appearances on the west coast; it is now shipped in from Hawaii, where it is called mahimahi. Market fish, however, have never matched those caught off that Florida boat. Dolphin is unique; try it if it is good and fresh.

Flounder—see Sole and Flounder

Halibut

The four species of commercial importance in America are actually members of the flounder family. The best are the Atlantic and the Pacific halibut, similar fish with firm, delicately flavored white meat. These flatfish can grow to over six hundred pounds, but today halibut over three hundred are rarely caught. The Atlantic halibut ranges from waters off New Jersey northward, the Pacific species from central California northward. Cool, deep ocean is their habitat; seldom do they enter waters shallower than two hundred feet.

The Greenland halibut is inferior in texture and flavor to Atlantic and Pacific halibut. The dense musculature is not bad when cooked slowly in a fish soup, but it becomes dry and tough under direct heat. Sometimes inaccurately sold as "turbot," this fish ranges over Arctic and sub-Arctic regions of the Atlantic and the Pacific, going no further south than Cape Cod in the East and southern California in the West.

The California halibut is found from central California to northern Mexico. The meat is similar to the Pacific halibut but less tasty. It is much smaller, usually weighing between four and twelve pounds.

Herring

Vegetarians that feed on tiny plankton and migrate widely in huge schools far out at sea, herring were once the world's most abundant food fish. So great was their commercial importance that wars were fought over control of the Baltic Sea's herring grounds. The Hanseatic League, formed by merchants from the Hansa towns of northern Germany, controlled these grounds in the late 1300's; some forty thousand boats fished the Baltic then, until the herring population center moved to the North Sea, likely because of depletion. Well into the nineteenth century, much of the history of northern Europe, England, Newfoundland, Spain, and Portugal was influenced by conflicts over the herring trade. More recently, conflict over exploitation by fleets of ships from the Soviet Union and other Communist countries led the United States in 1977 to extend coastal control of fishing rights to two hundred miles.

Two species of herring are of prime commercial importance. The Atlantic herring is found on both sides of the North Atlantic and as far south as North Carolina. The Pacific herring is found throughout the northern Pacific, and as far south as northern California. Typical length seen at market is ten inches, though herring grow to about eighteen and a weight of a pound and a half. The Pacific species spawns in shallow bay waters, while the Atlantic spawns offshore at depths down to one hundred feet.

Fresh herring is relished in Europe, but here there is little demand and usually it is seen pickled in wine sauce or sour cream. Fresh herring is prime when fat content is highest, about 15 percent in peak season, which varies in different seas. That sold in markets here has generally been imported frozen from Iceland.

Two other types of herring that enter rivers and streams in eastern America to spawn in spring and summer are the alewife and the blueback herring. Very similar, they are not nearly so tasty as Atlantic and Pacific herring. In New England, smoked alewives are sold as corned alewives when packed in brine, and as pickled alewives when packed in vinegar cure.

Herring have been packed in metal containers for well over one hundred years. Herring two to three inches long are referred to as sardines; many brands packed in olive oil are imported from southern Europe, but they are heavily salted, and the olive oil is not of the highest quality.

Mackerel

Many mackerel species occur in both the Atlantic and Pacific Oceans. Mackerel rapidly lose flavor if not iced immediately upon being caught.

Quite oily, they are rich in EPA. Fat content varies with species and is highest in autumn.

Mackerel has in common with tuna distinctly separate red and white musculature. The outer lateral band of red meat is composed primarily of slow twitch muscle fibers which sustain continuous swimming; these pelagic species never stop. The inner portion of lighter colored meat is composed primarily of fast twitch fibers which provide bursts of speed. The red and white layers correspond respectively with the fibers in a human being's muscles that adapt to endurance exercises such as long distance running and to power exercises such as weight lifting or sprinting; but in humans the fibers are intermixed.

Atlantic mackerel, found from Newgoundland to Cape Hatteras, is the most common northern species. Atlantic and king mackerel have more red muscle, are fattier, and are more strongly flavored than other popular species. King mackerel, commonly called kingfish, ranges from North Carolina to Brazil, and reaches 100 pounds. Twenty to forty pound fish are commonly caught off party boats in southern waters; great fighters, big kings are quite a thrill to land.

Kings are good eating. Their southern range keeps them clear of more polluted northeastern coastal waters. They may be filleted or cut into steaks; to minimize the oil flavor, marinate in lime juice and a little tamari for a few hours and then broil with butter.

More delicately flavored mackerel include cero, Spanish mackerel, and wahoo. All are leaner and have less red muscle than Atlantic and king. Cero and Spanish mackerel range north to Cape Cod. Cero are generally marketed in the five to ten pound range, Spanish, in the two to four pound range.

Wahoo is leanest of the three and largest, averaging thirty pounds when caught. Known in Hawaii as "ono," which means sweet, wahoo are found in all tropical and subtropical seas and have white, softly textured flesh. Seldom caught in adequate numbers for marketing, wahoo is considered by gourmets to be among the finest eating fish in the world.

Pompano

Pompano is considered by some connoisseurs the finest saltwater fish. Seldom over two pounds, with firm, delicate white flesh, they range as far north as Massachusetts, but are most popular along the southern Atlantic and Gulf coasts. A larger but very similar fish called the permit is sometimes seen in northeastern markets; when weighing less than about eight pounds, they are similar in taste to pompano.

Salmon

Sculpted in the floor of the Grotte du Poisson near Les Eyzies, France, is a carefully detailed bas-relief of a salmon done by an ancient caveman. Salmon bones have been found in caves used by Old Stone Age man twenty-five thousand years ago. North American Indians of the Columbia River basin in prehistoric Oregon thirteen thousand years ago had ceremonies honoring the salmon; the fish played an important role in their mythology. The people of these disparate cultures did not need the discovery of EPA to make salmon central in their nutrition and their lives.

There are seven distinct species of salmon. Born in rivers, all spend most of their lives at sea before returning to the river of birth to spawn. Salmon do not eat during the trip upriver and the flesh becomes pale and waterlogged. Fish caught and eaten fresh, or canned near the end of this trip, are distinctly less flavorful than those caught in open sea or earlier on the upriver journey.

Only Atlantic salmon are native to the Atlantic Ocean. Once abundant in rivers of northeastern America, Canada, and Europe, the Connecticut River salmon had been eliminated by dams and pollution from sewage and textile mills by 1815. Fisheries throughout New England followed, and by the 1870's even the rivers of northern Maine had been suffocated in sawdust and effluents of the lumber industry. The Atlantic salmon was largely gone from America; only a few remain in rivers in northeast Maine. Industrialized Europe suffered the same fate. Atlantic salmon in American markets are mostly from Canada and rural areas of Europe.

There are five North American Pacific salmon. Chinook or king is the largest (recorded up to 120 pounds), the fattiest (about 16 percent fat when prime), and the tastiest. When ocean caught, the flesh is deep red, rich in oil, and soft in texture. Coho or silver salmon is much smaller, often caught in the five to ten pound range. Their flesh is pink to red, but always lighter and less oily than that of king, though their flavors are comparable. Sockeye or red salmon, also called blueback, usually has deep orange-red flesh nearly as oily as that of king and a delicate flavor. Sockeye and king are the most expensive salmon; coho is a little less so.

Chum and pink salmon are lowest in fat content, most reasonably priced, and least flavorful. There is a dramatic difference between their taste and that of king, coho, or sockeye. Unspecified canned salmon invariably is chum or pink. Quality of canned salmon varies widely with the time of year the fish was caught, and is usually reflected by price.

Gonads of the male (white roe) and bright orange roe of the female may be lightly poached, eaten raw, or made into a caviar substitute. Rich in iodine and enzymes, roe were a staple of native Americans, especially children and pregnant women.

The bones, head, and skin may be used to make fish soup or stock. If the fish is baked or grilled whole, a smallish piece of meat just beneath the gillcover may be eaten; it has a delicate, slightly sweet, unique flavor.

Salmon is as rich in eicosapentaenoic acid (EPA) as any fish readily available. Most of its life is spent far out in northern seas, away from areas of coastal pollution. Smaller salmon, five to ten pounds, are quite low on the food chain and not as likely to concentrate pollutants as the larger king salmon. Fresh coho (silver) and small king are available throughout the Pacific Northwest and are widely shipped. Except in the Pacific Northwest, fresh sockeye is seldom seen. Fresh Atlantic salmon from Canada and Europe are widely available in the northeast. Both coho and sockeye are generally good canned, though canned salmon does not compare with fresh.

Sardines

The word sardines refers to small fish from any of several species, including two to three inch long herring, pilchards, and sprat. Sprat is called brisling sardines.

The Maine coast is the chief source of sardines in America, where in most places they are found only canned and packed in soybean oil, olive oil, or mustard sauce. An imported variety packed in sild (the Scandinavian word for herring) sardine oil is found in some markets, lightly smoked and salted. Sild oil is not too strong and is tasty on salads with vinegar and a little olive oil, and it is rich in the unsaturated fatty acids concentrated in fish oils. Sardines may also be found packed in water.

As is often the case with herring, whitebait, smelts, and alewife, when one eats sardines, one eats internal organs, skin, and bones; they are thus rich in certain nutrients, especially nucleic acids, found only in small quantities in most other foods. Raw shellfish also provide such nutrition, and additionally provide enzymes found only in raw foods.

Sardines were a major item in Dr. Benjamin Frank's "no aging diet," popularized in his book of that title several years ago. His thesis is that sardines and other foods rich in nucleic acids —shellfish and organ meats in particular—help slow down the aging process.

Sea Trout

Sea trout are brown trout that spend most of their lives at sea. More numerous in northern Europe, small numbers breed in Canadian and American rivers, and fish in the three to ten pound range occasionally appear in New England markets. The meat is similar to salmon, pink to red, quite fatty, and very tasty. The name is not to be confused with seatrout (one word), which refers to several members of an entirely different family of fish, the drum family.

Shad

Shad enter coastal rivers and bays seasonally on both coasts. Native to the east coast, shad run there from December in the south, to May in the north. This member of the herring family has been introduced on the west coast and now thrives from central California into British Columbia. The Columbia River run supplies a large market in May and June.

Shad typically weigh one to three pounds. The meat is white, sweet, and tasty, and the roe are considered a delicacy. As with all anadromous fish, the quality of the river water in which these fish are born and spend much of their lives affects the quality of the fish.

Shark

Shark and swordfish taste similar; mako shark is often substituted for swordfish. While the flavor and texture are similar, the flesh of mako is more whitish than the pinkish gray of sword. Both the blacktip shark of semi-tropical waters and the blue shark have snow white meat. The dogfish shark has been likened to halibut, and indeed the dogfish is called harbor halibut along the coast of Maine.

England's famous fish and chips is most commonly made with shark, often the spiny dogfish or the porbeagle. Shark has always been popular in most parts of the world and remains so today, though not in America. Even here, however, prices have risen, indicating increased demand. But at less than half the price of swordfish, mako remains a bargain.

Soaking the flesh in either an acid or a salt solution before cooking is the key to enjoying shark. The flesh has a high concentration of urea; this is one reason the meat, which overlies a skeleton of cartilage, does not keep long. Enzymes convert urea to ammonia, which strongly flavors the fish if allowed to remain. Soaking steaks or fillets in a salt or vinegar solution leaches out the ammonia. Use half a pound of salt to a gallon of water to submerge a large fillet or several steaks, and soak for several hours. Alternatively, lemon or lime juice, or vinegar with water, may be used to marinate small pieces for several hours prior to cooking or use as sushi or sashimi. Like swordfish, the meat is firm and excellent raw; when cooked, it is best broiled.

Smelt

Like salmon and striped bass, smelt once entered hundreds of rivers and bays on both coasts, coming seasonally in legion numbers each year to breed. To a lesser extent, these small anadromous fish still do, though they no longer abound in waters along the shores of Manhattan and Boston's Back Bay as they did in the latter half of the nineteenth century.

In many of the rivers where smelt still run, the waters are heavily polluted. Rainbow smelt is most common in American waters. Found on both coasts, populations exist also in the Great Lakes and in lakes across New England, New York, and southeastern Canada. Oceangoing fish enter rivers and bays in the spring.

The eulachon is the variety of smelt important in the Pacific Northwest, from Oregon to Alaska. The Kwakiutl Indians of coastal British Columbia, said to have been a strong and healthy people, used eulachon in some manner at every meal. In winter, the fish and its oil were mixed with summer-cut greens as a fishcake. Eulachon is also called candlefish; it is so oily the Indians dried the fish and, with a cedar bark wick, used them as candles.

Eulachon is marketed both fresh and smoked. On the west coast the surf smelt, a smaller and less oily fish, and several other varieties of smelt sold as whitebait are also marketed.

Smelt is usually sold in the six to eight inch range, frozen or fresh. They are easily cooked and eaten ungutted, with heads, tails, and organs; cook as with whitebait. The uninitiated will find this is most easily done with the smaller fish.

Snapper

Fifteen snapper species are found in American waters from North Carolina to Texas. Red snapper, the most popular, is found in the Pacific as well. The habitat of snapper is coastal waters sixty to two hundred feet deep. Fish seen at market usually weigh four to six pounds.

Red snapper is quite lean. Texture and fat content are similar to that of small cod. The flavor, though stronger than cod, is still quite mild.

Yellowtail is considered by many the most finely flavored snapper. Distinctively different from other snapper (it is of a different genus), the meat is white, sweet, and finely flaked. Freshly caught yellowtail—it loses its flavor quickly—is a favorite in many fine restaurants on Florida's Atlantic coast and on the Gulf from Key West to Texas.

Sole and Flounder

Flounder is the term for any one of three families of flatfish in the Atlantic and Pacific Oceans; over two hundred species are represented. Fish referred to as sole in America are actually varieties of flounder, as are halibut. The only members of the true sole family found in American waters are tiny and of no economic importance. But several of our flounder—in particular, lemon sole, gray sole, and Rex sole—are similar to the European dover sole (a true sole) used for classic fillet of sole dishes.

One last point of confusion—dover sole is also the common name of a species of Pacific flounder found from California to Alaska and widely sold in western America. Having distinguished sole from flounder from halibut, we turn now to individual species.

Winter flounder is the most abundant and popular flatfish in eastern America. This fish is marketed as flounder if weighing three pounds or less, and as lemon sole if weighing more. The meat is very sweet, finely flaked and, especially in the smaller sizes, fragile in texture. This is fish people often say doesn't taste like fish.

Delicate texture and flavor have made European dover sole and North American winter flounder, gray sole, and Rex sole central in seafood creations of chefs. Spices, herbs, sauces, fruits and vegetables, and contrasting seafoods are used with these fish to create scores of entrées.

Winter flounder ranges from Newfoundland south to the Chesapeake Bay, in coastal zones and bays as well as in deeper offshore grounds. Fish caught generally range in size from one to five pounds.

Much of this fish's habitat is polluted waters, but it is low in fat, and pollutants in fish concentrate in the fats. Still, a flounder spending half its life in a northern New Jersey bay carries highly undesirable substances. Winter flounder range widely; wherever caught, they spent a good part of life in shallow coastal waters of unknown quality.

Summer flounder, marketed as fluke, is similar in texture and taste to winter flounder, though somewhat larger. It too is a shallow water species, as is its smaller cousin the southern flounder, caught from North Carolina to Texas.

American plaice, marketed as dab, sanddab, long rough-dab, and rough-back, ranges from Cape Cod to the Grand Banks and across the Atlantic to Europe. This deepwater flounder is found at depths from 120 to 2,000 feet. The usual market fish weighs from two to three pounds. Their small size, deepwater habitat, and a northern range along lightly populated coasts combine to make this fish ideal food. This important commercial species is generally available in northeastern United States.

Petrale sole, rex sole, butter sole, sand sole, and Dover sole are among the Pacific varieties of flounder, in the order of usual ranking for flavor. All range north as far as Alaska. Pacific dover sole (as mentioned above, not to be confused with European dover sole, a true sole) is a deepwater variety. Pacific flounder caught in waters off northern California, Oregon, Washington, British Columbia, and Alaska have likely lived mostly or entirely in relatively unpolluted waters. Rex, butter, and sand sole are quite small; dover sole goes as much as about ten pounds, and petrale sole is somewhat larger.

Steelhead

Steelhead is the ocean-going form of the rainbow trout, returning to rivers to breed. Found seasonally throughout the Pacific Northwest, steelhead is pink, soft, almost salmon-like, and somewhat comparable in flavor. Fillets from fish as small as a pound are often seen, though fish up to ten or twelve pounds are not uncommon.

Striped Bass

Striped bass are most common from Cape Cod to South Carolina, though they are found north to the Gulf of St. Lawrence and south to the Gulf of Mexico. Like salmon, stripers live in saltwater but depend on fresh-water rivers to reproduce. Most fish now caught along the East coast have been spawned in tributaries of the Chesapeake Bay and the Hudson River, two bodies of water not particularly clean, especially the latter. Striped bass populations have proven highly resistant to pollution, but flavor suffers noticeably in fish taken in polluted waters; as an oily species they concentrate toxins. Some of the finest stripers are caught in waters off Montauk Point (the eastern tip of Long Island) and the New England coast.

Flavor is also dependent upon how quickly the fish was gutted and iced when caught. Skin is sparkly and silvery if the fish is fresh, becoming more reddish and dull with time. The tastiest stripers weigh no more than five to six pounds. Broiling or poaching suits fillets, and the whole fish is excellent baked in a wine sauce. Striper from clean waters makes fine sushi and sashimi.

Striped bass were transplanted to the Pacific Coast in the late 1800's, and many Oregon and California rivers support substantial populations. Striper is seasonally available commercially in these areas.

Descriptions of our eastern waters by early settlers make apparent the incredible multitude of striped bass, bluefish, mackerel, Atlantic salmon, and other species gracing our coasts in years past. Destruction of coastal breeding areas, and overfishing, particularly by huge Japanese and Russian vessels, have together eliminated or made scarce many species. Pollutants have tainted remaining fish; one best asks where a fish was caught, though one never knows where it was the week before. Those who value a clean environment and abundant fish and wildlife, have so far been unable to restrain forces of ignorance and greed threatening the destruction of what remains of our wilderness heritage. Modern life has paradoxes; a man urinating on a public beach may be arrested and jailed, yet he may pour thousands of gallons of toxic chemicals into public waters and go unpunished. The battle will be won or lost in our courts.

Swordfish

Like tuna, swordfish are found around the world in tropical and temperate seas, and those taken off American shores are tastiest in late summer and fall. The meat is firm, with a distinctive flavor, and is excellent for sushi and sashimi.

Swordfish has been shown to concentrate mercury and PCB's, and has the additional problem of being very large; large fish concentrate these toxins in higher concentrations than smaller fish. Nevertheless, occasional broiled or raw swordfish is for the author impossible to resist; one reasons that the benefits of this otherwise outstanding food will outweigh the liabilities.

Tilefish

This rather ignored species has distinct advantages—habitat and flavor. Requiring very cold water and feeding on bottom-dwelling crustaceans, tilefish live at depths of three hundred to over one thousand feet, from Nova Scotia to Florida, and also off the Pacific coast. When they do come into shallow water, they feed differently, which apparently results in a harmless but rather bitter flavor. The deep dwellers taste similar to lobster or scallops, sweet and tender; the flesh is firm and makes fine sushi and sashimi.

The common tilefish inhabits more northern Atlantic waters, the blackline tilefish more southern. The Pacific species is called ocean whitefish. Reasonably priced, marketed tilefish are generally six to eight pound fish sold as fillets, and make a good choice when seeking a tasty and clean fish.

Tuna

The geography of ancient Europe was much influenced by tuna. In pre-Christian times, crude spruce observation posts built atop coastal cliffs were used to spot tuna migrations from afar; a cry would go up, and fishermen would set to sea to row out and spread their nets. Around these posts grew various cities, all about the Mediterranean and Atlantic coasts. Many of the names derived from the root word "cete," meaning locations where tuna were caught.

Every part of the tuna was utilized by ancient fishermen; roe in particular were long considered a great delicacy. In Mediterranean cultures, specific cuts of the often very large bluefin tuna are known for superior culinary qualities. Tuna makes excellent sushi and sashimi.

Tuna is quite fatty, but the amount of fat varies greatly seasonally—they are fattiest and tastiest in late summer and early fall. The meat of different species is classed as white, light, or dark; flavor is strongest in darker species.

Six species come to American markets fresh, frozen, or canned. Most delicately flavored and valuable is albacore, the tuna with the lightest colored flesh. Found in tropical and temperate waters of both the Atlantic and the Pacific, albacore are caught from several to one hundred miles or so offshore, and typically weigh ten to fifteen pounds. A mainstay of the California canning industry, they seldom are seen in markets.

Blackfin is also a small tuna, typically eight to ten pounds. Like the albacore, the meat is delicately flavored and light in color. Though a favorite of tuna connoisseurs, it too is seldom seen in American markets. Blackfin is an Atlantic species and ranges from Cape Cod to Brazil.

Yellowfin is the key species for the California canning industry. It is found all around the world in tropical and subtropical waters. Fresh yellowfin steaks are generally cut from ten to twenty pound fish; the meat is a little less light than albacore, and very tasty.

Skipjack tuna too is a tropical and semitropical species, with light meat comparable to the yellowfin. The average size is six to eight pounds.

The largest tuna is the bluefin, ranging to over one thousand pounds, though four to six hundred is considered large today. Meat darkens as the size increases; usually fish over 120 pounds are too dark to be classed as light. Popular in Europe and Japan, the lighter, smaller fish make excellent sushi and sashimi; raw bluefin has no strong fish flavor and is very softly textured. Bluefin is found in all temperate and subtropical seas.

Canned tuna is labeled in one of three ways: solid pack or "fancy" (large pieces with no fragments); chunks or "standard" (three pieces of solid meat, filled in with flakes); or salad or "flakes" (crumbs or finely divided meat, packed down solid). Only albacore may be labeled white meat tuna. Yellowfin, skipjack, and small bluefin are the other tuna used for canning in this country, and are labeled light meat tuna.

Albacore is the smallest of commercially caught tuna and is available canned, packed in water; unfortunately it is salted. Yellowfin tuna is very tasty broiled lightly with a little butter and lemon, or used for sushi and sashimi.

Toxic residues make one hesitate to use much tuna; because they are fatty, highly carnivorous, and often grow large, tuna has higher concentrations of mercury and PCB's than most other fish. Tuna has the further disadvantage of not being a cold water species; the eicosapentaenoic acid (EPA) content is thus considerably lower than that of salmon, mackerel, and several other fatty species that have not been reported to concentrate mercury and PCB's.

Whitebait

As served seasonally in some fine seafood restaurants, whitebait consists of very small specimens (usually less than three inches) of some or all of several species—young silversides, sardines (herring), anchovies, surf smelts, and sand launce—that have been floured and flash fried. These fish when marketed as whitebait, either fresh or frozen, are sold whole and ungutted. They may be fried quickly in butter or olive oil, or broiled quickly in a hot oven.

These fish are often seen at the edge of the surf, and may easily be netted by two people working a short length of fine meshed net. Silversides and sand launce are especially numerous in New England.

SHELLFISH

Abalone

Of the world's approximately one hundred species of abalone, eight occur along our Pacific coast, mostly in California, which prohibits the canning or shipping of abalone out of state. Vast quantities of this once abundant shellfish were formerly shipped to the Orient.

Relative scarcity, high demand, and succulent, sweet meat make abalone an expensive, but unforgettable entrée. White meat steaks are sliced from flesh that has been pried away from colorful shells. Gentle pounding with a mallet on a wooden board tenderizes the steaks, which are then cooked quickly and lightly. Overcooked, they become tough.

Univalve vegetarian mollusks, west coast abalone average four pounds; they feed with tiny teeth on seaweed. Because they do not filter water as bivalves do, abalone do not concentrate bacteria in polluted waters and are immune to red tide. They are excellent for sushi and sashimi.

A dried Japanese abalone product, brined, smoked, and dried in the sun, is available in many markets specializing in Oriental foods. Shredded, this is called kaiho; powdered, it is called meiho.

Clams

Many widely divergent species of clams abound along all American coasts. Both hardshell and softshell clams are found in shallow eastern waters from the Arctic Ocean to Cape Hatteras. Hardshells, or quahaugs (pronounced co-hogs), usually eaten raw on the half-shell or in chowder, are classed by size. Smallest is the Little Neck (three to four years old, up to two inches across); a bit larger is the Cherrystone (about five years old); and larger still (over three inches), too big to eat on the half-shell and without the delicate flavor of smaller clams, is the chowder clam, often called simply the quahaug.

Softshell clams are also found on the coast of the Pacific Northwest, along with razor clams, littlenecks, and butter clams. Pacific littlenecks are unrelated to eastern Little Necks, and are not really good raw; usually they are steamed. Butter clams are usually found small, on gravelly intertidal beaches. They look and taste about the same as east coast Little Necks—tender, succulent, and absolutely marvelous fresh out of the sand.

Softshell clams are called steamers. Boil them in a half inch of water until opened—just a minute or two. Lemon juice and butter complete the broth.

Razor clams are too tough to be eaten raw, unless very small. They are usually steamed.

Live softshell or razor clams constrict their necks when the neck is touched; hardshells whose shells are open will close tightly. Throw away any dead ones. Clams will live at forty degrees in a refrigerator for several days, but they lose some freshness and flavor. If bought shucked in a container (preferably glass), the liquid should be clear, the clams plump. Like fresh clams in the shell, they are best eaten within forty-eight hours. If a little old, rinse with cold water before eating; this also freshens up jarred oysters.

Bivalves are safest and tastiest in months with an "r" in them. Toxic plankton overgrowths such as red tide are most likely during warm months—May through August (no "r"). September through April are all "r" months, and generally safe. Bivalves taste best during these times, and some enthusiasts eat them several times a week. Abstaining in the warmer months seems to make clams, oysters, and mussels taste better than ever by September. Fresh raw shellfish of good quality is among the most strengthening of foods.

Crab

The many varieties of crabs inhabiting our coastal zones differ markedly in habitats. Some species live in shallow water just offshore and in bays and estuaries; others live far offshore, at depths well beyond one thousand feet.

The blue crab is the most common on the east coast. Warmer months find it in shallow waters from New England to Florida. Females are full of eggs much of this time; she-crab soup is made from their meat and roe.

The jonah crab of the northeast is a more deep water species. Though in some areas it appears in shallows, and even in intertidal zones in the spring, generally the jonah stays in open waters, often at great depths. Typically five or six inches across the shell, the jonah crab has appeared commerically with the development of deep water crabbing operations now harvesting the Continental Shelf. The red crab too usually lives at great depths on the outer Shelf, though it may be found in waters as shallow as 150 feet. Once taken only during deep water lobstering, the red and the jonah have assumed greater commercial importance with the development of specialized traps. Both are delicious and are often compared to the king crab.

The king crab of the northern Pacific is usually called the Alaska king crab. They average ten pounds but, as with all crabs, the yield of meat is only about 25 percent. The most important other Pacific coast species is the dungeness crab, found from Alaska to southern California. Like the jonah it is a type of rock crab, spending most of the year at considerable depths and venturing into shallow waters and intertidal zones seasonally. Dungeness crabs are excellent eating and popular on the west coast.

The snow crab is worthy of mention because it is widely available canned and lives at depths beyond one thousand feet. Also known as the tanner crab, it is a northern Pacific species and lives along the Continental Shelf. Most taken are found in king crab traps off the coast of Alaska. A favorite easy dinner: snow crab in a salad of leafy greens with a little olive oil, vinegar, and lemon juice.

The lady crab is the little crab felt nipping at one's feet and seen scampering in shallow water on Atlantic beaches. Rarely more than three inches across the shell, they are tasty and easily netted. Many a fine meal has been made of whitebait and lady crabs cooked over an open fire on the beach.

The oyster crab is found living within some oysters. Seldom more than an inch across the shell, they are collected by some oyster wholesalers during shucking operations for sale to the few retailers who carry them. Seldom seen, oyster crabs are softshelled and, like the lady crab, need not be dressed; cook them as they are, or use in crab soup.

A crab periodically sheds its shell as it grows; until the soft covering underneath toughens, we have a softshell crab. Usually crabs are captured a few days before shedding and marketed afterward at a premium. Softshell blue crab is the common commercial species.

Lobster

Lobster species are found in oceans all over the world. Maine is the traditional home of the American lobster, though it is found as far south as North Carolina. Although still most abundant in the cold waters off the Maine and eastern Canadian coasts, the catch in Maine has declined to a third of what it was in the 1950's.

Maine (American) lobster usually weigh from one to five pounds, but may grow to fifty. Their usual habitat is ocean bottom at depths of ten to two hundred feet, though they have been captured at depths up to six hundred feet one hundred miles offshore. Lobsters are omnivores, eating slow-moving, bottom-dwelling sea animal life and seaweed. Their range is very limited, and they feed mostly in warmer months.

Beware the lobster's claws! The two are different; one is larger and for crushing, the other a lighter biting claw, and the lobster can be very quick with it. Bands seen around the claws in lobster tanks prevent cannibalism.

When picking out a live lobster, select a lively one, for a listless lobster may have been captive quite some time. Lobsters lose weight in captivity; one may notice this when cracking a lobster open after cooking. Select from a busy market with a rapid turnover. When buying precooked lobster, if in doubt about freshness, extend the tail out straight; if it snaps back to a curled position when released, the lobster was alive until cooked.

Females are preferred by those who enjoy the roe, called coral; it cooks to a bright red. Females have a broader abdomen than males of the same size, and the first pair of tail appendages are reduced in size.

Surprisingly, the size of a lobster gives no indication of tenderness and even the largest lobsters may be tender. But as with all seafood, younger and smaller individuals accumulate the smallest amount of pollutants in any given environment. Lobsters from 1 to 1 1/2 pounds are called quarters, and are adequate for most appetites, though some people prefer a large (1 1/2 to 2 1/2 pounds). Jumbos are over 2 1/2 pounds, chickens are under a pound and are often missing one claw.

Nearly all of a lobster is edible. The green pasty material inside the body cavity is called tomalley and is the lobster's liver; rich but not quite as sweet as the firm white meat of the claws, tail, body, and legs, it is quite delicious in its own right. Roe or coral of the female also has a unique taste. The shells, like those of all crustaceans, are rich in carotene (giving them their color), protein, and calcium. Shells may be used in making a stock that lends a distinct flavor to a soup or sauce.

Lobster is most easily cooked by boiling or steaming. Plunge headfirst into actively boiling water, cover, and keep heat on high to return the water to a boil; this will take a few minutes. Begin timing when the water has returned to a boil. When cooking more than one lobster, for a given lobster, allow ten minutes for the first pound and three minutes more for each additional pound.

Steaming causes less loss of nutrients. Boil an inch or two of water; then place the lobster in the pot and keep the pot covered. A perforated plate may be used in the bottom to keep the lobster above water. When steam reappears, begin timing as above.

Lobster is also wonderful baked. Stuffings are made with tomalley and coral; other ingredients may include crab meat. The claws are cracked; the lobster is split, stuffed, and then baked.

From North Carolina through Florida, and around the Gulf, the spiny lobster (also called rock lobster or sometimes crawfish, not to be confused with crayfish) makes its home. This lobster has no claws. Related species are found in many parts of the world; the South African lobster tails seen on many menus are from one such species.

Several other members of the lobster family have in recent years made an appearance in American markets. Collectively called lobsterettes, or sometimes langoustines or Danish lobsters, they are similar to the American lobster but smaller and very brightly colored. Their meat is mostly in the tail, and they live in deep water at depths from six hundred to over six thousand feet, making them less proximal to coastal pollutants.

Mussels

Mussels have never enjoyed in America the popularity they do in Europe, though they taste much like steamers and are considerably less expensive. Found from Canada to North Carolina clinging to rocks and seawalls in intertidal zones, mussels are most numerous in New England and can be gathered on many beaches. The blue or edible mussel is the most common species (not all saltwater mussels are edible); it is found on the Pacific coast also, along with the California mussel.

Rich in nutrients, mussels like clams and oysters are tastiest and least susceptible to toxic algae growths in fall, winter, and early spring. After spawning in late spring, they become watery and lose some of their flavor.

Unlike steamers, live mussels may open up when removed from the refrigerator and exposed to a temperature change; this does not mean they are dead. Try to slide the two halves of the shell laterally across one another; a live mussel holds quite rigidly. If the shells move much, the mussel is dead. Cook mussels similarly to steamers. Discard any that do not open in cooking, for they may have been dead beforehand.

Octopus

A mollusk in the same class as squid, the octopus too is a predator, living largely on shellfish; this makes its flesh very tasty. Octopuses are caught off both coasts, generally about a mile offshore in one hundred to two hundred feet of water. The usual size is one to three pounds.

Most demand in this country is from people of Mediterranean or Oriental origin. Scarcer than squid, octopus is also considerably more expensive. It is considered a great delicacy by those who enjoy it. Octopus is very popular as sashimi.

Oysters

Oysters grow best in bays and river mouths where the salinity of sea water has been diluted. Vegetarians, they feed on tiny unicellular plants filtered from the gallon of water their bodies process each hour. The flavor and color of oysters reflect the type and quality of these plants; these influences are in turn determined by the quality and temperature of the water, salinity and proximity to fresh water, nutrients available, and a host of other immeasurable contributory elements.

Cultivation of oysters has been successfully accomplished since Roman times, and among the finest oysters are cultivars from Cape Cod Bay in New England and Tomales Bay in California. Cultivars begin growth when oyster larvae catch on scallop shells that are threaded on strings suspended from racks; they grow until harvesting, far from the bottom and safe from predators.

Natural oyster beds are found in intertidal zones. The Atlantic coast, particularly the Chesapeake Bay with its thousands of rivers, bays, and streams, is the home of the most common North American oyster. Among its many names are the Blue Point, the Chincoteague, the Apalachicola, and the Cape Cod. Best known of Pacific coast oysters is the Olympia, bred in brackish waters of the Puget Sound near the capitol of Washington. Other oysters are native to the Gulf coast.

Oysters spawn during the warm months, and during that time produce excessive glycogen (the form in which glucose is stored in muscles), causing a milky look and poor taste. In northern areas oysters are best in fall, winter, and early spring; in southern, in winter.

Oysters vary greatly in size; the smaller have the finest flavor. Shells should be tightly closed, and there should be no hint of strong odor. If not very fresh, oysters do not taste quite right. If purchased already shucked, the container should be glass so one can see if the liquid is clear; if it is cloudy or milky, the oysters are not completely fresh. This liquid, which runs off the half-shell when oysters are shucked, is excellent to drink or use in oyster cookery. Particularly along the Gulf coast, oysters are a popular item in many gourmet dishes.

Scallops

Of hundreds of species throughout the world, only a few are used commercially. Only the adductor muscle is used in America, though the entire content is edible. The two species most often seen are the bay scallop and the sea scallop, both east coast natives. Several others are found on the west coast, but except in Alaska, not in sufficient quantities to be of much commercial importance.

The bay scallop is a shallow water species found in grassy lowlands from Virginia to the Gulf of Mexico. The adductor muscle—what we call a scallop—is rarely more than an inch across. The sea scallop is much larger, up to about four inches across, and is taken from waters as deep as one thousand feet off the coast from New Jersey to northeastern Canada. Maine is the center of the sea scallop trade. Another deep water species is the calico, taken off Florida's east coast.

Scallops are perhaps the sweetest of all seafoods and are outstanding lightly broiled, or sautéed in butter and herbs. Distributors sometimes soak scallops in fresh water for a few hours to increase bulk, much to the detriment of their flavor. Color is the clue; this process whitens them, and fresh scallops should be beige or cream colored. Excellent when raw in sushi or as sashimi, scallops need only minimal cooking; like all fish, they turn tough when overcooked. Quick broiling in a hot oven or sautéing in a hot skillet seals in the juices.

Shrimp

The ubiquitous shrimp cocktail has made shrimp the seafood of greatest commercial importance. Hundreds of freshwater and saltwater species exist. Several very similar species are taken in waters off our southeastern coast and in the Gulf of Mexico and several others, off the Pacific coast, mainly in Alaskan waters.

Though the word prawn is used for any large shrimps, prawn actually means freshwater species, while shrimp means saltwater species. Shrimp are classed by size; so-called prawns or jumbo shrimp are generally considered to number fifteen or fewer to a pound.

Fresh shrimp should be firm and clean smelling, with no offensive odor. Shrimp taken offshore may smell and taste of iodine because the organisms they feed on in waters of normal ocean salinity tend to concentrate iodine, making them a rich source of this nutrient. In the less saline water of bays, shrimp feed on organisms less rich in iodine, and rarely concentrate sufficient iodine for the odor and taste to be noticeable. However, sulfites are often sprinkled on shrimp and other fish as a preservative (a section on preservatives sometimes used on fresh fish and shellfish concludes this appendix) and sodium bisulfate in particular causes an iodine taste or magnifies any that may be present. So while offshore shrimp may be more desirable in areas where bay waters are of questionable cleanliness, one may not know if any iodine taste is natural or chemically induced. As always, the best safeguard is dealing with merchants aware of the source and handling of one's food.

Small or medium sized fresh shrimp are often available whole—complete with shells, tails, heads, and roe—quite reasonably priced. When very fresh, they may be sautéed in a hot skillet in a quarter inch of wine, butter, and their own juices, then served over brown rice or vegetables. Though not suited to everyone's taste, the entire shrimp is edible and this is indeed a sweet and succulent dish. Nutrients minimally supplied by the meat alone are richly supplied by the organs, roe, and heads.

When estimating how much shrimp to purchase, consider that two-fifths of the weight is lost in shelling and deveining. Steamed shrimp compared to boiled are equally firm but more tender, and flavor is not lost into the cooking water as it is when shrimp are boiled.

Squid

This ten-armed mollusk exists in scores of varieties, from one inch to sixty feet, and is found in oceans throughout the world. Important in the cuisine of many countries, especially in the Mediterranean and the Orient, squid is firm, tender when not overcooked, and gently flavored. Squid is a highly nutritious and tasty food, though rarely used simply because of its unfamiliarity.

As usually marketed, squid weigh a few ounces each. The white firm flesh turns yellow in cooking. Over three-quarters of the total weight of the animal is edible; even the ink is used in many European dishes. Ink, incidentally, is discharged as the squid propels itself away from predators, jetting water out of a funnel in its body. The ink leaves a cloud, and perhaps an image of itself to serve as a decoy, behind which the squid rapidly disappears.

FRESHWATER FISH

The problems of the oceans discussed in chapter 12 under the heading "Water Pollution" are being compounded in rivers, lakes, and streams by the increasing acidity of rainwater in many parts of the country. Sulfur dioxide emissions from coal combustion at power plants, and nitrogen oxides from automobile exhaust and various industrial sources, are converted into sulfuric and nitric acids in the atmosphere. These compounds are then precipitated in rain and affect the acidity of freshwater ecosystems.

As a result, freshwater fish even in relatively unpolluted areas in the eastern part of the country have been affected. In areas of concentrated population, freshwater fish have long been of questionable value because of pollution problems. Still, particularly in the west, there are vast unspoiled areas with high mountain lakes, free running streams, and good fishing.

While freshwater fish do not contain the high amounts of eicosapentaenoic acid found in many saltwater species, they provide excellent nutrition, and are available commercially in some parts of the country. Most of us have a limited selection of freshwater fish, especially fish from a clean environment. Comments here will be limited to bass, trout, and whitefish.

Bass

Freshwater black bass is unrelated to black sea bass and striped bass. Members of the sunfish family, they have meat that is lean and white. Not sold commercially, largemouth and smallmouth bass are popular game fish, and those under two pounds are firm and sweet, much tastier than larger ones. Bass survive and reproduce in many polluted waters; the taste depends on the quality of the water and deteriorates markedly in less than clean waters.

Trout

A popular game fish, trout is found on many restaurant menus and in most seafood markets. But trout on the menu, or in the market, must by law be hatchery raised, unless it is lake trout or steelhead. Trout caught by fishermen in more populated parts of the country are also hatchery raised; wild trout are found primarily in lakes, rivers, and streams of the Rocky Mountains.

The meat of hatchery raised trout is white; its flavor, even if from the better hatcheries, does not compare with that of the red to pink or orange flesh of wild trout. Carotenoids are found in crayfish, shrimp, and other crustaceans. Wild steelhead and rainbow trout of the American west feed upon them, causing the red tinge of their flesh. Wild brook trout, native to eastern North America and transplanted throughout the rest of the continent, has more of a yellow to orange flesh.

Wild brook, rainbow, and cutthroat trout of the west are, at their best, comparable to the anadromous steelhead trout discussed earlier. Lake trout is larger, usually ten to twenty pounds, and much oiler than other trout species. Quality varies greatly; in the Great Lakes they feed mainly on alewives, hence the flavor suffers. Quality of hatchery raised trout also varies greatly; some are quite tasty, while others are mealy and without flavor.

Whitefish

Whitefish refers to a variety of species found in lakes across northern America and throughout Canada. Abundant in Alaska, more may turn up in markets in the forty-eight states in the future. In the past they were of greater importance in the Great Lakes region; their numbers have dwindled.

SOME GENERAL CONSIDERATIONS

Sushi and Sashimi

Sashimi is the Japanese word for raw fish, carefully cut, and eaten with tamari and wasabi (grated horseradish root). Sufficiently fresh fish is delicate in taste and firm in texture; the aroma has a hint of sweet freshness with none of the strength of some cooked fish. The finest quality sashimi is made from fresh fish no more than a day out of the water.

Raw fish was central in the diets of traditional seacoast cultures everywhere; each culture had special ways of preparing species important to it. Special techniques of cutting different species of fish for sashimi prepare each in the best form for enjoyment raw. While the home chef does not have the training and knowledge of the skilled Japanese sashimi artist, the application of a few principles in cutting raw fish enables one to enjoy raw many fish that are commonly cooked. Parts of fish to be broiled or otherwise cooked may be prepared to eat as sushi or sashimi prior to the main course.

Very firm fish such as tuna, swordfish, shark, squid, octopus, tilefish, and abalone are usually cut into cubes. Those a little less firm, like striped bass, cod, and red snapper, are cut into paper-thin slices. A variety of cuts are used on fish of more delicate texture to produce slices about one-quarter inch thick.

Sushi refers to raw fish used together with rice, the seaweed nori, and sometimes other vegetables. While the finer points of sushi and sashimi are best accomplished by one with the skill and time to be creative, the incorporation of raw fish into the diet may be simple; one need not feel bound by the conventions of sashimi. Lemon juice and other ingredients are useful in marinating raw fish; cuts may be determined in part by a desire to accomplish the job quickly.

Parasites occasionally infect saltwater fish, but are reported (by A.J. McClane in *The Encyclopedia of Fish Cookery*) to be harmless varieties that do not infect humans. Freshwater fish, however, may harbor various disease-causing parasites, and should never be eaten raw or undercooked.

If one has or can develop a taste for raw fish and shellfish, using them is a major step in developing a diet for optimizing health, resistance to disease, and longevity. While this may be accomplished with other foods, fish and shellfish are for most people the most readily available.

Smoked and Salted Fish

Substances in smoked and grilled foods have been found to cause cancer in test animals, and some investigators have linked the use of smoked and salted fish and meat products with increased incidence of stomach cancer. And yet, traditional cultures often preserved fish and meats with smoking and salting, and among these people cancer of all forms was rare. Modern medicine blames skin cancer on the sun's rays, yet contemporary primitive people exposed daily to the sun apparently get no skin cancer.

A plausible explanation is that the degree of susceptability to all carcinogens is largely determined by the quality of the entire diet. Many substances in the environment and in food that can cause cancer in individuals with insufficient immunity do not cause cancer in those on more adequate diets. This has been demonstrated in dietary experiments with animals, and surveys designed to examine human susceptability to lung cancer have recently shown smokers eating more green vegetables have a significantly lower incidence of lung cancer than smokers eating fewer green vegetables.

The emphasis on carcinogenic effects of the use of smoked fish may thus be misplaced. Ancestral humans and later our more immediate forefathers cooked and smoked fish and game over open fires for perhaps four hundred thousand years. Salt is another issue; while excessive amounts may or may not be carcinogenic, there are other good reasons to minimize its use, as do some methods of smoking.

Many kinds of fresh smoked fish are available regionally; salmon and cod are seen almost universally. A wide variety of smoked fish and shellfish are available canned, usually packed in oil—herring, mussels, clams, sardines, and many more.

Many influences affect the smoking of fish: the lengths of time at which various temperatures are maintained, kinds of wood used, and amounts of salt. Salt is applied first, either as a brine solution of a specific strength, or by direct application. Salt removes fluids from the flesh by osmosis; bacteria are inhibited by lack of water, as the fluids drained are replaced by salt to a certain extent. Smoke adds flavor by dehydrating the fish further, and firms the flesh by strengthening connective tissues. If temperatures are kept low enough to prevent coagulation of all protein in the tissues, the flesh becomes firm yet remains somewhat moist.

Hot-smoking and cold-smoking are the two extremes of this process. In the former, the temperature range is from 120 to 180 degrees F and the smoking time, from six to twelve hours. Considerable coagulation of protein occurs during curing; still, the product remains firm. Without refrigeration, hot-smoked fish keeps only a few days. Hot-smoking and barbecuing are somewhat similar, but in barbecuing, the fish is placed closer to the heat and cooked slowly at about two hundred degrees F. A smoked flavor is imparted, but the fish crumbles easily and will not keep, for it has not been cured.

Cold-smoking is the traditional method that was used by coastal and northern Indians to preserve vast quantities of fish and meat for winter use. The fish is not cooked, for temperatures are kept around eighty degrees F, and the flesh is cured through drying. Protein coagulation is minimal; the fish is essentially preserved raw. This method requires minimal brining and at least two days of smoking, though the fish may be smoked two or three weeks to make a product that will keep a long time. These methods can produce a superior product, moist, not too salty, firm, and easily sliced.

Variations on cold-smoking are used by commercial smokehouses in the Pacific Northwest, and in England and Scotland, to produce superior smoked salmon. For salmon smoked in the British Isles, "Scotch smoked salmon" refers to Atlantic salmon, while "smoked salmon" refers to coho and chinook imported fresh from Washington and Alaska. By the time these fish are smoked and returned to America for sale, they may have logged more air miles than ever they did ocean miles. Perhaps this is why they cost fifteen dollars a pound.

Roe

The ovaries of female fish are two elongated sacs, usually a shade of yellow or orange, with visible, round, clear eggs covered by a membrane. The male gonads are long white sacs, small, and white with sperm in the sexually mature male. They were considered important foods for men in primitive cultures, and Weston Price reported they were eaten raw. Other reports confirm that coastal North American Indians ate the gonads raw, believing this increased virility. Even today this "white roe" is a great delicacy in many cuisines around the world.

Most modern palates prefer roe slightly cooked; some simple methods include poaching in water with lemon juice and butter, quick broiling for a minute or so, and sautéing in butter. Some fish already discussed with edible roe that is sometimes available commercially include salmon, flounder, cod, haddock, halibut, tuna, mackerel, dolphin, herring, and shad. Roe of most fish are edible, though those of some species (none described in this appendix) are toxic.

Stocks

From both a culinary and a nutritional standpoint, the head is the key to good fish stock. The brain is very fatty, full of the fatty acids EPA and DHA. The gelatin-like texture that the head contributes makes for stock that may be frozen, perhaps after reducing, and used for poaching, soups, or fish stews.

The bones too contribute much nutrition and flavor to a stock. Adding a little vinegar to the simmering pot helps leach calcium from bones.

Preservatives Sometimes Used on Fresh Fish and Shellfish

Regulations have recently been proposed, and in some places adopted, concerning use of preservatives, particularly sulfites, on fresh vegetables. Sulfites are commonly used to keep greens and other raw vegetables looking fresh at restaurant salad bars. The move for regulations governing their use began when they were found to cause in susceptible individuals severe allergic reactions, occasionally including asthmatic attacks and anaphylactic shock in several cases resulting in death.

Still, proposed regulations do not affect the fishing industry. Sulfites are sometimes sprinkled on clams, lobsters, crabs, scallops and, especially, shrimp. Sodium benzoates known to cause adverse reactions in sensitive individuals are commonly used to kill bacteria. Polytrisorbates are commonly used to control yeasts and molds and polyphosphates, to control moisture content of fish.

These substances are seldom used when fish is sold locally, but are often used when fish is shipped any great distance. Some fish retailers display signs stating their fish has not been treated with any of these chemicals; this assures that whatever fish is not locally caught has been efficiently and rapidly shipped, and that what appears fresh truly is.

*L*aboratory tests are a useful tool for gathering information, but too often may fail to indicate problems in areas where attention is needed. A broad range of relative wellness exists between optimal health and overt illness; tests do little to indicate where in that range one lies. An awareness of the limitations of laboratory tests allows their use within the broader framework established by the medical history and the physical exam. Results of laboratory tests and special diagnostic procedures seldom surprise the discerning physician; rather, they usually confirm what was suspected after the history and physical.

Discussions of some routine blood and urine tests follow. The objective is to provide a simple and clear understanding of their purpose and meaning.

Complete Blood Count (CBC)

The CBC and an analysis of the urine (urinalysis) are basic screening tests routinely done to check for abnormalities. The CBC determines the number of red and of white blood cells per milliliter of blood. Red blood cells (RBC's), with their hemoglobin, carry oxygen to all tissues of the body. White blood cells (WBC's) are part of the immune system; among other things, they attack bacteria and other foreign invaders. A significant increase in the WBC count usually indicates inflammation or infection.

Anemia is defined as the failure of the blood to deliver adequate oxygen to the tissues. The RBC count may be depressed in anemia, but in some types of anemia it never becomes depressed. Tests for hematocrit and for hemoglobin, also part of the CBC, are used to screen for anemia. The hematocrit test measures the percentage of the blood volume made up by RBC's. The hemoglobin test measures the amount of hemoglobin carried by the RBC's, thus determining the oxygen-carrying capacity of the blood. Both hematocrit and hemoglobin may also be normal in early stages of anemia.

On the other hand, the RBC count, hematocrit, and hemoglobin may all be below normal in a person with no signs or symptoms of anemia, and in good health. This is typical in those getting a great deal of endurance exercise—running, swimming, bicycling, cross-country skiing, or walking. Endurance exercise can cause the body's total volume of blood to increase dramatically, reportedly up to 30 per cent over time. With this increase, there are fewer RBC's per unit of volume. Still, because of the increased volume, the overall capacity of the blood to deliver oxygen to the tissues is increased. The three tests may be low simply because the blood volume has increased.

True anemia occasionally occurs in such individuals, and may be difficult to diagnose. If suspected, anemia can be confirmed by further tests involving levels of iron and iron-carrying molecules in the blood.

The CBC also may include a differential, the description of a blood smear made on a glass slide that is examined microscopically. The relative number of different types of white blood cells is determined, both white and red blood cells are examined for abnormalities, and the number of platelets is estimated.

Leukemia, bone marrow failure, adverse drug reactions, various types of anemia, inflammation, and the presence of malarial parasites are some of the many problems detectable by the CBC.

Urinalysis

Urine is routinely tested in several ways and examined under a microscope. Specific gravity (density) is a measure of the number of particles suspended in the urine, and indicates the ability of the kidneys to concentrate urine adequately. Sediments are concentrated by centrifuging a small sample of the urine specimen. They are then examined microscopically for presence of cells indicating problems of the kidneys, bladder, and associated anatomy.

Other tests are performed by dipping a paper strip into a sample of the urine. Small squares on the strip have been treated chemically to react individually to glucose (the form of sugar in the blood), protein, blood, and several other substances that may be found in the urine. Reactions cause color changes of the small squares that are read by the physician or medical technologist performing the test, giving approximate levels of the various substances. Abnormalities—for example, the presence of blood, sugar, or proteins—may be followed up by more quantitative tests. Abnormalities may also arouse suspicion about certain problems and indicate need for other tests and diagnostic procedures.

Erythrocyte Sedimentation Rate (ESR)

Erythrocytes are red blood cells. The ESR measures the extent to which erythrocytes settle toward the bottom of a thin glass tube in one hour, which is a function of the relative amounts of proteins, antibodies, and other substances in the blood. In health, they settle very little. This is a nonspecific screening test, frequently done; the result is elevated in many diseases, and often in a normal pregnancy.

The ESR is commonly used as a relative measure of the activity of autoimmune diseases in which the body reacts adversely to its own tissues, such as rheumatoid arthritis and lupus. In general, the more severe the problem, the greater the elevation.

The normal sedimentation range is up to ten millimeters per hour in men and twenty in women. In very healthy individuals, the ESR may approach zero. Although the blood may be thin due to endurance exercise, in an individual with proper diet the red blood cells scarcely settle at all in the test. Readings consistently between zero and one are commonly seen over the years in such individuals.

Blood Chemistry: Cholesterol, Triglycerides, Fasting Glucose, Glycohemoglobin, Glucose Tolerance Test, and Thyroid Hormones

Many substances normally found in the blood may become elevated or depressed in disease. Some are nutrients used by cells throughout the body; their levels may give indications about grossly inadequate nutrition. Others are by-products of the metabolism of certain specific cells and, if elevated, give indications about disease in the organs in which those cells predominate.

This section does not attempt to discuss all routine blood chemistry tests. Rather, both salient and a few subtle points about tests of concern to many individuals are explained.

Cholesterol.   The laboratory result most frequently discussed is the serum cholesterol (serum is the fluid portion of the blood remaining after the red blood cells and clotting factors have been removed). Cholesterol is found throughout the body and is used in a wide variety of normal metabolic reactions. It is a constituent of many common foods and is found in the fatty plaque which builds up in the arteries (including those to the heart, the coronary arteries) of an individual developing heart disease. Cholesterol has long been suspected to be a major cause of heart disease.

Many foods recommended in previous chapters are rich in cholesterol: liver and other organs, eggs, shellfish, dairy products, meat. Evidence was presented demonstrating that when of the proper quality, these foods may be part of an extremely healthy diet.

The human body makes, on the average, about three times as much cholesterol each day as the average diet contains. Cholesterol is as normal to human metabolism as any other nutrients found in foods. High blood cholesterol does occur in many individuals who develop heart disease, and it is likely that this contributes to the development of the problem. However, there is little indication that dietary cholesterol itself necessarily causes high blood cholesterol and heart disease. High blood cholesterol has been correlated with the development of heart disease, but high blood cholesterol has not been shown to result necessarily from eating a cholesterol-rich diet.

The fat composition of conventionally raised meat and, by inference, dairy products and eggs, was shown in chapters 4 and 14 to be very different from that of naturally raised animals and their dairy products and eggs. The former are much fattier; the fats are much more saturated and contain almost no EPA. These are among the real reasons such foods contribute to the development of heart disease, rather than their cholesterol content. The meat of wild game and of commercial animals has the same amount of cholesterol. Primitive people eating large amounts of wild game, including cholesterol-rich organs, did not develop high blood cholesterol and heart disease. Cholesterol is clearly not the difference between traditional and modern meat, and it is not the culprit in heart disease.

So while cholesterol-rich conventionally produced animal source foods are best avoided, there are nevertheless cholesterol-rich foods one may enjoy, secure in the knowledge they are among the healthiest of foods. Though a bit paradoxical, the logic of this conclusion should be clear in light of information presented in this book. When one follows a traditional diet, blood cholesterol generally falls into and remains in the 150 to 200 range, considered excellent by all authorities.

HDL cholesterol also causes some confusion. HDL stands for "high-density lipoprotein," and HDL cholesterol seems in general to be beneficial. At least two different types of HDL cholesterol have been identified; one is thought to be much more beneficial than the other. Excessive amounts of LDL (low density lipoprotein) cholesterol and VLDL (very low density lipoprotein) cholesterol are thought to be harmful. Consequently, increases in HDL cholesterol accompanied by decreases in total cholesterol are generally considered good. Vigorous exercise enhances HDL cholesterol, in particular the more beneficial type.

A noteworthy finding about HDL cholesterol emerged in a study on the effects of fish oils versus the effects of vegetable oils on volunteer patients (detailed in chapter 7). When eating the diet rich in vegetable oils, volunteers experienced significant *increases* in HDL cholesterol, along with moderate decreases in total cholesterol. When eating the diet rich in fish oils, they experienced slight *decreases* in HDL cholesterol, along with large decreases in total cholesterol and triglycerides. These results confirm the author's clinical experience. Consistently, individuals using quantities of vegetable oils have higher HDL cholesterol levels and lower total cholesterol to HDL cholesterol ratios than those who do not, especially when the latter eat considerable fish.

HDL cholesterol levels, and total cholesterol to HDL cholesterol ratios, should be viewed in light of this; while increased HDL levels, and a decreased total cholesterol to HDL ratio, are generally associated with decreased risk of heart disease, changes in these directions do not necessarily indicate optimal events are happening in the body. HDL increases associated with the use of vegetable oils may well prove to be of the less beneficial type of HDL, while the slight decrease in HDL associated with fish oil consumption may also be in the less beneficial HDL. Should this prove to be true, we would have a reasonable partial explanation of why fish oils generally benefit health while vegetable oils generally do not. Several conflicting influences are at work affecting HDL and total cholesterol levels.

Triglycerides.   Triglycerides are blood fats proving to be increasingly significant in the development of heart disease. They are the body's chief storage form of fat, and triglyceride molecules in the bloodstream transport fats throughout the body. Dietary fats break down in the intestines, pass through the intestinal wall, and are reassembled as triglycerides as they are absorbed into the blood.

The major source of serum triglycerides is not necessarily dietary fats. Because dietary carbohydrates are converted into substances that can be made into triglycerides in the liver, carbohydrates can greatly increase serum triglycerides. This is especially true of refined sugar (sucrose), refined (white) flour, concentrated fructose (as in fruit juice), and dried fruits. Because all are absorbed and enter the blood quickly, an excessive amount of carbohydrates must be metabolized rapidly. As a result, much more conversion to triglycerides occurs than when the complex carbohydrates of whole grain and vegetables are consumed. Alcohol too causes rapid elevation in the blood of metabolites (substances formed in the body from precursors) that are converted by the liver into triglycerides. Because fruits contain simple sugars, they too may contribute to increased serum triglycerides.

In recent years, research has indicated that elevated serum triglycerides are statistically correlated with heart disease. These metabolic pathways for dietary fats, carbohydrates, and alcohol indicate why so many Americans have high triglycerides. Overconsumption of alcohol and refined foods obviously contributes. But other foods commonly used and considered nutritious also contribute to the problem. Fruit juice, as mentioned, is an example. Furthermore, fruit juice provides calories without fiber, and valuable raw food enzymes are denatured in pasteurization. The vitamin C provided is better supplied by fresh raw vegetables, fruits, and lightly cooked meat and fish.

Fasting Glucose.   Fasting blood glucose (the sugar level in the blood after a twelve-hour fast), measured in the standard blood chemistry screen, like serum triglycerides is influenced by the amount of refined flour, sugar and other sweeteners, fruit, fruit juice, and alcohol in the diet. This test screens for diabetes; a fasting level above the upper limit of normal (which differs from laboratory to laboratory, ranging from 110 to 130), should be repeated, and confirmation of elevation calls for further evaluation. A glucose tolerance test is often done in borderline cases to determine if the individual is diabetic.

The upper limit of normal for the fasting blood glucose test has risen in the last twenty years by up to 20 percent, depending on the laboratory performing the test. Normal values for any given laboratory are based on averages for the population it serves. Average fasting blood glucose levels have risen, and laboratories have established higher new upper limits of normal. Levels formerly considered indicative of possible or probable diabetes now often fall within the normal range.

Regardless of a laboratory's upper limit of normal, the range from 100 to 130 should be considered borderline. A fasting blood sugar in this range should prompt a careful check for a diabetic or pre-diabetic condition. A blood test called glycohemoglobin is helpful; since the late 1970's it has been routinely used to determine the average blood sugar in diabetics, and it may be used in screening a potential diabetic.

Glycohemoglobin.   Glycohemoglobin molecules form in the blood when glucose and hemoglobin combine. A normal number form when the average blood sugar (glucose) level is normal. If glycohemoglobin is high, the blood sugar has on the average been high. Thus a physician may periodically determine if a diabetic is adequately controlling his blood sugar. The test may be routinely used in the initial evaluation of older individuals, or others in whom diabetes or borderline diabetes is suspected.

The glycohemoglobin test is of limited use in diagnosing hypoglycemia (low blood sugar); results are consistent in nonreactive hypoglycemia but inconsistent in reactive hypoglycemia. For both types, symptoms occur when blood sugar is low, but blood sugar in reactive hypoglycemia (hypoglycemia occurring in response to food) varies widely and may indeed at times be high. As a result, average blood sugar and glycohemoglobin may be high, low, or average. In chronic, nonreactive hypoglycemia, blood sugar is nearly always low, and glycohemoglobin is thus low.

Glucose Tolerance Test.   The glucose tolerance test (GTT) is routinely used in diagnosing diabetes and hypoglycemia. After a twelve-hour fast, a sample of blood is taken for determination of the fasting glucose level. The individual then drinks a standardized sugar solution, and blood sugar levels are periodically determined for up to six hours.

Many people subjected to this test become acutely ill and may feel poorly for as long as a few days. Use of the GTT is unnecessary in most cases, since either diabetes or hypoglycemia may be diagnosed from symptoms, physical findings, and other laboratory tests. A two-hour post-prandial blood glucose determination may be useful; the individual comes to the laboratory for a blood glucose test two hours after completing a carbohydrate-rich meal. Approaching the diagnosis in this manner avoids putting the individual through the metabolic insult of the glucose tolerance test.

Thyroid Hormones.   A determination of thyroid hormone levels is commonly ordered along with a CBC and a chemistry screen, particularly if the physician suspects under- or overactivity of the thyroid gland. The routine tests are called T_3 and T_4 (triiodothyronine and thyroxine), and while they may confirm a condition of myxedema (grossly underactive thyroid function) or thyrotoxicosis (grossly overactive thyroid function), these tests often show normal values in people suffering from chronic low thyroid function.

T_3 and T_4 replaced the basal metabolism rate test in the 1950's as the standard laboratory procedure for evaluating thyroid function. Since then, researchers and clinicians have often emphasized in the medical literature that these tests may fail to determine adequately thyroid status, and that the physician must primarily consider symptoms, signs, history, and physical findings (rather than laboratory results). In the author's experience, hundreds of people in whom T_3 and T_4 tested normal suffered from conditions related to a chronically underactive thyroid gland. Though this is not the prevailing view of thyroid problems, it is an important one, well expressed by Dr. Broda Barnes in his 1975 book, *Hypothyroidism: The Unsuspected Illness.* Barnes's work, and the evaluation and treatment of thyroid problems, were discussed in chapter 10.

Food Irradiation

*The Latest Threat
to Our Foods*

*T*he National Food Processors Association, the U.S. Department of Energy, the U.S. Food and Drug Administration, and several congressmen from districts with nuclear power facilities have joined in an organized and well financed plan to create a multi-billion-dollar-a-year industry to irradiate nearly half the food Americans will eat by 1990.

Massive doses of radiation (from five thousand to four million rads, depending on the food product; a chest X-ray gives off less than one rad) from cobalt-60 or cesium-137 would be used for food preservative effects—to control sprouting of onions and potatoes; to kill insects, bacteria, and fungi on stored grains and seeds; and to extend the shelf life of fresh fruits and vegetables, meats, and processed foods. Food does not become radioactive from irradiation; rather, chemical changes involving the formation of little understood chemical compounds in food called "unique radiolytic products" occur as part of the preservative effect.

At the time of this writing, bills pending in the House and Senate would legalize food irradiation and would finance the conversion of wastes from the production of nuclear weapons at the Hanford facility in Washington state into cobalt-60 and cesium-137. These materials would be used in the over one thousand food irradiation plants that food processing industry analysts predict will be operating in America by 1995.

As with nuclear power plants, radioactive materials would be stored in large pools of water when not in use. Leaks of radioactive water have been a common problem in nuclear power plants; even minor leaks in food irradiation plants could easily make great quantities of food radioactive. Would this always be detected? Might such contaminated food, when detected, be used as livestock feed? At what level of radioactivity would this be deemed unacceptable? Who would do the monitoring? There are no satisfactory answers to these questions.

The bills referred to above would change the intent of the Cosmetic Act-Food Additive Amendment of 1958 by allowing irradiation of food. The bills are sponsored by the congressman whose district includes the Hanford facility. The U.S. Department of Energy supports these efforts. Attempts to reprocess waste materials from nuclear weapons production into fuel rods for power plants have failed; both plants built for this purpose had so many leaks and incidents of worker contamination that they were permanently closed. The problem of what to do with these waste materials is very real for the Department of Energy, which in 1985 joined forces with the National Food Processors Association in plans to build a food irradiation research and demonstration plant in Dublin, California. The Department is thus the largest government subsidizer of food irradiation; the creation of a food irradiation industry would effectively solve their nuclear waste disposal problem.

Little careful research has been done into the health effects of food irradiation. The U.S. Army has done a number of studies over the past twenty-five years, but only three measured up to the FDA's criteria for acceptable research. Those three showed questionable findings. FDA rejection of numerous Army studies led the Army to use a private company called Industrial Biotest, and some studies done by this company have been cited by the FDA in the agency's claims for the safety of food irradiation. But in 1983, officials of Industrial Biotest were convicted of fraud for suppressing unfavorable research findings. The Army would very much like to use irradiation in the storage and preservation of food, and the company was apparently giving the Army results the Army wanted.

What responsible studies have been done make the prospect of food irradiation frightening. *The Journal of Food Science* in 1973 reported that aflatoxin production increased following irradiation of foods containing spores of fungus. Aflatoxin is a toxin normally made by a particular type of fungus often found on stored foods, especially grains and nuts. Animal tests have shown aflatoxin is a potent carcinogen, and it is suspected strongly to be the cause of the extraordinarily high incidence of liver cancer among Africans eating large amounts of inadequately stored and moldy corn and ground nuts. Levels of aflatoxin production on wheat increased with increasing doses of irradiation in a series of studies in India from 1976 to 1979; the studies also found that irradiation stimulated aflatoxin production in many other grains and vegetables.

In 1983, the U.S. Department of Agriculture sponsored a study by a division of Ralston-Purina. Mice fed irradiated chicken had a shorter lifespan, and an increased incidence of testicular cancer, than control animals fed nonirradiated chicken. Male dogs similarly tested weighed less and females showed a tendency to reproduce larger litters. Fruit flies, on the other hand, showed decreases in the number of offspring reproduced when fed irradiated foods. The size of the decrease corresponded with the amount of irradiation used on the food. Many results of this study relate to little understood effects on the reproductive system.

An article in *Consumers' Research Magazine* in 1982 reported that irradiation of food destroys significant amounts of some vitamins, especially A, C, E, and some of the B-complex. Other research done by the Department of Energy and the Pentagon into long-term effects of food irradiation is classified as military research, and has not been released to the public. One must assume that if this research supported the case the Department of Defense is attempting to make for food irradiation, it would have been declassified and released.

"Unique radiolytic products" referred to above are formed from free radicals (charged and highly reactive particles) produced by ionizing radiation. A 1980 FDA report stated that food irradiation at the proposed levels may create enough of these radiolytic products to warrant "toxicological evaluation."

Dr. John Gofman is professor emeritus of medical physics at the University of California at Berkeley and a world renowned authority on low level radiation. In 1984, he told the FDA that an epidemiological study researching the effects of a diet of irradiated food on human cancer rates and genetic injuries would require controlling the diets, and following the health histories, of many thousands of people for at least thirty, and preferably fifty, years. This amplifies how little is currently known about the effects of food irradiation.

The FDA has proposed that there is no need for a special label on irradiated foods. If current plans proceed, we will not be told which foods have been irradiated. In July of 1983 the FDA approved radiation doses of up to one million rads to control bacteria in spices and seasonings, and these foods are now sold nationwide without any explanatory labels.

Upon learning this information, one is tempted to conclude that the insanity of the entire plan is such that it cannot possibly go forward, that its very unreasonableness insures its defeat. We must not make this error. The forces behind the move to irradiate food are powerful. A great deal of money is involved; reason may well not prevail unless an aroused and informed citizenry makes its voice heard. As with most issues, the wallet's vote will be heard loudest; do not buy irradiated foods, and let food retailers know why.

Appendix   4

*An Explanation
of California's
Organic Food Act
of 1982*

*T*he California law states that the terms "organic," "organically grown," "naturally grown," "wild," "ecologically grown," or "biologically grown" may not be used for the advertising or labeling of a raw agricultural commodity, processed food product, or meat, poultry, fish, or milk, unless the food complies with the following conditions:

—Raw agricultural commodities must be in their unpeeled natural form, except for rapid heating or chilling, and with no applied coloring or synthetic materials. They must have been produced, harvested, distributed, stored, processed, and packaged without application of synthetically compounded fertilizers, pesticides, or growth regulators. No such materials may have been used on the fields for at least twelve months prior to the time the commodity was grown.

— Processed foods must be made only from foods grown as described above; only ascorbic acid, sodium ascorbate, calcium ascorbate, and citric acid may be used as preservatives.

— Meat, poultry, or fish must be produced without the use of any chemical or drug to stimulate or regulate growth or tenderness. No drugs or antibiotics may be injected or ingested, except for treatment of a specific disease and, if this is done, it must not have been within ninety days of the slaughter of the animal. At least the final 60 percent of the sale weight of the animal must be raised on organically grown feed (as defined above), with no medication or any other drug or chemical added.

— Milk must be from animals raised on organically grown, additive-free feed, unmedicated except for the treatment of a specific disease. If medications are used, they must not have been used within thirty days of the production of the milk.

Raw agricultural foods, processed foods, and meat, poultry, fish, or milk meeting these criteria may be labeled "Organically Grown (or "Organically Grown and Processed," or "Organically Grown and Produced") in Accordance with Section 26569.11 of the California Health and Safety Code."

That is the gist of California's law; Oregon's is similar. The California law has a clause specifically stating it does not apply to use of the term "natural" in labeling or advertising of a food; many food producers use this word, which has no clear meaning. Some animal products advertised as natural are raised without the use of antibiotics and hormones, but the animal feed used is commercially grown with pesticides and chemical fertilizers. In states where the term "organic" is not legally defined, these products may even be claimed to be organically raised.

Appendix 5

Exercise and Sports

*T*hroughout evolution, human beings have been hunters, food gatherers, and eventually agriculturists. Traditionally, people have spent each day working at physical tasks, walking, and sometimes running. Entertainment as well revolved around vigorous exercise, primarily in games and dance. Physical activity is as natural to us as breathing.

These things are missing from most lives today. Instead, we exercise for its own sake, if at all. And yet, the intense use of one's body in sport, game, or dance may give great satisfaction. So too may the simpler pleasure of a walk. Many of us allow little time for these things. We may take an occasional walk or a run after work, or perhaps play a weekend round of golf, but everyday pressures on our time seem to preclude doing more. Periodically, we may strive for regularity in our exercise in an attempt to "get in shape." At best, we take what exercise we can in what time we have.

Excercise that is enjoyed may most easily become a habit. Children may play until exhaused; time is suspended, and all life centers on the action of the play itself. Adults too may enjoy and benefit from vigorous physical play. The development of skills makes an activity fun; commitment and practice lead to enjoyment. The play of games and the often solitary enjoyment of activities such as walking may work well together for those who make the time for both.

Walking and Running

Walking and running require no team, partner, appointment, or court. The setting is outdoors, and for walking street clothes are appropriate. A pair of shoes is the only equipment needed.

Regular walking keeps one fit for occasional running, and occasional running keeps one fit for most other sports. Regular running keeps one fit for occasional racing.

People often ask if running is good for you. This depends on the individual. Approached reasonably and adapted to personal needs, running may be both fun and of lasting value.

All exercise initially fatigues muscles, tendons, and joints; when one stops, he is weaker than when he started. As the body recovers during the ensuing period of rest, strength returns. Given sufficient rest, the body's natural response to exercise is to become stronger. This is the physiological basis for increasing strength and endurance.

Thus a runner or walker becomes progressively weaker if he attempts so much at each session that his body cannot fully recover by the next session. Injuries eventually and inevitably result. In the excitement of getting involved, most of us begin in just that way.

For most people, the surest and safest way to become involved in running is to begin by walking. If interested in becoming a fit walker and runner, follow this plan.

Begin with two daily walks of five to fifteen minutes each, depending on previous exercise levels. This is more than it appears. The great marathoner Bill Rogers wrote that even a trained runner can never increase his total workload by more than 10 percent in one week without risking injury. For most people, adding five to fifteen minutes of walking twice a day to the total current amount of steady daily walking represents at least a 10 percent increase. So ease into this. Don't push the pace, and if ever stiff, sore, or just plain tired, skip a day and consider that too much may have been attempted.

Once ten to thirty minutes a day becomes effortless, with no stiffness or soreness, add five minutes a day to the total each week, building up to thirty minutes twice a day. The pace should have one just short of breathing hard, with the pulse in the 90 to 120 beats per minute range. Even the athletic individual is wise not to push harder than this in the beginning, for if one has not recently walked or run regularly, the muscles and joints easily become sore in the beginning.

Most people start out moving faster, but for shorter periods of time; running a mile or two in ten or twenty minutes is typical. This may be quite easily done, but the risk of injury is usually high. The heart and cardiovascular system can in most people take more strain than the joints. A preliminary walking program strengthens and trains the muscles, tendons, and joints to stand the strain of regular running. This beginning period builds a foundation for enjoying injury-free running. The body adapts slowly but very surely. As soon as an hour a day of walking becomes easy, some light jogging may easily be intermixed. A gradual buildup to thirty to sixty minutes of jogging on some days may follow.

A principle well known among runners is that of hard days and easy days. The body does not fully recover from a taxing effort in twenty-four hours. Days when one puts in extra effort (in distance or speed) are best followed with a day of easy or no effort. Very hard efforts may require more than one subsequent easy day. A hard-easy pattern is more natural, more interesting, and more fun than doing the same thing every day, and more rapid conditioning results.

Hard running that leaves one out of breath (anaerobic running) is best avoided the first few months. Such running rapidly conditions the heart for faster running, but the musculoskeletal system at this early stage is rarely able to handle the strain. Injuries usually result.

For the Serious Runner.   The individual interested in becoming a runner capable of covering several miles quickly may have difficulty proceeding slowly in the early stages. The adult previously involved in other sports, and with the cardiovascular fitness to run at a rapid pace, finds this especially true. Distance running is unlike most other sports, however, in that continuous stress is placed on the muscles and joints. Both the accomplished runner and the person seeking to become one should understand that musculoskeletal fitness lags behind cardiovascular fitness during the first few years of running. Most runners are thus capable of routinely running a given distance much faster than the muscles and joints can regularly stand.

This is why so many runners hurt so often. The sports medicine business has grown by treating runners with injuries through surgery, special shoes, physiotherapy, and a host of other methods, mostly because people insist on running too much too soon. We are built to run, indeed to run very fast, but not to run very fast continuously. The adaptations the body must make to do so without injury take time. Many champion runners have never hurt themselves running, so we know it is possible to reach one's potential without creating injuries. Indeed, development proceeds most rapidly when the demands placed on the body are the maximum that remain shy of causing injury.

Running that becomes a natural and balanced part of life will not cause injuries, especially if one eats a traditional diet. Poor nutrition makes runners more susceptible to injuries.

The challenge of competitive running is to discover what a concerted effort of body and mind can accomplish. Most people who race compete primarily against themselves; the other runners serve to spur one on to the exhilaration of one's own best effort. It is a unique satisfaction.

How Sports Can Help You

We balk at least a bit at the salaries of today's professional athletes. But pay is determined by supply and demand; we collectively place a premium on their skills.

Can we help but envy a bit the man or woman paid handsomely to play a game? Most of all, we admire the winners, those who through some combination of gifts and hard work have become what we sometimes would like to be—rich, famous, admired, and successful.

Those of us with an interest in sports occasionally live vicariously through athletes. Their victories and defeats are to an extent ours. Their lives are more like those of our primitive ancestors; they succeed or fail by the performance of their bodies. They know intimately the excitement of physical competition, the fear of injury, the thrill of winning.

For most of us, these things are a more subtle part of our lives; we miss the directness of sport. We compete instead for jobs, money, spouses, cars, prestige, houses...but inside we miss the more elemental competition of the athlete, the warrior, the primitive hunter.

Playing at a sport need not become all of these things. But personal sports and competition may fill a real and natural need. If we competed more ourselves in our own sports we might have less need to compete so viciously (as we sometimes do) economically, and less need for million-dollar-a-year heroes.

Athletic events may have marvelous moments. The way a person wins or loses may tell us a great deal about him. The way some teams work together like a family—or a tribe—calls to mind a not so distant past when survival depended on such cooperative but exhilarating effort. In our serious approach to the business of life, we often forget to laugh and have fun. Playing helps keep the child inside us alive.

Bibliography

The bibliography is arranged by chapters. For some chapters, two listings are presented—general and technical. The first is of material, mostly books, of potential interest to most readers. The second is of other references used in writing this book—journal articles and books of a more technical and specialized nature.

1   Traditional Diets and Natural Health Care

Darwin, Charles. *On the Origin of Species: A Facsmile of the First Edition.* Cambridge: Harvard University Press, 1975.
Hippocrates. *Hippocratic Writings.* Ed. by G. Lloyd, translated by J. Chadwick and W. Mann. Cambridge: Penguin Books, 1978.

2   Dr. Weston Price and Traditional Societies

General

Ashley-Montagu, F.M. "The Socio-Biology of Man." *Scientific Monthly,* June 1940.
Price, Weston. *Nutrition and Physical Degeneration.* La Mesa, California: The Price- Pottenger Nutrition Foundation, 1945 (originally published by The American Academy of Applied Nutrition, Los Angeles, 1939).

Technical

Price, Weston. "Why Dental Caries With Modern Civilizations?," Parts I—VI (I—IV: Field Studies; V: An Interpretation; VI: Practical Procedures For the Nutritional Control of Dental Caries). *Dental Digest,* March—August 1933.
————. "The Experimental Basis for a New Theory of Dental Caries, with Chemical Procedures for Determining Immunity and Susceptibility." *Dental Cosmos,* December 1932.
————. "New Light on Some Relationships between Soil Mineral Deficiencies, Low Vitamin Foods, and Some Degenerative Diseases Including Dental Caries with Practical Progress in Their Control." *Oral Health,* August 1932.
————. "New Light on the Cause of Tooth Decay in Man from Field Studies of Primitive Districts Providing Immunity." *The Australian Journal of Dentistry,* December 1, 1933.
————. "Acid-Base Balance of Diets Which Produce Immunity to Dental Caries Among the South Sea Islanders and Other Primitive Races." *Dental Cosmos,* September 1935.
————. "Studies of Relationships Between Nutritional Deficiencies and (a) Facial and Dental Arch Deformities and (b) Loss of Immunity to Dental Caries Among South Sea Islanders and Florida Indians." *Dental Cosmos,* November 1935.

―――――. "Eskimo and Indian Field Studies in Alaska and Canada." *Journal of the American Dental Association*, March 1936.

―――――. "Changes in Facial and Dental Arch Form and Caries Immunity in Native Groups in Australia and New Zealand Following the Adoption of Modernized Foods." An address to the Connecticut State Dental Association, Hartford, on May 12, 1937.

―――――. "Field Studies Among Primitive Races in Australia and New Zealand." *The New Zealand Dental Journal*, March 1938.

3   Benefits of Raw Foods

General

McCarrison, Sir Robert. *Nutrition and Health*. London: Faber and Faber, 1953.

Pottenger, Elaine, and Robert Pottenger Jr., eds. *Pottenger's Cats: A Study in Nutrition* (edited writings of Francis Pottenger). La Mesa, California: The Price-Pottenger Nutrition Foundation, 1983.

Technical

Pottenger, Francis M. Jr. "Hydrophilic Colloidal Diet." *American Journal of Digestive Diseases*, April 1938, Vol. 5, No. 2.

―――――. "Clinical Evidences of the Value of Raw Milk." *Certified Milk*, July 1938.

―――――, and Simonsen, D. "Deficient Calcification Produced by Diet: Experimental and Clinical Considerations." *Transactions of the American Therapeutic Society*, 1939.

―――――, and Simonsen, D. "The Influence of Heat Labile Factors on Nutrition in Oral Development and Health." *Journal of Southern California State Dental Association*, November 1939.

―――――. "Heat Labile Factors Necessary for the Proper Growth and Development of Cats." *Journal of Laboratory and Clinical Medicine*, December 1939.

―――――. "The Clinical Significance of the Osseous System." *Transactions of American Therapeutic Society*, 1940, Vol. 40.

―――――. "The Importance of a Vital, High Protein Diet in the Treatment of Tuberculosis and Allied Conditions." *Bulletin of the American Academy of Tuberculosis Physicians*, July 1941.

―――――. "Nutritional Aspects of the Orthodontic Problem." *The Angel Orthodontist*, October 1942, Vol. 12, No. 4.

―――――. "The Therapeutic Value of a Thermo-labile Factor Found in Fats, Particularly the Lecithins, in Dermatoses." *Transactions of the American Therapeutic Society*, 1943. *Southern Medical Journal*, April 1944, Vol. 37.

―――――. "The Effect of Heat-processed Foods and Metabolized Vitamin D Milk on the Dentofacial Structures of Experimental Animals." *Journal of Orthodontics and Oral Surgery*, August 1946, Vol. 32, No. 8.

―――――, and F.M. Pottenger, Sr. "Adequate Diet in Tuberculosis." *American Review of Tuberculosis*, Sept. 1946, Vol. 54, No.3.

―――――. "The Responsibility of the Pediatrician in the Orthodontic Problem." *California Medicine*, Oct. 1946, Vol. 65, No. 4.

―――――, I. Allison, and W. Albrecht. "Brucella Infections." *Merck Report*, July 1949.

―――――. "The Use of Copper, Cobalt, Manganese, and Iodine in the Treatment of Undulant Fever." *Annals of Western Medicine and Surgery*, September 1949.

―――――, and Bernard Krohn. "Influence of Breast Feeding on Facial Development." *Archives of Pediatrics*, October 1950, Vol. 67.

————, and Bernard Krohn. "Reduction of Hypercholesterolemia by High-fat Diet Plus Soybean Phospholipids." *American Journal of Digestive Diseases*, April 1953, Vol. 19, No. 4.

————. "The Effects of Disturbed Nutrition on Dento-Facial Structures." *Southern California State Dental Journal*, February 1982.

————. "Essentiality of Fats in Nutrition." *Journal of Applied Nutrition*, Autumn 1956, Vol. 9, No. 2.

————. "Therapeutic Effect of Lamb Fat in the Dietary." *Journal of Applied Nutrition*, Spring 1957, Vol. 10, No. 2.

————. "Milk—The Importance of Its Source." *Modern Nutrition*, November 1961.

————. "Applied Nutrition—President's Address." *Journal of Applied Nutrition*, 1965, Vol. 18, Nos 1—4.

4   *Evolution, Food, and Health: From Ancient Ancestors to Contemporary Hunter-Gatherers*

General

Bronowski, Jacob. *The Ascent of Man*. Boston: Little Brown & Co., 1974.

Darwin, Charles, introduced and abridged by R.E. Leakey. *The Illustrated Origin of Species*. New York: Hill & Wang, 1979.

Leakey, Richard E., and Roger Lewis. *Origins: The Emergence and Evolution of Our Species and Its Possible Future*. New York: E.P. Dutton, 1977.

Shute, Wilfrid E., and H. Taub. *Vitamin E for Ailing and Healthy Hearts*. New York: Pyramid, 1972.

White, Paul Dudley. *Heart Disease*. New York: Macmillan Co., 1943.

Technical

Allen, C.E., M.A. Mackey. "Compositional Characteristics and the Potential for Change in Foods of Animal Origin." In: Beitz, D.C., R.G. Hansen, eds. *Animal Products in Human Nutrition*. New York: Academic Press, 1982.

Angel, J.L. "Paleoecology, Paleodemography, and Health." In: Polgar, S., ed. *Population, Ecology, and Social Evolution*. The Hague: Mouton, 1975.

Bunn, H.T. "Archaeological Evidence for Meat-eating by Plio-Pleistocene Hominids from Koobi Fora and Olduvai Gorge." *Nature* 1981; 291.

Byerly, T.C. "Effects of Agricultural Practices on Foods of Animal Origin." In: Harris, R.S., and E. Karmis, eds. *Nutritional Evaluation of Food Processing*. Westport, Connecticut: Avi, 1975.

Cavalli-Sforza, L.L. "Human Evolution and Nutrition." In: Walcher, D.N., and N. Kretchmer, eds. *Food, Nutrition, and Evolution: Food as an Environmental Factor in the Genesis of Human Variability*. New York: Masson, 1981.

Cohen, M.N. *The Food Crisis in Prehistory: Overpopulation and Origins of Agriculture*. New Haven: Yale University Press, 1977.

Eaton, S.B., and M. Konner. "Paleolithic Nutrition." *The New England Journal of Medicine* 1985; 312.

Enos, W.F. et al. "Coronary Disease Among United States Soldiers Killed in Action in Korea." *The Journal of the American Medical Association* 1953; 152.

Foley, R. "A Reconsideration of the Role of Predation on Large Mammals in Tropical Hunter-Gatherer Adaptation." *Man* 1982; 17.

Gaulin, S., and M.Konner. "On the Natural Diet of Primates, Including Humans." In:
    Wurtman, R., and J. Wurtman, eds. *Nutrition and the Brain*, Volume 1. New York: Raven
    Press, 1977.
Hayden, B. "Subsistence and Ecological Adaptations of Modern Hunter-Gatherers." In:
    Harding, R., and G. Teleki, eds. *Omnivorous Primates: Gathering and Hunting in Human
    Evolution*. New York: Columbia University Press, 1981.
Howells, W.W. *Evolution of the Genus Homo*. Reading: Addison-Wesley, 1973.
Kay, R. "Diets of Early Miocene African Hominoids." *Nature* 1977; 268.
Lee, R. "What Hunters Do For a Living, or, How to Make Out On Scarce Resources." In:
    Lee, R., and I. De Vore, eds. *Man the Hunter*. Chicago: Aldine, 1968.
Lee, R., and I. De Vore, eds. *Kalahari Hunter-Gatherers: Studies of the Kung San and their
    Neighbors*. Cambridge: Harvard University Press, 1976.
MacNeish, R. "A Summary of the Subsistence." In: Byers, D., ed. *The Prehistory of the
    Tehuacan Valley*, Volume 1. Austin: University of Texas Press, 1967.
Moodie, P. *Aboriginal Health*. Canberra: Australian National University Press, 1973.
Nickens, P. "Stature Reduction as an Adaptive Response to Food Production in Mesoam-
    erica." *Journal of Archaeological Science* 1976; 3.
Potts, R., and P. Shipman. "Cutmarks Made by Stone Tools on Bones From Olduvai Gorge,
    Tanzania." *Nature* 1981; 291.
Rendel, J. "The Time Scale of Genetic Change." In: Boyden, S., ed. *The Impact of Civilization
    on the Biology of Man*. Canberra: Australian National University Press, 1970.
Schaefer, O. "Medical Observations and Problems in the Canadian Arctic." *Canadian Med-
    ical Association Journal* 1959; 81.
Schoeninger, M. "Diet and the Evolution of Modern Human Form in the Middle East."
    American Journal of Physical Anthropology 1982; 58.
Stini, W. "Body Composition and Nutrient Reserves in Evolutionary Perspective." In:
    Walcher, D., and N. Kretchmer, eds. *Food, Nutrition, and Evolution: Food as an Environ-
    mental Factor in the Genesis of Human Variability*. New York: Masson, 1981.
Trowell, H. "Hypertension, Obesity, Diabetes mellitus and Coronary Heart Disease." In:
    Trowell, H., and D. Burkitt, eds. *Western Diseases: Their Emergence and Prevention*. Cam-
    bridge: Harvard University Press, 1981.
Truswell, A., and J. Hansen. "Medical Research Among the !Kung." In: Lee, R., and I. De
    Vore, eds. *Kalahari Hunter-Gatherers*. Cambridge: Harvard University Press, 1976.
Velican, D., and C. Velican. "Atherosclerotic Involvement of the Coronary Arteries of
    Adolescents and Young Adults." *Atherosclerosis* 1980; 36.
Walker, A. et al. "A Possible Case of Hypervitaminosis A in Homo Erectus." *Nature* 1982;
    296.
Watt, V., and A. Merrill. *Composition of Foods* (Agriculture Handbook #8). Washington,
    D.C.: U.S.D.A., 1975.
Wehmeyer, A. et al. "The Nutrient Composition and Dietary Importance of Some Vegetable
    Foods Eaten by the !Kung Bushmen." *South African Medical Journal* 1969; 43.

5   *Long-Lived People of Vilcabamba, Hunza, and Georgian Russia*

General

Clark, John. *Hunza, Lost Kingdom of the Himalayas*. New York: Funk and Wagnalls, 1956
Davies, David. *The Centenarians of the Andes*. Garden City, NY: Anchor, 1975.
Leaf, Alexander. "Every Day Is a Gift When You Are Over 100." *National Geographic*, January
    1973.
Pearson, Durk, and Sandy Shaw. *Life Extension: A Practical Scientific Approach*. New York:
    Warner Books, 1982.

Taylor, Renee. *Hunza Land: The Fabulous Health and Youth Wonderland of the World.* New York: Award Books, 1964.

Technical

McCarrison, Robert. "Faulty Food in Relation to Gastro-Intestinal Disorder." *Journal of the American Medical Association* 1922;1.
————. *Studies in Deficiency Diseases.* London: Oxford Medical Publications, Henry Frowde and Hodder & Stoughton, 1945.

6   *Protective Characteristics of Traditional Diets*

General

Bland, Jeffrey. *Historical Use of, Biological Basis For, and Preparation of Glandular-Based Food Supplements.* Tacoma: 1979.
Passwater, Richard A. *EPA—Marine Lipids.* New Canaan, Connecticut: Keats Publishing, 1982.

Technical

Crawford, M.A. "Fatty-acid Ratios in Free-living and Domestic Animals." *Lancet* 1968; 1.
Culp, B.R. et al. "The Effect of Dietary Supplementation of Fish Oil on Experimental Myocardial Infarction." *Prostaglandins* 1980; 20.
Dyerberg, J. et al. " Eicosapentaenoic Acid and Prevention of Thrombosis and Atherosclerosis." *Lancet* 15.7.78.
Hemmings, W.A., and E.W. Williams. "Transport of Large Breakdown Products of Dietary Protein Through the Gut Wall." *Gut* 1978; 19.
Hornstra, G. et al. "Fish Oils, Prostaglandins, and Arterial Thrombosis." *Lancet* 17.11.79.
Jakubowski, J.A., and N.G. Ardlie. "Modification of Human Platelet Function by a Diet Enriched in Saturated Fat or Polyunsaturated Fat." *Atherosclerosis* 1978; 31.
Moncada, S., and J.L. Amezcua. "Prostaglandins, Thromboxane A2 Interactions and Thrombosis." *Haemostasis* 1979; 8.
Sanders, T.A., and K.M. Younger. "The Effect of Dietary Supplements of Omega-3 Polyunsaturated Fatty Acids on the Fatty Acid Composition of Platelets and Plasma Choline Phosphoglycerides." *British Journal of Nutrition* 1981; 45.

7   *Fish, Fat-Soluble Nutrients, and Health*

Technical

Bang, H. et al. "The Composition of the Eskimo Food in North Western Greenland." *American Journal of Clinical Nutrition* 1980; 33.
Bang, H. et al. "Plasma Lipids and Lipoproteins in Greenlandic West Coast Eskimos." *Acta Med. Scand.* 1972; 192.
Bronsgeest-Schoute, H. et al. "The Effect of Various Intakes of Omega-3 Fatty Acids on the Blood Lipid Composition in Healthy Human Subjects." *American Journal of Clinical Nutrition* 1981; 34.
Connor, W. et al. "A Comparison of Dietary Polyunsaturated Omega-6 and Omega-3 Fatty Acids in Humans: Effects Upon Plasma Lipids, Lipoproteins and Sterol Balance." *Arteriosclerosis* 1981; 1.

Connor, W. et al. "Dietary Deprivation of Linolenic Acid in Rhesus Monkeys: Effects on Plasma and Tissue Fatty Acid Composition and on Visual Function." *Transactions of the Association of American Physicians* 1985.

Dyerberg, J. et al. "Eicosapentaenoic Acid and Prevention of Thrombosis and Atherosclerosis?" *Lancet* 1978; 2.

Exler, J. and J. Weihrauch. "Finfish: Comprehensive Evaluation of Fatty Acids in Foods." *Journal of Am. Diet. Assoc.* 1976; 69.

Fehily, A. et al. "The Effect of Fatty Fish on Plasma Lipid and Lipoprotein Concentrations." *American Journal of Clinical Nutrition* 1983; 38.

Goodnight, S. Jr. et al. "Polyunsaturated Fatty Acids, Hyperlipidemia, and Thrombosis." *Arteriosclerosis* 1982; 2.

Goodnight, S. Jr. "The Effects of Dietary Omega-3 Fatty Acids Upon Platelet Composition and Function in Man: A Prospective, Controlled Study." *Blood* 1981; 58.

Harris, W. et al. "The Mechanism of the Hypotriglyceridemic Effect of Dietary Omega-3 Fatty Acids in Man." *Clinical Research* 1984; 32 abstract.

Harris, W. et al. "The Comparative Reductions of the Plasma Lipids and Lipoproteins by Dietary Polyunsaturated Fats: Salmon Oil Versus Vegetable Oil." *Metabolism* 1983; 32.

Hirai, Aizan et al. "Eicosapentaenoic Acid and Platelet Function in Japanese." *Lancet*, Nov. 22, 1980, letter to ed.

Holman, R. "Significance of Essential Fatty Acids in Human Nutrition." In: Paoletti, R. et al, eds. *Lipids*, Vol. 1. New York: Raven Press, 1976.

Hornstra, G. et al. "Fish Oils, Prostaglandins, and Arterial Thrombosis." *Lancet* 1979; 2.

Iritani, N. et al. "Reduction of Lipogenic Enzymes by Shellfish Triglycerides in Rat Liver." *Journal of Nutrition* 1980; 110.

Keys, A. *Seven Countries: A Multivariate Analysis of Death and Coronary Heart Disease.* Cambridge: Harvard University Press, 1980.

Kromhout, D. et al. "The Inverse Relation Between Fish Consumption and 20-Year Mortality From Coronary Heart Disease." *New England Journal of Medicine* 1985; 19.

Lossonczy, T. et al. "The Effect of a Fish Diet on Serum Lipids in Healthy Human Subjects." *American Journal of Clinical Nutrition* 1978; 31.

Neuringer, M. et al. "Dietary Omega-3 Fatty Acid Deficiency and Visual Loss in Infant Rhesus Monkeys." *Journal of Clinical Investigation* 1984; 73.

Phillipson, B. et al. "Reduction of Plasma Lipids, Lipoproteins, and Apoproteins by Dietary Fish Oils in Patients With Hypertriglycidemia." *New England Journal of Medicine* 1985; 19.

Sanders, T. et al. "Cod Liver Oil, Platelet Fatty Acids, and Bleeding Time." *Lancet* 1980; 1.

Siess, W. et al. "Platelet-Membrane Fatty Acids, Platelet Aggregation, and Thromboxane Formation During A Mackerel Diet." *Lancet*, March 1, 1980.

8   *A Review of Several Well-Known Diets*

General

Atkins, Robert, and Ruth West Herwood. *Dr. Atkins' Diet Revolution.* New York: Bantam Books, 1972.

Haught, S.J. *Has Dr. Max Gerson A True Cancer Cure?* North Hollywood, California: London Press, 1962. Retitled *Cancer? Think Curable! The Gerson Therapy.* Bonita, California: The Gerson Institute, 1983.

Kinderlehrer, Jane. "Liver May Hold the Secret of Cancer Prevention." *Cancer Control Journal* 1975, Vol. 3, Nos. 1 & 2.

Kushi, Michio. *The Macrobiotic Approach to Cancer.* Wayne, New Jersey: Avery Publishing, 1981.

Kushi, Michio, and Alex Jack. *The Cancer Prevention Diet*. New York: St. Martin's Press, 1983.

Pritikin, Nathan, and Patrick McGrady, Jr. *The Pritikin Program For Diet and Exercise*. New York: Grosset & Dunlap, 1979.

Sattilaro, Anthony, and Tom Monte. *Recalled By Life: The Story of My Recovery From Cancer*. Boston: Houghton-Mifflin, 1982.

Straus, Charlotte Gerson. "The Gerson Therapy." *Cancer Control Journal* 1975, Vol. 3, Nos. 1 & 2.

Tarnower, Herman, and Samm S. Baker. *The Complete Scarsdale Medical Diet*. New York: Bantam Books, 1978.

Walker, N.W. *Fresh Vegetable and Fruit Juices*. Phoenix: Norwalk Press, 1978. Originally *Raw Vegetable Juices*, 1936.

Technical

Gerson, Max. *A Cancer Therapy: Results of Fifty Cases*. Del Mar, California: Totality Books, 1958. Now published by The Gerson Institute, Bonita, California, 1986.

9 Creating a Traditional Diet for Health and Longevity

General

Lieb, Clarence W. "The Effects of an Exclusive Long-Continued Meat Diet, Based on the History, Experience and Clinical Survey of Vilhjalmur Stefansson, Arctic Explorer." *Journal of the American Medical Association*, July 23, 1926.

Stefansson, Vilhjalmur. "Adventures in Diet," Parts I—III. *Harper's Monthly Magazine*, November 1935—January 1936.

————. "Food of the Ancient and Modern Stone Age Man." *Journal of the American Dietetic Association*, July 1937,Vol.13, No. 2.

————. *My Life With the Eskimo*. New York: The Macmillan Co., 1951.

————. *The Fat of the Land*. New York: The Macmillan Co., 1957.

10 Recovery Through Nutrition: Dietary Considerations For Specific Conditions

General

Barnes, Broda, and Lawrence Galton. *Hypothyroidism: The Unsuspected Illness*. New York: Thomas Y. Crowell Co., 1976.

Harrower, Henry. *Practical Organotherapy: The Internal Secretions in General Practice*. Glendale, California: The Harrower Laboratory, 1922.

————. *An Endocrine Handbook*. Glendale, California: The Harrower Laboratory, 1939.

Hooten, Ernest A. *Apes, Man and Morons*. New York: Putnam, 1937.

————. *Up From the Apes*. New York: The Macmillan Company, 1946.

Moss, Ralph. *The Cancer Syndrome*. New York: Grove Press, 1980.

Page, Melvin. *Degeneration-Regeneration*. Page Foundation, 1949.

————, and H. Leon Abrams, Jr. *Your Body Is Your Best Doctor* (originally *Health Versus Disease*). New Canaan, Connecticut: Keats Publishing Company, 1972.

Passwater, Richard. *Supernutrition*. New York: Dial Press, 1975.

————. *Cancer and Its Nutritional Therapies*. New Canaan, Connecticut: Keats Publishing Company, 1978.

Schachter, Michael, and David Shienken. *Food, Mind and Mood.* New York: Warner Books, 1980.
Shelton, Herbert. *Fasting For Renewal of Life.* Tampa: Natural Hygiene, 1974.
Warmbrand, Max. *The Encyclopedia of Health and Nutrition.* New York: Pyramid Books, 1974. Originally *The Encyclopedia of Natural Health.* The Julian Press, 1962.

11   Relationships: Individuals, Physicians, and Health Goals

Baynes, C.F., and R. Wilhelm, trans. *I Ching or Book of Changes.* Princeton: Princeton University Press, 1967.
Degowin, E., and R. Degowin, *Bedside Diagnostic Examination.* New York: Macmillan, 1981.

12   Fish and Shellfish

Abelson, P. "Oil Spills." *Science* 195: 1977.
Ahmed, A. "PCB's In the Environment." *Environment* 18: 1976.
Blumer, M. "Scienfific Aspects of the Oil Spills Problem." Paper presented to the Oil Spills Conference Committee on Challenges of Modern Society, NATO. Brussels, 1970.
Blumer, M. et al. "A Small Oil Spill." Contribution No. 2630 of the Woods Hole Oceanographic Institution. *Environment* 13: 1971.
Gerber, W. "Coastal Conservation." *Editorial Res. Rep.* 1: 1970.
Goto, M., and K. Higuchi. "The Symptomatology of Yusho (Chlorobiphenyls Poisoning) in Dermatology." *Fukuoka Acta Med.* 60: 1969.
Grant, N. "Mercury in Man." *Environment* 13: 1971.
Hammond, H. "Mercury in the Environment: Natural and Human Factors." *Science* 171, 1971.
Jensen, S. "The PCB Story." *Ambio* 1: 1972.
Krebs, C., and K. Burns. "Long-Term Effects of an Oil Spill on Populations of the Salt-Marsh Crab Uca Pugnax." *Science* 97:1977.
Kuratsume, M., et al. "Yusho, a Poisoning Caused By Rice Oil Contaminated With Polychlorinated Biphenyls." *HSHMA Health Rep.* 86: 1971.
Maugh, T. "Polychlorinated Biphenyls: Still Prevalent, But Less of a Problem." *Science* 178: 1972.
Pimentel, D. "Effects of Pollutants on Living Organisms Other Than Man." In: *Restoring the Quality of Our Environment.* Report of the Environmental Pollution Panel, President's Science Advisory Committee, Appendix Y10. Washington, D.C.: November 1965.
Stallings, D., and F. Mayer Jr. "Toxicities of PCB's to Fish and Environmental Residues." *Environmental Health Perspectives* 1: 1972.

13   The Production of Modern Meat, Fowl, and Eggs

The Humane Farming Association. "Consumer Alert: The Dangers of Factory Farming." San Francisco, 1985.
Schell, Orville. *Modern Meat: Antibiotics, Hormones, and the Pharmaceutical Farm.* New York: Random House, 1984.

14   Naturally Raised Meat, Fowl, and Eggs

Brewington, C., Branch Chief, Labeling Branch, Standards and Labeling Division, Meat and Poultry Inspection Technical Services, Food Safety and Inspection Service, USDA,

Washington, D.C. Correspondence to Coleman Ranch verifying that Coleman Natural Beef label was approved by USDA.

California Legislative Counsel's Digest. Chapter 914, Assembly Bill No. 443. "California Organic Foods Act of 1982."

Coleman Natural Beef, Inc. "Coleman Certified Chemical Free Meats From the Colorado Rockies." Collection of letters from government officials, veterinarians, and feed suppliers, dated 1983–1986, verifying Coleman meats are completely chemical free and organically grown, as verified by USDA.

The Cook's Magazine: The Magazine of Cooking in America. "Dream Meat." May/June 1984 (article about Brae Beef of Stamford, Connecticut).

Industrial Laboratories Co. "Analysis Report" on Coleman beef. All tests negative (for DES, antibiotics, and drugs and chemicals commonly used in beef production).

Oregon Homegrown Meats. "Fat Content and Lean Yield By Boneless Primal Cut." Comparison of grass-fed and grain-fed beef by Oregon State University scientists, in private correspondence from Oregon Homegrown Meats. Eugene, March 1, 1986.

Thompson, Kevin. "Chemical-Free Meat: Is it a 'natural' or just another gimmick." *Meat Industry,* January 1986.

See also references for Lieb, Clarence W., and Stefansson, Vilhjalmur, under chapter 9.

15   Conventional Milk and Milk Products

Brehm, Wayne. "Potential Dangers of Viosterol During Pregnancy With Observations of Calcification of the Placenta." *The Ohio State Medical Journal,* September 1937, Volume 33, No. 9.

Dong, Collin H., and Jane Banks. *New Hope For the Arthritic.* New York: Ballantine Books, 1975.

The National Enquirer, March 11, 1975 (quoting Drs. Kurt Oster and Kurt Esselbacher).

16   Certified Raw Milk, Butter, and Raw Milk Cheeses

See references on food and evolution in chapter 4 and on certified raw milk in chapter 6.

17   Chemical Versus Organic Farming

California Certified Organic Farmers. "Improve Your Life For Good." Santa Cruz, 1985.

Fredericks, Carlton. *Look Younger, Feel Healthier.* New York: Simon and Schuster, 1972.

Rodale, J.I. *Organic Gardening.* Garden City, New York: Hanover House, 1959.

Squire, Mark. *Organically Grown: A Consumer's Guide to Sustainable Agriculture.* Fairfax, California: Good Earth Natural Foods, 1984.

18   Vegetables

Bland, Jeffrey. "Lecture on Calcium Metabolism, May 12, 1979." In: Schmid, Ronald F., ed. *Lectures of Dr. Jeffrey Bland: Nutrition, Exercise, and Health.* Portland, Oregon: The National College of Naturopathic Medicine, 1980.

19   Whole Grain Foods   *20   Fruits, Nuts, and Seeds*

See references on food and evolution in chapter 4.

21   Other Foods, Seasonings, and Beverages

Alcoholics Anonymous. *Alcoholics Anonymous.* New York: Alcoholics Anonymous World Services, Inc., 1955. Originally published in 1939.

Alcoholics Anonymous. *Pass It On: The Story of Bill Wilson and How the A.A. Message Reached the World.* New York: Alcoholics Anonymous World Services, Inc., 1984. Originally published by Princeton University Press in 1953.

Dadd, Debra. *Nontoxic and Natural.*Los Angeles: Jeremy P. Tarcher, Inc., 1984.

Thomsen, Robert. *Bill W.* New York: Harper & Row, 1975.

22   Vitamins, Minerals, and Food Supplements

Squire, Mark. "How Natural are Natural Vitamins." Fairfax, California: Good Earth Natural Foods, 1977.

Czap, Al. "Take Two Tablets of BHT and Call Me in the Morning." *Townsend Letter for Doctors.* June 1984/Issue No. 16.

———. "Are Vitamin Companies Solvent; A Non-Pecuniary Review." *Townsend Letter for Doctors,* July 1984/Issue No. 17.

Appendix 1   Seafood: Characteristics and Habitat of Popular Fish and Shellfish

McClane, A.J. *The Encyclopedia of Fish Cookery.* New York: Holt, Rinehart & Winston, 1977.

Detrick, Mia, *Sushi.* San Francisco: Chronicle Books, 1982.

Omae, Kinjiro, and Yuzuto Tachibana. *The Book of Sushi.* New York: Kodansha International Ltd., 1981.

Appendix 2   Understanding Laboratory Tests

Berkow, Robert, ed. *The Merck Manual.* Rahway, New Jersey: Merck, 1982.

Appendix 3   Food Irradiation: The Latest Threat to Our Foods

The Marin Coalition to Stop Food Irradiation. *Food Irradiation: Protect Your Right to Know.* Novato, California: 1986.

Rauber, Paul. "Irradiation: What Are the Risks?" *Coop News: The Bay Area Consumer Weekly,* December 9, 1985.

Appendix 4   An Explanation of California's Organic Food Act of 1982

The California Health and Safety Code, Section 26569.11.

Appendix 5   Exercise and Sports

Rodgers, Bill. *Marathoning.* New York: Simon & Schuster, 1982.

Index

Abalone, 221

Abkhazia, 54. *See also* Georgian Russia

Aborigines, 22–23; photographs of, 30, 32, 33

Acid rain, 228

Acne, 124

Activator X, 9

Adrenal glands, 14

Advertising, of vegetable oils, 80

Aflatoxins, and food irradiation, 242

Africa, 18–21

African tribes, 19–20

Africans, photographs of, 30,33

Agricultural revolution, 45, 48

Agricultural tribes, 20

Agriculture: modern, 70, 172–73; organic, 173–74

Agriculturists, and chronic diseases, 46

Alcoholic beverages, 191–93; and centenarians, 55; and gastrointestinal diseases, 125; health effects, 192–93; and migraines, 128; toxic ingredients in, 193; use by immune groups, 66

Alcoholics Anonymous, 191

Alcoholism, 191–92

Allergies, 108–110; and butter, 169; and dairy products, 163–64; and cheeses, 169; to sulfites, 233

Alpha-linolenic acid: and EPA, 76,83; in sprouts, 177

America, pre-industrial, 64

American Medical Association, 4

Amino acids, 71

Anchovies, 207

Anemia, 234–35

Angina pectoris, case history, 192–93

Animal Welfare Act, 155

Animals: conventional feeding of, 150–51; natural diet for, 157; treatment of, 155

Antibiotics: in acute illness, 94; and dairy products, 164; in meat production, 146–47, 152, 153; resistance to, 146; and viral diseases, 107

Antibodies, 117

Antioxidants, 198–99

Anxiety, 128–29

Arachidonic acid, 76,77,78

Archeological evidence (skull), photograph of, 31. *See also* Skulls

Arginine, 124

Arrhythmias, 116

Arteriosclerosis, 114

Arthritis: absence in primitive cultures, 10, 14, 23; and calcium metabolism, 114; incidence in modernizing primitive cultures, 11, 14–15, 16, 17, 23; symptoms, causes, and treatment, 112–14; and vitamin D₂, 165

Arthritis, rheumatoid: and alfalfa sprouts, 177; and dental decay, 24; and refined foods, 14–15; among Seminole Indians, 16; treatment of, 122–23

Ashley-Montagu, F.M., 21

Assessment, medical, 132

Atherosclerosis: and calcium metabolism, 114; and raw foods, 40

Australopithecus, 47–48

Autopsies, 46

Back problems, 113

Baptismal records, in Vilcabamba, 53–54; of centenarians, 53

Barnes, Broda, 240

Bass, freshwater, 229

Beef, fat composition of, 158. *See also* Meat; Foods, animal source

Beer, 193. *See also* Alcoholic beverages

Behavior, abnormal, 39

Biopsies, 119

Birth control, 60

Birth defects, and caffeine, 194

Blood pressure, and traditional diets, 116

Blood sugar, and sweeteners, 188. *See also* Glucose

Bluefish, 207–208

Bones: as a calcium source, 167; fish, 11, 214, 233; in soups, 8, 214, 233

Bone marrow, 14,34

Brain, and DHA, 159

Breads, whole grain, 182

Breast enlargement, from DES, 149

Bronchitis, and pork production, 152

Brucellosis, 43–44

Buckwheat, 180–81

Bursitis, 40

Butter: and fat-soluble nutrients, 83–84; in Loetschental Valley, 8,9; quality of, 169; raw, laws prohibiting, 170

Butterfish, 208

Caffeine: and caffeinism, 193–94; and heart problems, 116–17
Calcium: in egg shells, 158; in hunter-gatherer diets, 49; in immune groups' diets, 70; and periodontal disease, 113; in the Pottenger Cat Study, 37; and pregnancy, 104; sources, 161, 167, 200; and sugar consumption, 189; and traditional diets, 115
Calcium deficiency: and colitis, 125; and hypertension, 168
Calcium metabolism, 112–13; and chronic diseases, 114–15; and raw foods, 40–41; and vitamin D₂, 165–66
Calcium supplements, 200; for heart problems, 115
Cancer: absence of in primitive and traditional cultures, 7, 10, 15, 24, 54, 55–56; 60–61; accepted treatments and statistics, 118; in beef cattle, 153; and caffeine, 194; controversy over treatment, 119; and DES, 148; and EPA, 85; Hodgkin's disease, 108; and hormones, 148; incidence of, and dietary fiber, 69; incidence of, among whites in Torres Strait Islands, 24; lung, case history, 96; lung, and green vegetable consumption, 231; melanoma, case history, 120–21; nutritional therapy for, 90–92, 119, 120, 121; in poultry, 154; prevention of, 122; recovery from, 91; and smoked foods, 231; skin, 231; and vegetable oils, 80
The Cancer Syndrome, 119
A Cancer Therapy, Results of Fifty Cases, 91
Cancer? Think Curable—A Cancer Therapy, 91
Candidiasis, 129
Candlefish, 216
Carcinogens, 153, 231–32
Cardiovascular diseases, absence in centenarians, 55. See also Heart disease
Carotene, 225
Carotenoids, 186
Case histories: angina pectoris, 192–93; cancer, lung, 96; cancer, melanoma, 120–21; ear infections, 109; hemorrhoids, 126; migraines, 128
Castration, in meat production, 145
Cataracts, 40, 124
Cats (Pottenger's), 34, 35–38, 39
Cayenne, 190
Cellular infiltration, 115–16
Centenarians: diets of, 56–57, 57–59; fishermen, 59; life habits, 54; records of, 52; status and habits, 56
Centenarians of the Andes, 53
Character, 100–101
Cheese: allergies to, 168; fat-soluble nutrient content, 83–84; life-giving qualities, 9; in the Loetschental Valley, 8–9; and migraines, 128; natural, 169; salt content, 169; raw milk, 168,169

Chemotherapy, 91, 118
Chesapeake Bay, 218, 226
Children: and caffeine, 194; of centenarians, 56; spacing of births, 60, 104
Chloramphenicol, 151–52
Chlorophyl, 186
Chloroplasts, and EPA, 76, 77–78
Cholesterol: in animal source foods, 236–37; and fish oils, 79–80; and fish and shellfish, 114; and heart disease, 236–37; laboratory test for, 236–38; and the thyroid gland, 115–16; total to HDL ratio, 238
Cholesterol, HDL: and exercise, 237; significance, 237–38
Churchill, Winston, 204
Cigarettes. See Smoking
Civil registers in Vilcabamba, 54
Clams: characteristics and habitat, 221–22; and red tide, 222
Clark, John, 61, 62–63
Clotting of blood, and EPA, 82
Cod, 208–209; roe, 233
Cod liver oil: EPA content, 83; and hemorrhoids, 126; nutrient content, 85; and serum EPA, 83; supplements of, 200
Coffee, 125. See also Caffeine
Colds, 106–107
Colitis: and fruit, 184; treatment of, 125–26. See also Gastrointestinal disease
Colloids, 42
Competence of physicians, 5
Complete blood count (CBC), 234–35
Constipation: and calcium supplements, 115; and fiber, 69; and food selection, 99
Cooking: advantages of, 34; of bluefish, 208; of cod, 209; and digestion of protein, 69; effects on digestive tract, 42; effects on protein, 42; of lamb, 160; of lobster, 224–25; of shrimp, 228; of whole grains, 181
Cortisone, 123
Crab, 222–23
Cultures: primitive, 6 (See also Hunter-gatherers); traditional—See America, preindustrial; Gaelics; Georgian Russia; Hunter-gatherers; Hunza; Peru; Swiss; Vilcabamba
Curricula of medical schools, 4
Customs, dietary, 66. See also Wisdom, traditional; Diets, traditional; Foods, traditional

Dart, Raymond, 47
Davies, David, 53
Darwin, Charles, 3
Dairy products: and acute illnesses, 108; and allergies, 167,168; arguments against, 163–66; and arthritis, 113; controversy over, 166; EPA content, 68; and evolution, 168; historical use of, 167; raw, restrictions on, 170; recommended usage, 168–69; and sal-

monella outbreaks, 170; vitamin content of, 8–9, 67. *See also* Butter; Cheese; Milk

Death, 132

Decay, dental: absence of in primitive people, 7, 8, 10, 11–12, 14, 16, 19, 20, 23–27; and Aborigines, 23; and Africans, 18–19; and agriculture, 47; and Amazon Jungle Indians, 27; and ancient Peruvian skulls, 26; and Andes Mountain Indians, 27; and calcium-phosphorous metabolism, 189; cessation of, 8; in children, 6; and Gaelics, 10; and New Zealand Maori, 25; and North American Indians, 15; in modernizing primitive people, 9, 10, 11–12, 15, 17, 19, 20, 23, 24; protection against, 6; reversal of, 67; and South Seas Islanders, 17; and Swiss, 9; and Torres Strait Islanders, 24

Dental arches
—broad, photographs of, 29–31
—misshapen: absence of in primitive people, 7, 11–12, 15, 16, 19, 20, 22–27; in modernizing primitive people, 9, 11, 15, 17, 19, 20, 23–25; and changes in nutrition, 6; photographs of, 32–33

Diabetes: causes and treatment, 126–27; and the Gerson diet, 90; and glycohemoglobin, 240; and hypoglycemia, 240

Diagnosis, 134–35

Diet: of animals, and EPA, 68, 157; Atkins, 89; balanced, 102; fatless, 161; Gerson, 90–91; high-protein, at Pottenger Sanatorium, 34, 41; high-protein weight-loss, 89; macrobiotic, 94–97; all meat and fish, 103, 160–62; "no-aging," 214; optimal, dynamic aspect of, 99–101; Pritikin, 87–89; raw foods, 93, 94; rotation, 117; Scarsdale, 89; vegetarian—*See* Vegetarianism. *See also* Diets, traditional

Diethylstilbestrol (DES): and cancer, 148; in chicken production, 148–49; illegal use of, 149, 150; and meat production, 148

Diets, traditional: American, 64; of Aborigines, 23; of Amazon Jungle Indians, 27; of ancestral humans, 47–48, 63–64; in ancient Peru, 26; of Andes Mountains Indians, 27; calcium content of, 115; of centenarians, 56–57, 58–60; of Eskimos, 12; and fiber, 69–70; of Gaelics, 10; of hunter-gatherers, 49–50; of Hunzas, 61–62, 63, 182; individual variations, 103–104; of Masai, 19; and minerals, 70; post-agricultural, 50; of Pottenger, 41; and raw foods, 72; of South Seas Islanders, 17; of Torres Strait Islanders, 23. *See also* Diet

Digestion, and cooking, 42

Digestive system, and raw foods, 41–42

Disease: acute, 106–108; acute, in Hunza, 62; autoimmune—*see* Arthritis, rheumatoid; cardiovascular, 55 (*see also* Heart disease); causes of all, 130; gastrointestinal—*see* Gastrointestinal disease; heart—*see* Heart disease; rice oil, 141; skin—*see* Skin disease; as an unnatural phenomenon, 132. *See also names of individual diseases*

Diseases, chronic degenerative: absence of in Gaelics, 10; absence of in America around 1900, 64; absence of in Georgian Russia, 55; absence of in primitive cultures, 27–28; absence of in Vilcabamba, 54, 55; and arachidonic acid, 77; causes of, 12–13, 130; general treatment of, 130; immunity from, 7; 18–19; increased incidence of, 64–65; in Pottenger's cats and modernized humans, 39; and raw foods, 41; recovery from, 68; and refined foods, 20; and thyroid function, 111. *See also* Diseases, chronic and acute; *names of individual diseases*

Diseases, chronic and acute: in Pottenger Cat Study, 36–37; immunity from, among primitive Africans, 18–19

Docosahexaenoic acid (DHA): sources, 76; and vision, 82

Dolphin (mahimahi), 210; roe, 233

Down's syndrome, 130

Drug therapy, 5, 133, 150

Dulse, 177

Ear infections, 109

Eastman-Kodak, 197

Eaton, Boyd, 46

Eczema, 124

Eggs: naturally grown, 157–58; production of, 152

Eicosapentaenoic acid (EPA): amounts consumed, 80–81; blood levels, 81; and the diet of animals, 68; effects, 68; in fish, 78–79, 80; and heart disease, 78–79; immune-stimulating effect, 85; and intellectual function, 82; metabolism of, 75–78; and platelet aggregation, 81; in salmon, 214; sources, 67, 68, 77, 78; supplements of, 85; in tuna, 220; and vision, 82

Emotional disturbances, 128–29

Encyclopedia of Fish Cookery, 207, 231

Enemas: in acute illness, 107; in cancer therapy, 121

Enzymes: in alcoholic beverages, 192; in fruit, 183; and raw foods, 71

Epilepsy, 130

Erythrocyte sedimentation rate (ESR), 236

Eskimos: and fish consumption, 79; photographs of, 30, 32, 33; modernized and primitive, 11–12; and vitamin C, 161–62

Essential fatty acids: and EPA, 75–78. *See also* Alpha-linolenic acid; Gamma-linolenic acid; Linoleic acid

Eulachon, 216

Eutrophication, 139

Evolution: of ancestral humans, 47–48; cultural, 97; and diet, 3, 45–50
Examination, physical, 133, 134–35
Exercise: and bowel regularity, 99; endurance, and blood volume, 235; endurance, and HDL cholesterol, 237; and the heart, 117; and longevity, 53, 55; physiological effects, 247; and play, 246; in traditional cultures, 246; walking and running, 246–48

Farmers, Japanese, and EPA, 80–81
Farming: chemical, 172–73; organic, 173–74
Fasting: and acute illness, 94; author's experience, 103; case history, 107; and chronic disease, 93–94; and raw foods diets, 93–94; when and how, 106–108
Fatigue, chronic, 110
Fats, in hunter-gatherer diets, 50
Fats, animal: in Eskimo diet, 12–13; influences on quality, 159
Fat-soluble vitamins. See Vitamins, fat-soluble
Fat-soluble nutrients. See Nutrients, fat-soluble
Feminization, from DES, 149
Fertility, 39
Fertilizers: and meat production, 145; as water pollutants, 139–40
Fiber: and bowel regularity, 99; in hunter-gatherer diets, 49; in traditional diets, 69; in whole grains, 180
Fire, early use of, 34
Fish: flavor of, 218; cold-smoked, 232–33; freshwater, 228–30; raw, 103, 161 (see also Roe; Sushi and sashimi); saltwater, 207–222; smoked and salted, 231–32. See also Fish and shellfish
Fish and chips, 215
Fish and shellfish, 207–229; as dietary staples, 9–10, 17, 24, 25; and EPA, 75, 76; fat content, 142; and heart disease, 78–79, 114; least polluted species, 141–42; in the macrobiotic diet, 96–97; and pollution, 139–42; and pregnancy, 104; preservatives used on, 233; quality of, 141–42
Fish consumption: and arthritis, 114; effects on platelets, 81–82; and heart disease, 78–79; in evolution, 48; of Japanese fishermen and farmers, 80–81; optimal levels, 81
Fish liver oils, 198. See also Cod liver oil; Fish oils
Fish oils: and HDL cholesterol, 237–38; influence on blood fats, 79–80. See also Cod liver oil; Fish liver oils
Fishermen: photographs of, 29; Japanese, and EPA, 80–81; centenarians, 59
Fitness, musculoskeletal versus cardiovascular, 249
Flaxseed oil, 83
Flour, refined, 195; loss of nutrients in, 181–82. See also Foods, refined

Flounder, 216–17; roe, 233
Flu, 106–107
Food and Drug Administration (FDA): and alcoholic beverages, 193; and DES, 149; and food irradiation, 242, 243
Food supplements, 200–201; glandular products, 201. See also Vitamin supplements
Foods. See also names of individual foods
—animal source: and cholesterol, 237–38; and biological strength, 97; essentiality of, 49, 102; and height, 46; proportions of, 162; quality of, 144; and teeth, 59; in Vilcabamba, 57–58
—classification, in groups, 101–102
—indigenous, 66, 176
—raw: in the Arctic, 103; and arthritis, 113–14; and calcium metabolism, 40–41; in cancer therapy, 121; and chronic diseases, 41; diets of, social aspects, 94; and the digestive system, 41–42; essentiality of, 102; of Indians of the north, 14; and optimal health, 73; in the Pottenger Cat Study, 35, 36, 37, 38; in prehistory, 34; proteins and enzymes in, 71; safety of, 42–43; of South Seas Islanders, 17; in traditional cultures, 34, 72. See also Butter; Cheese; Meat; Milk
—refined: avoidance of, 195–96; and carbohydrate metabolism, 126–27; and chronic diseases, 20, 28, 47; and dental problems, 9, 10, 11–12, 15, 17, 19, 20, 23–25; effects of, photographs of, 32–33; history of, 47; imported into South Seas, 16; and loss of biological strength, 97; in primitive cultures, 7; problems associated with use of, 27–28
—traditional: and cancer prevention, 122; changing to, 195–96; displacement by refined foods, 13; versus vitamin and mineral supplements, 201–203. See also Diets, traditional; Wisdom, traditional
Foramen magnum, 47
Fowl: and antibiotics, 147; naturally raised, 157; production of, 154
Frank, Benjamin, 214
Fructose, 188, 189
Fruit, 183–185; and arthritis, 113; dried, 184, 188; in immune groups' diets, 67; juices, 183–84, 188
Fungicides, 172

Gaelics, 9–10
Gallstones, 40; and calcium metabolism, 114
Gamma-linolenic acid, 71
Gas, intestinal, 100, 184
Gastrointestinal disease: and caffeine, 184, 194; treatment of, 125–26
Gerson, Max, 90–92, 118
Gerson therapy: and lung cancer, 96; and pso-

riasis, 124; and rheumatoid arthritis, 123.
  See also Diet, Gerson
Genetic conditions, 130
Genetic material, non-nuclear, 130
Georgian Russia, 54–57; average blood pressure, 116; diet of oldsters, 57, 63–64; geography and population, 52; longevity in, 63; marriage in, 56; smoking in, 60; vigor of oldsters, 53
Glandular products, 201
Glaucoma, 130
Glucose: fasting, laboratory test for, 239; in honey, 188
Glucose tolerance test, 240
Glycohemoglobin, laboratory test for, 239
Goals, in health, 132, 135–36
Goiter, 26, 201
Gofman, John, 243
Grains
—as animal food, and EPA, 77
—refined, 181. *See also* Foods, refined
—whole, 180–82; cooking method, 181; as dietary staples, 10–11; foods made from, 181–82; organic, legal definition of, 244
Great Barrier Reef fisherman, photograph of, 29
Green leaf juice, 92. *See also* Juice, raw vegetable
Greens: cooked, 176; importance as animal feed, 77, 84, 157, 158

Haddock, 209; roe, 233
Hake, 209
Halibut, 210; roe, 233
Haught, S.J., 91
Hawaii, 16
Headaches: causes and treatment, 127–28; migraines, 128
Healing power of nature, 3
Health: and attitudes, 204; optimal, 68, 73; and resistance to disease, 43
Healing, natural, 4
Health care, alternative, 5
Hearing, 55
Heart, beef, 159
Heart Disease, 46
Heart disease: and caffeine, 194; causes and treatment, 114–17; and cholesterol, 237–38; and EPA, 68, 81; and fat-soluble nutrients, 84; and fish consumption, 78–79; and homogenized milk, 165; and prostaglandins, 76
Heat-labile nutrients. *See* Nutrients, heat-labile
Height, 45–46
Hematocrit, 234–35
Hemmings, W.A., 71
Hemoglobin, 234–35
Hemorrhoids, 125–26
Herbal medicine, 94
Herbicides, 172

Herbivores, African, 50
Herbs, 189–90
Heredity, intercepted, 12
Herpes, 123–24, 185
Herring, 211; roe, 233
High blood pressure. *See* Hypertension
Hippocrates, 4
Hippocrates Institute, 93
History, the medical, 134–35
Hodgkin's disease, 108
Hoffmann-La Roche, 197
Homo sapiens and *Homo species*, 47–48
Homogenization, 164–65
Homosexuality, 37, 39
Honey, 188–89
Hormones, in meat industry, 145, 147–150
Hudson River, 218
Hunter-gatherers: and chronic diseases, 46; contemporary, 46, 48–50; and the killing of animals, 155; strength of, 47. *See also* Aborigines; African tribes; Eskimos; Indians; Maori; Melanesia; Polynesia; Torres Strait Islanders
Hunza, 52, 60–63; conclusions about, 63; dietary staples, 62; diseases in, 61; geography and population, 52
Hunza Land, 61
Hunza, Lost Kingdom of the Himalayas, 61
Hyperactivity, 194
Hypercalcemia of infancy, 165–66
Hypertension: and caffeine, 116; and calcium, 115, 168; and hypothyroidism, 115–16
Hypoglycemia, 126–27, 184
Hypothyroidism: and hypertension, 115–16; and iodine deficiency, 201; symptoms of, 110

Illness, acute, 106–108
Immune groups: diets of, 66–67, 70. *See also* Decay, dental, absence of in primitive people
Immune system: and allergies, 117; in cancer, 118; in rheumatoid arthritis, 122
Immunity, from acute and chronic diseases, 18–19
Incan civilization, 26
Indians: Amazon Jungle, 27; Andes Mountain, 27; Kwakiutl, 216; North American, 13–16; northern, diet of, 13–14; northern, health of, 14–15; Seminole, 15–16
Industries, and water pollution, 140
Infants, treatment of acute illness in, 108
Influenza, 106–107
Insecticides, 145, 150
Intellectual function, and fish oils, 82
Iodine: and goiter, 200–201; in immune groups' diets, 70; in salmon roe, 12, 214; in shrimp, 227; sources, 201; supplements of, 201
Iron, 70

Irradiated ergosterol (vitamin D₂), 197
Irradiation of foods, 241–43
Isle of Harris, 9–10
Isle of Lewis, 9–10

Jesuits, 54
Journal of the American Dental Association, 7
Journal of the American Medical Association, 160
Juice: fruit, 183–84, 188; lemon, 216; raw liver, 92, 121; raw vegetable, 92, 179

Kasha, 180–81
Kelp: and iodine, 201; use by Peruvian Indians, 26
Ketones, 89
Kidney stones, 40; and calcium metabolism, 114
Kikuyu, 19–20
Konner, Melvin, 46
Kung tribe, 48–49
Kushi, Michio, 95, 97

Laboratory tests. *See* Tests, laboratory
Lamb, 159–160
Lasuria, Khfaf, 54–55
Laws: natural, and human health, 4; natural, and modern civilization, 21; nature's, and hereditary patterns, 12; about organic foods, 245–46
Leaf, Alexander, 54, 61–62
Leakey, Richard, 49
Lecithin, 186
Legumes, sprouted, 177
Lemon juice, 216
Lemons, 187
Leukemia, 92
Life expectancy, 64–65
Linoleic acid, 77–78
Linolenic acid. *See* Alpha-linolenic acid; Gamma-linolenic acid
Linseed oil, 83
Liver: importance of, 20; juice, 92, 121; in traditional diets, 13
Lobbies, political, 147
Lobster, 223–25; roe, 224
Loetschental Valley, 8, 9, 10–11
Longevity: and absence of disease, 54; in America, 64; conclusions about, 54, 63–64; in contemporary traditional cultures, 50–51; in hunter-gatherers, 49; and sex, 56; verification of, 52–53
Lutalyse, 146

Machhu Piccu, 26
Mackerel, 211–12; as exclusive diet, 81–82; roe, 233
Macrobiotics, philosophy of, 94, 97. *See also* Diet, macrobiotic
Macular edema, 130
Magnesium, 70
Malformations, dental, 39. *See also* Dental arches, misshapen
Maligancies, 117–122. *See also* Cancer

Maori, 24–25; and EPA, 82; fisherman, photograph of, 29
Maragoli, 20
Marriage, 56
Masai, 19
McCarrison, Robert, 38–39, 61, 62; and thyroid function, 111
McClane, A.J., 207, 230
Meat: consumption of by ancestral humans, 48; consumption of in Loetschental Valley, 8; desire for, 154–55; and EPA, 68, 162; exclusive diet of, 160–62; inspection of, 152–54; modern, EPA content, 68; modern, fat content, 50; modern, production of, 145–46; and mysticism, 49; naturally raised, 156–57; and northern Indians and Eskimos, 12–16; organic, legal definition of, 244; quality of, 145, 154–55; raw, organs, 159; raw, and prevention of scurvy, 103; raw, safety of, 43; from wild game, fat content, 50. *See also* Beef; Foods, animal source
Melanesia, 16
Melanesians, photograph of, 31
Melanoma, 120–21
Mental illness, 128–29
Mercury: in fish and other foods, 140; in swordfish, 219; in tuna, 220; in water, 139
Methylene chloride, 194
Mexico, 91
Migraines, 90
Milk
—breast, 41
—cultured, preparation of, 169
—in Loetschental Valley, 8
—organic, legal definition of, 244
—pasteurized, and osseous disturbances, 41
—processed, effects of in Pottenger Cat Study, 37–38
—raw: availability of, 171; certification and safety, 170; cultured, 168; and the dairy industry, 164; effects compared with other milks, 40–41; and pregnancy, 104; quality, safety, and legal status, 170–71; in traditional cultures, 9; versus pasteurized, 37–38
Milk products. *See* Butter; Cheese; Dairy products; Milk
Millet, 181
Mineral supplements, 202
Minerals: in butter, 9; deficiencies in brucellosis, 43–44; deficiencies in modern diets, 71; in traditional diets, 70; trace, in hunter-gatherer diets, 49
Modern Meat, 149
Mononucleosis, 107–108
Mortality, infant, 55–56, 59–60
Moss, Ralph, 119
Mucous, 99
Muhima, 20
Multiple sclerosis, 130; and calcium metabolism, 114

Muscular dystrophy, 130
Mussels, 225; and red tide, 222
Mysticism, and meat, 49
Myxedema, 201. *See also* Hypothyroidism

Natural hygiene, 93
Natural laws, 4, 21
Nature, healing power of, 3
Nature's laws, 12
Naturopathic medicine, 4
Neanderthal man, 48
Neurs, 20
New England Journal of Medicine, 46
New Zealand Maori. *See* Maori
Nightshade vegetables, 178–79
Nilotic tribes. *See* Masai
Nori, 178
Nucleic acids, 214
Nutrients
—fat-soluble, essentiality of, 10–11. *See also* Vitamins, fat-soluble
—heat-labile: in fresh versus dried greens, 38; and raw milk, 170
—protective: in animal life, 59; and animal source foods, 157; sources and significance, 72–73
Nutrition: and dental decay, 6; and doctor-patient relationships, 133–34; and mis-shapen dental arches, 6. *See also* Foods; Diet; Diets, traditional
Nutrition and Physical Degeneration: cultures studied, 7; photographs from, 29–33; reception on publication, 6; scope of Price's studies, 7; and traditional wisdom, 4
Nuts and seeds: and herpes, 124, 185; and intestinal gas, 185
Nystatin, 129

Oat meal, 181
Oats: as a dietary staple, 10; steel-cut, 181
Octopus, 225–26
Ohsawa, George, 95
Oil, as a water pollutant, 140
Oils, fish. *See* Fish oils
Oils, vegetable. *See* Vegetable oils
Olive oil, 80, 187
On the Origin of Species, 3
Optimal health, 68, 73, 101
Oregon Regional Primate Center, 82
Organ meats: in Pottenger's diet, 41; and pregnancy, 104; in primitive diets, 10, 11, 12, 13–14, 15; strengthening effects, 100; in therapy, 159
Organic farming, 173–74
Organic foods: California law defining, 244–45; legal status, 156
Origins, 49
Osteoporosis: and arthritis, 112; and calcium metabolism, 114–15
Oster, Kurt, 164–65
Outer Hebrides, islands of, 9–10
Oxalic acid, 176

Oysters, 226; and red tide, 222

Page, Melvin, 188–89
Pain, 113
Palpitations, 116
Pancreas supplements, 92
Parasites, 230
Passwater, Richard, 199
Pastas, whole grain, 182
Pasteurization, 163–64
Peking man, 34, 48
Personality, 100–101
Periodontal disease, 113
Peru, 25–27
Peruvians, photographs of, 29, 31
Pesticides, 164, 172
Pharmaceutical companies, 4
Physicians: relationships with patients, 132–35; as teachers, 133; naturopathic, 4, 5, 134
Plant growth, and nutrients in dairy products, 83–84
Politics, and meat inspection, 153
Pollution: and seafood, 139–42, 219; and fresh-water fish, 228–29
Polychlorinated biphenols (PCB's): in bluefish, 207–208; in Hudson River and in fish, 141; sources, 141; in swordfish, 219; toxic effects on fish, 140; toxic effects on humans, 141; in tuna, 220
Polynesia, 16
Polynesian, photograph of, 32
Pompano, 212
Pork, 152
Potassium, 183
Pottenger, Francis, 34–35; and lamb fat, 159–60; and raw foods, 72,159; and sweetened foods, 189
Pottenger Cat Study (Ten-Year Study), 34, 35–38, 39, 40
Poultry. *See* Fowl
Prawns, 228
Pregnancy: and caffeine, 194; danger from Lutalyse, 146; and DES, 148; exercise in, 104; megavitamin supplements in, 202; nutrition in, 19, 104; problems in, among reservation Indians, 15; problems in, and Vitamin D_2, 165
Preservatives: legally used in organic food, 244; on seafood, 227, 233
Price, Weston, 6; and fat-soluble vitamins, 8–9; and *Nutrition and Physical Degeneration*, 4; photographs by, 29–33; time in history, 7; travels of, 7, 18, 25
Price-Pottenger Nutrition Foundation, 6, 29
Primitive cultures. *See* Cultures, primitive; Hunter-gatherers
Pritikin, Nathan, 87, 88
Prostaglandins: and EPA, 68; metabolism and effects, 76–78
Protective nutrients. *See* Nutrients, protective
Protein: absorbtion of, 71–72; digestability of, 69; in hunter-gatherer diets, 49; in Hunza,

61; in Vilcabamba, 58. *See also* Foods, animal source
Psoriasis, 124

Radiation. *See* Irradiation of Foods
Raw meat. *See* Meat, raw
Recalled By Life, 96
Red tide, 222
Relationships, 132–36
Rice: brown, 181; wild, 181
Rice oil disease, 141
Roe, 232; lobster, 224; use by Peruvian Indians, 26; salmon, 12, 214; shrimp, 228
Romig, Josef, 15
Running: 246–48; and health, 101; injuries from, 247, 248; and pregnancy, 104

Salad, 175; dressing, 175
Saliva, 189
Salmon, 213–14; in Eskimo diet, 12; in prehistory, 213; roe, 213, 233; smoked, 232
Salmonella, 170
Salt, 190–91
Sardines, 214; in salad, 175
Sattilaro, Anthony, 95
Scallops, 226–27
Schell, Orville, 149; and meat inspection, 152–53, 154
Schweitzer, Albert, 90
Scurvy, 13–14, 161
Sea trout, 214–15
Seafood, 207–233. *See also* Fish and shellfish; *names of individual species*
Seasonings, 190–91
Seaweeds, edible, 177–78; as fiber source, 69
Seeds. *See* Nuts and seeds
Selenium, 199–200
Selenium as Food and Medicine, 199
Seton, Ernest Thompson, 204
Shad, 215; roe, 233
Shark, 215
Shellfish, 221–28; as a dietary staple, 9–10. *See also* Fish and shellfish
Shelton, Herbert, 93
Shrimp, 227–28
Skeletons, pre-Columbian, 15
Skin, redness of, 100
Skin disease, 124–25, 184
Skull, photograph of, 31
Skulls: Aborigine, 22; Maori, 24; Peruvian, 26; pre-Columbian, 15–16, 26
Smelt, 215–16
Smoking, 55, 60
Snapper, 216
Sodium, 49, 190
Sodium bisulfite, 227
Sodium chloride. *See* Salt
Solanaceae (nightshade) vegetables, 179
Sole, 216–17
Soup: chicken, 107; fish, 233
South Seas Islanders, 16–17; photographs of, 29, 31, 32.

Spices, 189
Spondylitis, 40
Sports, 248–49
Sprouts, 176–77; alfalfa, 123, 177; buckwheat, 176–77; in cancer therapy, 121; clover, 177; how to grow, 176–77; in Pottenger's diet, 41; sunflower, 176–77
Sprouted whole grain breads, 182
Squid, 228
Steelhead, 218
Stefansson, Vilhjamur, 103, 160–62
Stocks, fish, 233
Strength: biological, 97; and diet, among Africans, 18–19
Striped bass, 218
Strokes, 40
Studies in Deficiency Diseases, 61
Sucrose, 188–89
Sugar, 195–96; and arthritis, 112; in fruit, 184; and heart problems, 116–17; metabolism of, 188–89. *See also* Foods, refined
Sulfites: and allergies, 234; on shrimp, 227; on vegetables and fish, 233–34
Sunlight, 67
Surgery, 133
Sushi and sashimi, 230–31; abalone, 221; safety of, 43; scallops, 227; shark, 216; striped bass, 218; tilefish, 219; tuna, 219. *See also* Fish, raw
Sweeteners, 188–89
Swiss, 10–11; photograph of, 29
Switzerland, 8–9; 10–11
Swordfish, 219
Szent-Gyorgyi, Albert, 92

Tauhuanocan culture, 26
Taylor, Renee, 61
Teeth: crowding and malocclusion of, 12 (*See also* Dental arches, misshapen). *See also* Decay, dental
Ten-Year Study. *See* Pottenger Cat Study
Tests, laboratory: desirability of, 133; explanation of, 234–240; limitations of, 234. *See also* Cholesterol; Complete blood count; Erythrocyte sedimentation rate; Glucose, fasting; Glucose tolerance test; Glycohemoglobin; Thyroid gland, testing of; Triglycerides; Urinalysis
Thyroid gland: and cholesterol, 115–16; and metabolism, 112; and overweight, 127; testing of, 110–111, 115, 240
Thyroid glands, as food, 14
Thyroid supplements: in Gerson therapy, 92; natural versus synthetic, 111–12
Thyroxine, 240
Tilefish, 219
Tomatoes, 124, 178
Torres Strait Islanders, 23–24; photographs of, 29, 32
Toxic materials, as water pollutants, 140
Traditional cultures. *See* Cultures, traditional
Traditional diets. *See* Diets, traditional

Traditional foods. *See* Foods, traditional

Treatment: choices in, 133; pharmaceutical, 5; surgical, 5. *See also names of specific conditions*

Triglycerides: and fish oils, 79–80; and heart disease, 238; laboratory test for and influences upon, 238–39

Triiodothyronine, 240

Trout, freshwater, 229

Tuberculosis: absence of among primitive people, 8, 10; and dental decay, 24; in modernizing primitive people, 9, 10, 11, 15, 17, 23; and the Pottenger Sanatorium, 34; recovery from, 7, 15

Tuna, 219–20; roe, 233

Ulcers, 184

Unsaturated fatty acids, 159. *See also* Alpha-linolenic acid; Arachidonic acid; Docosahexaenoic acid (DHA); Eicosapentaenoic acid (EPA); Gamma-linolenic acid (GLA); Linoleic acid

Urinalysis, 235

Values: material, 204; moral, 21; spiritual, 8, 9

Veal calves, 151–52

Vegetable oils, 186–87; and aging, 80; and blood lipids, 79–80; and cancer, 80; manufacturing methods, 186–87; in Pottenger's diet, 41

Vegetables, 175–79

—green: amount desirable, 175; effect on guinea pigs, 38; effect on milk in Pottenger Cat Study, 38; in Loetschental Valley, 8; and protection from cancer, 231

—nightshade, 178–79

—organic, legal definition of, 244

—sea. *See* Seaweeds, edible

Vegetarianism: among *Australopithecines*, 47–48, 49; among primitive cultures, 17; and EPA, 78; and healing, 17–18; and the macrobiotic diet, 97; and raw foods, 73, 93

Vigor, in extreme old age, 53

Vilcabamba, 52, 57–59; and blood pressure, 116; problems in, 56, 60

Vinegar, 187

Vision: and fish oils, 82; in Georgian Russians, 55

Vitamin A: in fish tissues, 14; natural supplements, 198; in seal oil, 12

Vitamin B6, 202

Vitamin B12: deficiencies, 73; in leukemia, 92; natural supplements, 198

Vitamin B-complex: manufacturing of supplements, 198; megadoses in pregnancy, 202; natural supplements, 198

Vitamin C: in acute illness, 107; and Arctic Eskimos, 161–62; in fruits and vegetables, 183; megadoses in pregnancy, 202; and northern Indians, 14; supplements, 197–98, 199

Vitamin D: sources in ancient Peru, 26; synthetic—*see* Vitamin D2. *See also* Vitamin D3; Vitamin D-complex

Vitamin D2: and arthritis, 113; manufacturing process, 197; problems with, 165–66

Vitamin D3: function, 67; natural supplements, 198; and nightshade vegetables, 179; sources, 197; and the vitamin D-complex, 165–66

Vitamin D-complex: and calcium, 9; sources, 67; and vitamin D2, 165–66

Vitamin E: and oxidation, 182, 186, 199; supplements, 197, 198, 199; in traditional diets, 199

Vitamin F. *See* Essential fatty acids

Vitamin supplements, 197–98; megadoses versus traditional foods, 201–203; and pollutants, 202

Vitamins

—in immune groups' diets, 70, 199

—fat-soluble: in butter, 9; early measurements of, 8–9; sources of, 17, 67 (*see also* Foods, animal source)

Wahoo (mackerel), 212

Walking, 246–47; and pregnancy, 104

Warmbrand, Max, 121

Weight loss, 89, 90, 126–27

Wheat, 181

White, Paul Dudley, 46

Whitebait, 221

Whitefish, freshwater, 230

Wine. *See* Alcoholic beverages

Wisdom, traditional: and the art of medicine, 5; and EPA, 82; and fertility, 12; in food selection, 100; and health, 4; of North American Indians, 16; and scurvy, 14; and xeropthalmia, 14

Wisdom teeth, 12

Xanthine oxidase, 164–65

Xeropthalmia, 14

Yeast, nutritional, 198

Yin and yang, 100–101

Yogurt, 168

About the Author

Dr. Ronald Schmid is licensed to practice as a naturopathic physician in Oregon, Washington State, and Connecticut. A graduate of the Massachusetts Institute of Technology, he holds degrees in design, education, human biology, and naturopathic medicine. He has taught at naturopathic medical schools in Oregon and Washington, and is now in private practice in Connecticut. He lives in Stratford, Connecticut.

Acknowledgments

Many wonderful people provided invaluable assistance in the production of this book. Bruce Kauffman and Dr. Edward Alstat gave me early guidance in determining the substance and style of the material. Larry and Marie Slinn, Carol Cartaino, and Dr. Michael Schachter kindly read the early manuscript, encouraged me, and helped create its final shape. Michael LoSardo and Sally Sears Mack polished the many areas in need of their editorial talents.

Most authors wishfully dream of an opportunity to participate actively in the design and production of their books. My good fortune has been to collaborate with the editors at Ocean View Publications, with Gary Peirce, David Cammack, and Miriam El-Massri of Lettick Typografic, with Robert Abrams of Quinn-Woodbine, with our cover artist, Virginia Ryan Lauzon, and with our photographer, Marcus Halevi, on shaping my ideas and my writing into the final form of this book. Their efforts, creative skills, and enthusiasm, and those of the many people who work with them, were the substance of the making of this book. My deepest thanks go to all of these people who have helped make my dream—the chance to present my work to the public—a reality.

RON SCHMID